D1274505

MANAGEMENT
OF MEDICAL
FOODSERVICE

MANAGEMENT OF MEDICAL FOODSERVICE

Catherine F. Sullivan
Ph.D., R.D.

Second Edition

VNR Van Nostrand Reinhold
New York

Copyright © 1990 by Van Nostrand Reinhold

Library of Congress Catalog Card Number 89–5725
ISBN 0-442-31951-7

All rights reserved. No part of this work covered by the copyright hereon may be
reproduced or used in any form or by any means—graphic, electronic, or mechanical,
including photocopying, recording, taping, or information storage and retrieval systems—without written permission of the publisher.

Printed in the United States of America

Van Nostrand Reinhold
115 Fifth Avenue
New York, New York 10003

Van Nostrand Reinhold International Company Limited
11 New Fetter Lane
London EC4P 4EE, England

Van Nostrand Reinhold
480 La Trobe Street
Melbourne, Victoria 3000, Australia

Nelson Canada
1120 Birchmount Road
Scarborough, Ontario M1K 5G4, Canada

16 15 14 13 12 11 10 9 8 7 6 5 4 3 2 1

Library of Congress Cataloging-in-Publication Data

Sullivan, Catherine F.
    Management of medical foodservice / Catherine F. Sullivan.—2nd
ed.
      p.   cm.
    Includes index.
    ISBN 0–442–31951–7
    1. Health facilities—Food service—Management.   2. Hospitals–
—Food service—Management.   I. Title.
RA975.5.D5S85   1990
362.1'76'068—dc20   89–5725
                                                                 CIP

DISCARDED

WIDENER UNIVERSITY
WOLFGRAM
LIBRARY
CHESTER, PA.

Contents

APPENDIXES   373

Index   451

Foreword

It is a pleasure to write the foreword to the second edition of *Management of Medical Foodservice*. As a consultant in nutrition and food management, I have conducted surveys throughout the State of Michigan. This book provides a "ready" source of reference for most problems encountered by practitioners at various facilities. The reward for the practitioner comes in the application that can be developed from this book to help patients and residents.

The first edition of this book was published in 1985. Changes in concepts of dietetic service operations and requirements for licensure and certification necessitated a revision. The purpose of the book remains: adding updates to promote desired outcomes. The second edition covers proven dietetic guidelines, federal regulations, state rules, and related organizational requirements.

This book is the answer to challenging foodservice problems. Despite the progress made in dietetics, food-borne illness continues to be the major public health problem. The incidence of such illness can be reduced by following basic principles of food production and service as outlined.

With use of the systems approach to management, the medical foodservice facility can realize that a plan of operation is necessary to provide an intended level of service on a consistent and continuous basis. In health care facilities it is necessary for a Registered Dietitian, with support of qualified staff, to coordinate functions of the department; to attain the intended level of health care and outcome; and to provide for efficiency of operation. The readers will be pleased with the contents of this edition to use as a textbook and reference.

This book represents the commitment and dedication of Dr. Sullivan to the profession of dietetics in promoting practical guidelines and standards of practice to ensure positive outcomes for patients and residents.

Carlean Williams, M.S., R.D.

Preface

The second edition is designed, as was the previous edition, as a text for students in dietetics and as a reference for practitioners and administrators in health care and related facilities. Both groups need technical knowledge and practical management skills if they are to understand and utilize available resources fully. Major objectives are as follows:

1. To present information in a systematic and pragmatic manner so that the reader can get a macroview of medical foodservice management.
2. To emphasize the intra- and interdepartmental milieu in which the manager must work.
3. To concentrate on unique activities, functions, and problems pertinent to medical foodservice operations.
4. To provide essentials of medical foodservice management in a single book with emphasis on practical application.

The concept of the systems approach prevails, thus promoting the theory that the menu is the "hub" of the foodservice system, and all subsystems revolve around it. To reinforce the systems concept, subject matter relating to safety, sanitation, computer application, energy conservation, quality control, and quality assurance is treated as an integral part of each subsystem.

I have received numerous comments from colleagues in academia, practitioners in food management, and the food industry on the usefulness of information provided in the text. Many positive comments were made on the presentation of management principles prior to discussing foodservice systems.

The first chapter provides a comprehensive overview of the systems approach: how systems and subsystems interrelate and how systems theory applies to the management of medical foodservice. Management principles are presented in Chapters 2–8, providing a basis for understanding management concepts in a systematic manner. Since the first edition, major changes in federal regulations, and minor changes in other areas of food management have been made. New information includes Medicare and Medicaid Conditions of Participation and effects of mergers on employees in Chapter 3; an update on DRGs, professional ethics, malpractice, and patient rights in Chapter 4; and a case study to illustrate the functions of management in Chapter 5. The subject matter flows in a logical and practical order, beginning with developing objectives and goals as prerequisites to other management functions. The management chapters end with Time Management, a crucial resource for all managers. PERT-Time, a complex managerial tool, is shown to be applicable to medical foodservice management.

The remaining chapters discuss the subsystems as integral parts of a foodservice system; Menu Planning, Equipment, Food Purchasing, Food Production, Food Distribution and Service, Personnel, and Finance. The material is presented in sequential order to correspond with the flow of resources throughout the operation. Additions to the subsystems include nutritional analysis of menus and JCAH requirements for diet manuals in Chapter 9; a new convection combo oven in Chapter 10; changes in beef grades in Chapter 11; JCAH requirements for quality assurance in Chapter 13; and infection control training requirement for HIV, handling drugs in the workplace, and hazard communication on chemicals in Chapter 14.

A valuable section of the book is the appendixes. Users of the first edition have remarked on the usefulness of these materials in determining amounts to purchase and in extending recipes. Additional appendixes in the second edition include: JCAH Standards for Dietary Services, Long-Term Care Survey Guidelines, Conditions of Participation for Patient Rights, and Material Safety Data Sheets for Hazardous Chemicals.

Charts, graphs, and photographs are integrated throughout the text to illustrate and clarify the theory and the practical applications. This book is concise and comprehensive. All subject matter required for an effective and efficient operation is treated in a manner that can be easily understood by students and practitioners.

To assist instructors in food management and dietetics, a new feature of the second edition is a teacher's guide, which includes a proposed course syllabus, chapter objectives, key words, test questions and answers, and suggested class assignments.

━━ Acknowledgments ━━━━━━━━━━━━━━━━━━━━━━━━━━━━

Many people have contributed to the second edition of this book. Special thanks to Carlean Williams, M.S., R.D., Nutrition and Food Management Consultant, Michigan Department of Public Health, for valuable input of information and time spent in chapter review; Evelyn Jones, M.S., R.N., Acting Division Chief, Michigan Department of Public Health, for explicit information on licensing and certification update of health care facilities. To Cubie Watson, M.A., R.D., Director of Dietetics, Detroit Riverview Hospital, and Barbara Saulter, M.A., R.D., Director of Dietetics at Hawthorn Center, for providing input from a practical viewpoint; Joyce Moody, Ed.M., M.P.H., R.D., Senior Lecturer, Department of Internal Medicine and Department of Nutrition and Food Science, Wayne State University, for input from an academic perspective; Alethia Carr, M.A., R.D., for assistance with computer analysis of menus; Wanda Redmond, my daughter Kimberly, and my son John for many hours of word processing.

Catherine F. Sullivan

MANAGEMENT OF MEDICAL FOODSERVICE

PART 1

PRINCIPLES OF THE SYSTEMS APPROACH

Chapter 1

A Systems Approach

Conceptualizing the diverse, complex nature of medical foodservice management can best be accomplished through the use of the systems approach. As defined by Johnson, Kast, and Rosenzweig (1967), a systems approach is "a way of thinking." It is not a set of rules on how to organize and manage, but it is a way of looking at the various parts as they integrate to make an organized whole. The practitioner, functioning in an environment of different parts, must be able to analyze the inherent interrelationships. An understanding of how the various parts of the foodservice system are related and how effective outcome in one part is affected by outcome in another part is of paramount importance. Systems theory, as a frame of reference, facilitates this comprehension.

Complexity of Medical Foodservice

Although there are certain commonalities among various types of foodservice operations, such as medical, industrial, hotel, and school foodservice, there are also distinct differences. These differences are complex enough to warrant special attention. The uniqueness of medical foodservice begins with its primary objective, which is to provide direct, individualized, total nutritional care for patients on both regular and modified diets—a mission unlike that of any other type of foodservice operation. In addition to the primary objective, meals are provided for personnel, guests, and for special activities in a variety of settings. For example, in nonmedical foodservice operations the nutritional component may be subordinate to other objectives, such as profit and marketing of goods and/or services. The exception may be in the case of school foodservice, where partial nutritional care is provided by meeting one-third of the daily dietary allowance in the school lunch.

In most medical facilities of 300 beds or more, the foodservice manager may be involved in all forms of production and service found in other types of operations, as well as the following:

Patient foodservice (personalized diet–room service)
Cafeteria (employee and guest meals)
Vending (contract or independent)
Short order (coffee shop, snack bars)
Table service (special luncheons and dinners)
Banquet (special activities)
Tea service (retirement, promotion parties)

Another reason why management of medical foodservice requires special attention is the nature of the client. Most patients are not hospitalized by choice. Therefore, managers of medical foodservice must be able to deal with the psychological effects of providing nutritious meals to individuals in an unfamiliar atmosphere with consideration to other factors that may be associated with their state of health.

Special attention is also required because much of the information required for effective and efficient operation is scattered in a number of resources with little attempt to organize available knowledge into a cohesive, understandable whole. With the use of the systems approach to management, order can be brought to what often may be characterized as a frustrating, chaotic situation.

Systems Defined

The difficulty associated with defining a system is attributed to the broad use of the term and the manner in which it is used in the various disciplines. Early use of systems theory related primarily to the physical sciences and engineering. As applied in disciplines such as physics, biology, and engineering, the parts of the system were considered to be static, concrete, or mechanical. As all practitioners can attest to, management of a medical foodservice operation is far from static, inasmuch as subsystems interface inside and outside of the systems boundaries. A theoretical base, applicable to management, must recognize the difference in terms of parts or subsystems. Additionally, the systems approach as applied to management is concerned with people as well as machines and materials.

As defined in Barnhart and Barnhart's *The World Book Dictionary* (1983), a system is "a set of things or parts forming a whole: a mountain system, a railroad system." According to this definition, many natural man-made units, such as automobiles, rivers, planets, electrical units, plumbing units and organizations, can be classified as a system. One of the earlier investigators and founders of general systems theory emphasizes interaction with the environment and defines system as "a set of elements standing in interrelation among themselves and with the environment" (Von Bertalanffy 1972). The key word in this definition and one that is useful to our discussion is "environment." For our purposes, a combination of the two definitions is used to define a system as the *integration of parts into an organized whole that functions within a larger environment for a specific purpose.* In this definition, the parts are considered subsystems and the larger environment is the medical facility in which the system (foodservice) operates.

Closed and Open Systems

Systems may be classified as closed or open. In a closed system, there is little or no interaction with the environment. This type of system is primarily physical in nature. The reverse is true of an open system, which is characterized primarily as social. Systems, as related to management of a medical foodservice, are open because there is constant output into and input from the environment. An open system does not operate in isolation; it is interrelated and interdependent.

Input–Output Relationship

How inputs and outputs are viewed depends on the vantage point. Outputs from one system may be the inputs for another (Berrien 1968). This concept will be discussed later in this chapter under suprasystems. The input–output relationship for a medical foodservice system is illustrated in Figure 1-1. The inputs are

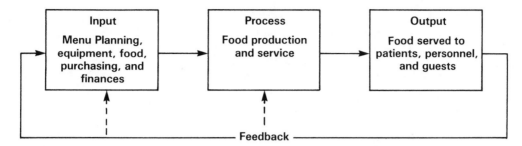

Figure 1-1. Input–output relationship.

the resources and the outputs are the finished products. In medical foodservice, the raw products are processed into acceptable meals for patients. In order for the system to survive, the outputs must be useful and acceptable to the larger environment (medical facility). When the output is unsatisfactory, the finished product is rejected and eventually the system will fail unless corrective action based on feedback is taken (Bertrand 1972).

The feedback loop provides control and is an important part of the system. Feedback, as shown in Figure 1-1, can be directed to input or process, and may be of a negative or positive nature. When the output is unsatisfactory, there will be a flow of complaints from the environment. In medical foodservice, the complaint may refer to an unacceptable entree (the meat is tough). The feedback loop for corrective action may go to input such as purchasing, or to process such as preparation technique in order to determine the problem area. The manager uses negative feedback as a point of corrective action and positive feedback as an opportunity to praise, encourage, and motivate employees. In a successful operation, it is desirable to have more positive than negative feedback.

Subsystems

A *subsystem is a component of a system and has a specific purpose of its own.* It is designed to operate within a system in an integrated manner in order to realize the primary purpose of the total system. In medical foodservice, the subsystems are identified as follows:

Menu planning
Equipment selection and design
Food purchasing
Food production
Foodservice
Personnel
Finances

Other components of a foodservice system such as sanitation, safety, quality control, and computer application are not considered subsystems and therefore are not presented as a separate entity. The conceptual view is that these components are an integral part of all subsystems.

System–Subsystem Relationship

The relationship between the system and subsystem is shown in Figure 1-2. The importance is placed on how effectively and efficiently the subsystems interact

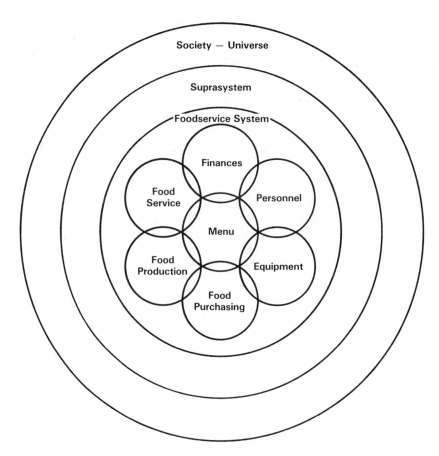

Figure 1-2. Conceptual model of system–subsystem relationship.

and are integrated into the system for purpose of achieving the goals of the system and the environment.

The menu is considered the *hub* of the system, with subsystems interrelated and interdependent on its purpose, process, and content. To view menu planning as the hub of the system is based on the concept that all of the activities taking place in the other subsystems are dependent on the purpose, process, and content of the menu. Examples of how the subsystems overlap in their relationships and dependence are described in the following:

1. Equipment is selected and designed according to the type and volume of food items on the menu. If baked potatoes are to be served with roast beef, then ovens (conventional, convection, or microwave) must be available for timely preparation of both items. The number of ovens required will depend on the volume needed for a given time. Since the purchasing of equipment is based on need, some pieces of equipment could be eliminated completely. For example, if no fried food items appeared on the menu, there would be no need to purchase a deep fat fryer.

2. Food is purchased according to dictates of the menu. Depending on the use of the food item, it may be desirable to vary the quality or grade of food purchased. For example, if canned peaches were served as a dessert, a higher quality would be required than if they were served in a jellied form as a salad.

3. The production of a food item is directly related to the intended use as indicated on the menu. Whether to fry, bake, broil, peel, or trim a food item will depend on the nature of the food and for whom it is intended. Food for patients on modified diets is prepared differently from food for patients on regular diets.

4. The service of food with reference to portion size, holding, and serving

temperatures are directly related to menu planning. For example, the portion size for stews, casseroles, and sliced meats are all different. In addition, there are some controlled intake diets in which specific ounce portions are prescribed. Holding and serving temperatures vary from frozen to the very hot, depending on the menu item.

5. Personnel skills required to prepare and serve food depend on the type and complexity of the food item. For example, if gourmet foods appear on the menu, more highly skilled employees are required.

6. Finances are related to menu planning in a number of ways. For example, the food cost will vary depending on menu offerings of seasonal foods, low versus high quality, the portion size, and so forth.

When the menu is accepted as the hub of the foodservice system, it is considered to be a catalyst that sets into motion the functions to be performed in other systems. It is important for managers to understand interrelationships that are dependent upon effective menu planning.

Suprasystems

A suprasystem is the environment in which systems function. The relationship between suprasystem and system is similar to that of system and subsystem since the outputs from systems serve as inputs for the suprasystem. Expressed another way, the foodservice system may be considered to be a system or subsystem, depending on how it is viewed. For example, when the foodservice system receives input from its subsystems, it is regarded as a system; when the foodservice system provides inputs for the larger system (medical facility), it may be considered a subsystem. As shown in Figure 1-3, the foodservice system is just

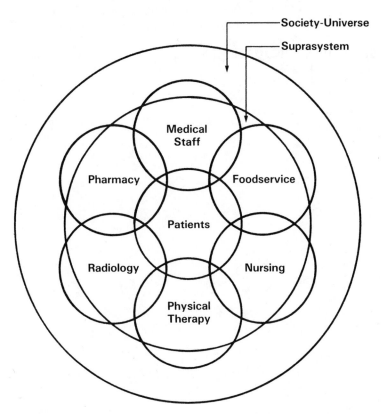

Figure 1-3. Conceptual model of suprasystem–system relationship.

one of the partial listing of interrelated parts. As noted, the patient is the hub of the suprasystem and the other systems interact to provide support.

The suprasystem is also part of a larger environment, with inputs from systems (foodservice) and outputs (healthy individuals) into the community. The outputs must be acceptable to the larger environment if the suprasystem is to survive. To use the illustration in Figure 1-1, the feedback loop may return to any one of the inputs such as foodservice, nursing, medical, or to the processing of inputs.

Medical facilities are complex organizations. Their degree of complexity depends on purposes, objectives, and goals, as will be discussed in the next chapter. The more complex the organization, the greater is the need for a systems approach. Some of the advantages of approaching the management of a medical foodservice from a systems viewpoint are as follows:

1. It provides the manager with an understanding of the basics necessary to operate in a milieu of dynamic interrelationships.

2. It requires the manager to look at all parts and discern the interdependence of each as a part of the whole.

3. It provides a conceptual framework for viewing the interrelationships of parts in a complex operation and how they overlap in meeting organizational goals.

4. It forces the manager to synthesize rather than isolate the various parts within the foodservice system.

References

Barnhart, C. L. and Barnhart, R. K., eds. (1983). *The World Book Dictionary*, Volume 2: L–Z. Chicago: Doubleday.

Berrien, F. K. (1968). *General and Social Systems*. New Brunswick, NJ: Rutgers University Press.

Bertrand, A. L. (1972). *Social Organizations*. Philadelphia: F. A. Davis.

Johnson, R. A., Kast, F. E., and Rosenzweig, J. E. (1967). *The Theory and Management of Systems*, New York: McGraw-Hill.

Von Bertalanffy, L. (1972). The History and Status of General Systems Theory. *Acad. Mgt. J.* 15(4), 407–426.

Chapter 2

Developing Objectives and Goals

It is appropriate that objectives and goals precede theory pertaining to organization since the structure and functions of an organization are based on its purpose. Additionally, when objectives and goals are defined, there are indications for functional levels and relationships within the organization. Not only must objectives and goals be defined, but they must be communicated in such a way that they will serve to direct action, motivate members of the organization, provide standards for measurable performance, and evaluate organizational effectiveness. At a time when accountability is increasingly necessary for those in managerial positions, statements in terms of what is to be achieved are of utmost importance.

Objectives and Goals Defined

Some writers prefer not to distinguish between objectives and goals (Terry 1978; Albanese 1975; Huse & Bodwitch 1977) and thus use the terms interchangeably. Other writers make a distinction not only between objectives and goals, but also between related terms such as purpose, mission, and target (Koontz & O'Donnell 1974). *Purpose* is considered the highest aim and relates to reasons why an organization exists. Statements at this level are broad and general in nature. *Mission* is also a broad term and similar to purpose, except that it is usually applied to nonprofit organizations such as military operations, churches, government, and medical facilities. *Goals* or *targets* are more specific and are usually stated in terms of quality or quantity, whereas *objectives* are used to indicate the endpoint of a management program. Objectives may be stated as long range, intermediate, or short range.

According to Carlisle (1976), objectives are a desired condition and refer in a general way to the results or conditions that an individual or organization wishes to attain in the future. His thesis is that the hierarchy of organizational aims, in descending order, is (1) purpose, (2) objectives, (3) strategy, (4) organizational goals, (5) subunit goals, and (6) individual goals. It is believed that aims should be established in this order to ensure goal compatibility. Application of this theory, as applied to medical facilities, is as follows:

1. *Purpose.* To be responsive to the needs of the community.
2. *Objective.* To meet health care needs by providing quality health care to individuals and groups.
3. *Strategy.* To gain support from both private and public sources.
4. *Organizational goal (medical facility).* To provide personalized and professional medical treatment for patients.

9

5. *Subunit goal (foodservice).* To provide total nutritional care for patients.
6. *Individual goal.* To perform challenging and creative work in a health care setting.

It can be seen that purpose and objectives are more general in nature than goals, and refer to the philosophy and ideals of the organization. You might expect to find statements of purpose and objectives posted in the lobby of an institution or included in annual reports issued by the organization.

Because objectives start at the top and filter down through the organization, the question may be asked, "Who is involved in the formulation of objectives?" Generally, the purpose and objectives are formulated by top administration with impact from vested interest groups. For medical facilities, the interest groups may include federal, state, and local governments; foundations or other private funding groups; owners; and the community in which the facility operates.

Strategy refers to the method or schemes used to achieve the objectives. Although financing is frequently part of the strategy, other resources such as personnel, equipment, and materials may well be included in the method stated for achieving the purpose of the organization. For example, in the use of methods, the strategy may be to promote organizational efficiency.

Goals, in contrast to objectives, are concrete statements that contain a certain amount of specificity for obtaining objectives. Put another way, goals are tools for translating the general statements pertaining to purpose, objectives, and strategy into meaningful guidelines for organizational activity. Therefore, organizational, subunit, and individual goals must be based on aims at the top of the hierarchy. Since the organization is made up of individuals, each with his or her own set of personal goals, conflict is more likely to occur at the individual level. How the organization and individuals adapt to goal conflict is discussed later in this chapter.

Goal Classification

Seldom will an organization have only one goal. To illustrate the variety of goals organizations seek, Perrow (1970) distinguishes five categories as follows:

1. *Social goals* refer to society in general, such as cultural values, maintaining order, and producing goods and services.

2. *Output goals* refer to the consumer toward which the product is directed. The importance placed on this category is an understanding of the organization's relationship to the environment. Examples of how conglomerates may add new products or services are discussed in detail. These include such actions as the diversification of products by Ford Motor Company when it took over Philco Appliances, provisions for job corps training to the unskilled or unemployed worker, and the attack on the Tennessee Valley Authority because it interfered with local competition.

3. *System goals* refer to the manner in which the organization functions, independent of the goods and services it produces or its derived goals. Some typical system goals are profit for the organization, high rate of growth, and emphasis upon a particular type of organizational structure.

4. *Product goals* refer to the characteristics of goods or services produced, such as quality or quantity, variety, styling, availability, uniqueness, or innovativeness.

5. *Derived goals* refer to how organizations use power in pursuit of other goals, independent of product or system goals. The power generated by organizations may be in the form of political aims, community services, employment development, investment, and plant location and relocation policies. For example, organizations can decide to move from one community and select a relocation site, thus affecting the lives of individuals in both areas.

Perrow used the case of the National Foundation for Infantile Paralysis to illustrate his goal clarification. For example, polio was practically eliminated as a result of research, thus leaving the foundation without concrete goals. The foundation considered several alternatives and finally decided to concentrate on childhood diseases in general. Although the shift was from polio to all childhood diseases, there was no change in output goals: to finance research and to treat human diseases. The system goals in support of health causes was not changed, nor was the highly centralized structure at the national level or the decentralized local leadership. In terms of derived goals, the new arrangement served as a means to an end, generating power and prestige in the health field.

Organizational goals, similar to those for individuals, are generally multiple in nature and may be pursued simultaneously or in sequential order. One of the problems associated with formulating objectives and goals is that often the stated goal is quite different from the goal pursued. According to Huse and Bodwitch (1977), the official goals are for public view, whereas the actual goals toward which the organization exerts its energy or effort are used as operating guidelines. On a lower level, the foodservice department may state its objective as providing optimum nutritional care; however, resources may be provided for only minimal care.

Goal Criteria

Since goals are more specific than objectives, it may be desirable to understand guidelines for ensuring goal validity. As proposed by Carlisle (1976), eight guides apply to establishing goals. In the following lists, questions were formulated in reference to each guide.

1. *Make goals specific*
     Do goals provide direction?
     Do goals imply action?
2. *Make goals verifiable*
     Are quantitative controls set?
     Are qualitative controls set?
     Are time limits set?
     Are cost controls set?
3. *Make goals action-oriented and result-centered*
     Do goals focus on results?
     Do goals imply action?
     Do goals serve to motivate?
4. *Make goals realistic*
     Are improvement areas included?
     Are goals reachable?
5. *Make goals problem-oriented*
     Do goals focus on low performance?
     Are goals ranked according to priority?

Subunit: Patient Tray Service

Objective: To reduce food costs

Goal: To reduce the number of unused trays delivered to wards by 90% from present level of 45 trays per day within a 30-day period.

Tasks: Consult with patient service personnel.
Monitor unused trays left after each meal.
Review census sheets.
Review standard operating procedures for diet changes
    (admissions, discharges, surgery, other).
Determine cause for excessive number of unused trays.
Communicate with nursing personnel.
Reinforce or rewrite standard operating procedure.
Train foodservice personnel, if needed.

Figure 2-1. Sample of subunit goal for foodservice unit.

   6. *Make goals restrictive in numbers*
        Are goals limited for each unit?
        Are goals limited for each individual?
   7. *Make goals participative*
        Do participants have input in goal setting?
        Do participants have authority comparable to assigned responsibility?
   8. *Make goals balance and integrate*
        Are goals consistent at all organizational levels?
        Do goals cover all major activities?

The most controversial of the guidelines listed above is the one related to restriction of the number of goals. Carlisle suggests limiting organizational goals to six or less. The number may be realistic when we consider that goals relate to major areas and not to the activities and tasks involved in attaining the goal. Furthermore, since goals are likely to be multiple at all levels of the organization, it is realistic for managers to pursue a number of goals simultaneously. According to Koontz and O'Donnell (1974), the number of goals established and pursued by a manager will depend on how much is delegated, thereby limiting the manager's role primarily to assigning, supervising, and controlling.

An example of a subunit goal and the associated tasks and activities are shown in Figure 2-1. The objective relating to this goal may be to lower food cost, which is a very broad and general statement, but the goal is specific both in quantity and time.

Goal Congruency

Organizations have goals. Individual members of the organization have goals. The optimal relationship is when organizational and individual goals harmonize in such a fashion that both are met. Frequently, this harmonizing calls for adjustment on both parts.

A new employee who enters the organization brings his or her own set of values, goals, and needs. The primary reason for joining the organization may be for monetary gain or security, but not necessarily. The employee may seek prestige, social interaction with others, and challenging and creative work—or there may be other reasons that may not be stated during the interview or written on job application forms. Attempts to integrate personal and organizational goals can result in situations varying from no conflict to workable conflict and cooperation (Albanese 1975).

1. *No conflict.* Though uncommon, mutual goals are more likely to be found between top executives and the organization than with employees at the lower level of the hierarchy. In such cases one can say that the executive's life and work are identical. It is further theorized that for most employees there is no conflict between some of the personal goals and the goals of the organization. For example, an employee who cannot satisfy any of his or her personal goals, though meeting the goals of the organization will probably leave.

2. *Destruction conflict.* This type of conflict develops when there is incongruence between the needs of the mature personality and the goals of the formal organization. Organizational interference may be in the form of rules, policies, controls, authority, and methods of supervision. Employees cope with this type of conflict in a number of ways: Some may leave the organization; some will work toward higher positions in the organization with the hope that the higher position will be less restrictive; others will increase absenteeism, decrease productivity, and withdraw from active involvement in organizational activities; and some may even cope by committing acts of sabotage and violence.

3. *Workable conflict and cooperation.* There is recognition on the part of the organization and the part of the employee that they need each other. Therefore, there is enough give and take on both sides to permit sufficient organizational survival and growth. The degree of conflict may be related to whether the individual views work as a central life interest. For individuals who value work as a partial—but not the total or central—life interest the restrictions placed on behavior are not too upsetting. Such employees simply find outside activities to fulfill their needs.

As practitioners, managers can probably cite a number of job-related incidents that reflect goal congruence or conflict. For example, when an employee talks about the organization in terms of *we*, there is inference of goal congruence. On the other hand, when an employee says, "This is not part of my job," we can infer that goal conflict is taking place. In the latter example, the employee either does not know or understand the organizational goal or may have lost interest or a sense of direction because of the growing complexity and bureaucracy of medical facilities. If the primary reason for existence of a medical facility is to promote patient well-being, then this criterion must be communicated to the lowest level of the organization.

Management by Objectives

One of the most effective systems that can be used to foster goal congruency is management by objectives (MBO). The concept of MBO was introduced by Drucker (1954) during the early fifties and was further developed by Odiorne (1965) a decade later. The system, which deals with individual and organizational goal setting, is widely used in both public and private organizations.

In practice, both the employee and the supervisor are involved in the assessment of the employee's job responsibilities and the ranking of tasks in the order of importance. If there are discrepancies—and there usually are—differences are discussed until mutual agreement is reached. The second phase is similar to a job performance appraisal in which both parties indicate strengths and weaknesses of job performance. Again, discussion follows to reinforce the employee's strengths and to suggest ways to improve in areas of weakness. After agreement has been reached in job improvement, performance standards are established for all major duties. During the final stage, when goals are agreed upon, resources required for implementing tasks are provided. Frequent feedback is an important part of the system and should be an integral part of the evaluation.

No system is perfect. Although the advantages far outweigh the disadvantages, there are some shortcomings. MBO, as any other system, requires adequate time for planning. The system cannot be put into effect overnight. In large organizations it may take several years before the program is integrated throughout the organization. All participants involved in goal setting should be thoroughly indoctrinated on the philosophy of the system and how to avoid pitfalls such as inflexibility and exclusive concentration on short-term goals. With adequate consideration to the above, benefits of using MBO may be as follows:

1. The system can be implemented and used throughout the organization.
2. Improved role clarification is realized for both managers and subordinates.
3. Management by objectives elicits commitment to concepts of participative management.
4. It encourages initiative and creativity on the part of the participants.
5. With its open environment, communication is improved.
6. The goal setting process improves morale.
7. The system improves coordination and planning of short- and long-range goals.
8. It promotes effective performance appraisals based on results.
9. Productivity is improved.
10. Feedback is provided through frequent progress reports.

There have been successes and failures in attempts to apply MBO in various organizations. The application of MBO has the greatest potential for success if there is proper atmosphere, organizational clarity, and an effective management information system (McConkey 1972). The importance of adequate preparation cannot be overemphasized, since the basic premise is that of accomplishing goals of the organization and individual in a more efficient and effective manner. This can best be realized if there is good structure, goal congruency, goal clarity, and goal commitment (Villarreal 1974).

Policies, Procedures, and Rules

Policies, procedures, and rules are part of the decision-making process that determines how the organization will function in meeting overall aims and objectives. The policy-making process for the *business for profit* type of operation is considerably less complicated than for organizations such as complex medical facilities. One of the reasons for the complexity of decision making in medical facilities is due to the multiple lines of authority, involving board of governors, medical boards and chiefs, and administrators. Rakich and Darr (1978) delineate policy-making responsibilities in hospitals as follows: (1) Governing boards make overall policy; (2) medical boards and chiefs recommend and implement policies related to medical service; and (3) administrators recommend and implement policies dealing with financial and support services and with the relationship of these services to medical service and other units within the organization. In addition, policies are influenced by external sources such as the American Hospital Association (AHA), Joint Commission on Accreditation of Hospitals (JCAH 1988), employee unions, and local, state, and federal agencies.

In practice, the terms *policy, procedure,* and *rule* are frequently grouped together and issued as the organizational or departmental policy manual. This grouping is due, in part, to the nature of some policy statements. Policy statements tend to limit or establish parameters for decision making. The degree to which alternatives are limited depends on whether the policy statement contains elements of a rule. In the following discussion, a distinction is made between the terms.

Policy

A policy is a broad statement used as a guide for managerial decision making. The individual responsible for carrying out a policy has some discretion in its implementation. A sample policy statement is illustrated in Figure 2-2.

This policy has elements of a rule but the manager of the foodservice unit has discretion in terms of the number of meals offered per day (three, four, or more) and the hours of meal service. The rule element is that the manager must conform to the time span as specified in the policy. Policies and procedures are often interdepartmental, with application to more than one department. In the example given in Figure 2-2 the policy must be adhered to by the medical staff, nursing, as well as the dietary department. Additionally, to illustrate the influence of external sources, the above policy is included in standards published for licensure by the Michigan Department of Public Health (1977) and for accreditation of hospitals by the JCAH (1988).

Procedure

A procedure is a step-by-step sequence of how an activity is to be performed. The procedure may include prescribed standards for time, quality, and quantity. A sample procedure, reference to the above policy, is shown in Figure 2-3.

In compliance with the policy for timespan between evening and morning meals, the procedure is specific in terms of meal hours. As in most procedures, there is a call for action rather than thinking on the part of those responsible for carrying it out.

Rule

A rule is specific action to take or not to take in a given situation. A rule leaves no discretion on the part of an individual responsible for carrying it out. It is a simple, straightforward, and explicit statement. A rule is able to stand alone without further explanation. An example of a rule is as follows:

Rule: *There shall be no smoking in the food preparation and service areas.*

To summarize, a distinction is made between the terms as follows: (1) A policy tells you what to do, with discretion; (2) a procedure tells you how to do it,

DATE: _____

POLICY NO.: _____

Unit: Foodservice Department

Subunit: Patient Tray Service

Policy: Not more than 14 hours shall elapse between the serving of the evening meal and the next substantial meal for patients who are on oral intake and do not have specific requirements.

Effective: Immediately

APPROVED BY:

_____   _____
Director, Foodservice   Administrator

_____   _____
Chief, Medical Staff   Chief, Nursing

Review dates: _____   _____

_____   _____

Figure 2-2. Sample policy for foodservice unit.

with no discretion; and (3) a rule tells you what you can or cannot do, with no discretion.

___ Oral vs. Written Policies, Procedures, and Rules ___

The decision to use oral or written forms of communicating policies, procedures, and rules is no longer left entirely to the discretion of the organization. The need to defend against possible lawsuits from employees and clients and the need to comply with standards posed by outside agencies make it imperative for written forms of communication to be in use. According to the Joint Commission on Accreditation of Hospitals (1988), policies and procedures should be in writing. Standard III, relating to dietetic services, is interpreted as follows:

> There are written policies and procedures concerning the scope and conduct of dietetic services. Administrative policies and procedures concerning food procurement, preparation, and service shall be developed by the director of the dietetic department/service. Nutritional care policies and procedures are developed by a qualified dietitian. When appropriate, concurrence or approval should be obtained from the medical staff

DATE: _____
PROCEDURE NO.: ____ _____

Unit: Foodservice Department

Subunit: Patient Tray Service

Reference: Policy No. FS 26

Purpose: To ensure that patient meals are served at proper intervals.

Procedure: 1. Meals will be served to patients at the following hours:

   Breakfast   7:00 A.M.
   Lunch   11:30 A.M.
   Dinner   5:00 P.M.

2. Observe the following rotation for tray service:

   East Wing
   South Wing
   West Wing
   North Wing

Effective: Immediately

APPROVED BY:

_____   _____
Director, Foodservice   Administrator

_____   _____
Chief, Medical Staff   Chief, Nursing

Review dates: _____   _____

_____   _____

Figure 2-3. Sample procedure for foodservice unit.

through its designated mechanism, and from the nursing department/ service. Policies and procedures are subjected to timely review, revised as necessary, dated and enforced.

As noted, the standard not only states that the policies should be in writing, but also by whom they should be developed and approved, and provides a procedure for review.

___ Advantages of Written Policies _____

In addition to making sure that major areas are covered, other advantages are that written policies:

1. Improve the communication process.
2. Can be checked for consistency with overall objectives and goals.
3. Can be used to orient and train new employees.
4. Can be used for objective performance rating.
5. Reduce confusion on the part of employees.
6. Can be used to measure standards of performance.
7. Aid delegation of authority.

It may be impossible to establish policies for all potential problem areas; however, in areas where problems continually arise in the absence of policy guidelines, clearly managerial attention is required.

References

Albanese, R. (1975). *Management: Toward Accountability for Performance.* Homewood, IL: Richard D. Irwin.

Carlisle, H. M. (1976). *Management: Concepts and Situations.* Chicago: Science Research Association.

Drucker, P. (1954). *The Practice of Management.* New York: Harper & Row.

Huse, E. F., and Bodwitch, J. L. (1977). *Behavior in Organizations: A Systems Approach to Managing.* Reading, MA: Addison-Wesley.

Joint Commission on Accreditation of Hospitals. (1988). *Accreditation Manual for Hospitals,* Chicago: JCAH.

Koontz, H., and O'Donnell, C. (1974). *Essentials of Management.* New York: McGraw-Hill.

McConkey, D. D. (1972). Implementation: The Guts of MBO. *SAM Adv. Mgt. J. 37*(2), 13–18.

Michigan Department of Public Health. (1977). *Rules and Minimum Standards for Hospitals.* Lansing: MDPH.

Odiorne, G. (1965). *Management by Objectives.* New York: Pitman.

Perrow, C. (1970). *Organizational Analysis: A Sociological View.* Belmont, CA: Wadsworth.

Rakich, J. S., and Darr, K. (1978). *Hospital Organization and Management.* New York: Halsted Press.

Terry, G. (1978). *Principles of Management.* Homewood, IL: Richard D. Irwin.

Villarreal, J. J. (1974). Management by Objectives Revisited. *SAM Adv. Mgt. J. 39*(2), 28–33.

Chapter 3

Organization Theory and Design

The starting point for organization design is to examine and understand why an organization exists. Concern should center around the following: (1) The stated *objectives,* (2) the *work* to be accomplished, (3) the *individuals* in the work place, and (4) the *environment* in which the organization operates.

An organization is formed when it is necessary to combine the efforts of two or more individuals in the process of meeting stated objectives. The primary purpose for organizing is to divide the work that must be accomplished; this can only be done after one has defined, examined, and understood the objectives. According to Barnes, Fogg, Stephens, and Titman (1970), when objectives are defined, a framework is provided within which the detailed organization structure can be built. In the process of dividing the work, determination is made on internal interactions such as lines of communication, authority, responsibility, control, and other patterns of human relationships necessary to accomplish objectives and goals. The approach to organization design varies from one organization to another. This text supports the open system theory to organization, as will be discussed later.

At this time it is appropriate to provide an overview of traditional theories to organization for a better understanding of modern concepts. The principles of traditional management, developed during the early part of the twentieth century, were sound, valid, and applicable to their time. Many of these principles can be found in organizations today, in varying degrees. The following discussion presents a brief description of three theoretical approaches to organization: (1) classical, (2) human relations, and (3) open system theory.

Classical Approach

Classical theory developed in three streams: bureaucracy, administrative theory, and scientific management (Hicks & Gullett 1975). The three theories were developed by different theorists, about the same time, and with essentially the same practical effects on management. Because of the similarity of basic assumptions, the theories are grouped as one approach.

Bureaucracy

This theory is characterized by extensive rules and procedures, rigid hierarchical structure of authority and responsibility, systematic division of labor, impersonal relationships, and centralized authority from top to bottom. To some individuals, the word *bureaucracy* is synonymous with red tape—the direct opposite of its intended purpose, which is to promote rational, competent, and efficient organization (Albanese 1975). As the major contributor to bureaucracy theory,

Max Weber concentrated on the internal workings of the organization and the efficiency therein. The main features of bureaucratic structure, as proposed by Weber (1967), are (1) systematic division of labor, (2) hierarchy of authority, (3) system of rules, (4) system of procedures, (5) impersonality, and (6) technical competence.

The extent to which the above characteristics are found in an organization will depend on the degree of bureaucratization. In studying the concepts of bureaucracy, Hall (1972) concluded that the degree of bureaucratization depends on the type of organizational activity. For example, in the ideal bureaucracy all of the factors would be present, whereas nonbureaucratic or simple organizations would have a low degree of all of the features present.

Administrative Theory

This theory focuses on the upper levels of the organization with emphasis on principles of management. According to Hicks and Gullett (1975), a bureaucratic theorist proposes what an organization should be, and an administrative theorist proposes how to accomplish or implement an effective organization.

The principles and functions of management, as proposed by Foyal (1949), Gulick (1937), Mooney and Reiley (1939), Urwick (1944), and others, were all centered on efficiency. *Division of work* is considered the foundation of organization for administrative theorists. If work is divided, then it must be coordinated. The *principle of coordination* means that the subdivision of work should be allotted to persons in a structure of authority so that orders can flow from superior to subordinate, reaching the bottom of the organization (Gulick 1937). Since persons in authority give orders, the principle relating to a structure of authority is known as the *scalar chain*. This principle implies that a hierarchy of authority exists in a series of steps from the very top to all subordinate positions and is necessary in order to promote effective communication and control.

In addition to defining the hierarchy of authority, a major principle also relates to the person to whom an individual is responsible. To avoid confusion and inefficiency, the principle of *unity of command* dictates that each individual should receive orders and be responsible to only one superior. More recently, this principle is interpreted to mean that each individual should know exactly to whom he or she is accountable for particular responsibilities (Albanese 1975). This generality is a particular problem due to the dual line of authority found in many complex organizations today, especially medical facilities.

Administrative theorists believe that there is a limit to the number of persons an individual can effectively manage. The principle that deals with this managerial problem is called *span of control*. Vytautas A. Graicunas (1937) used a mathematical formula to show the possible number of relationships between an individual and his subordinates. As subordinates increase in numbers, potential relationships increase geometrically. For example, for four subordinates there are 11 relationships with any one individual. A fifth subordinate will bring 20 new relationships, plus 9 more relationships to each colleague, for a possible 100 relationships in the unit. Although there are no absolute numbers of subordinates that a superior can manage, the number generally varies from 3 to 6 for upper levels of management, and up to 15 for lower levels. Factors affecting the optimum number relate to (1) the level of training of subordinates, (2) the nature of the job, (3) the complexity of the job, (4) location of jobs, such as widely dispersed or all in same location, (5) the difficulty of the job, and (6) the knowledge of the superior.

The *principle of line and staff* relates to the authority of individuals in the respective positions. The main difference between line and staff is that line personnel have the authority to give orders, whereas staff personnel tend to serve in an advisory or consultative capacity. In addition to line and staff, most organizations have individuals in positions with *functional authority*. In this capacity, the position holder may serve as both line and staff. For example, a personnel director may have direct supervision for an assistant personnel director, a secretary, and others in his area, and at the same time have limited authority over all departments in the organization in terms of personnel action.

Scientific Management

Scientific management marked the beginning of the scientific method as applied to organization. It was in direct contrast to bureaucracy and administrative theories, which used *good judgment* as a basis for arriving at managerial principles. Frederick Taylor is considered the father of scientific management because of his contributions to the theory. Taylor, along with other theorists such as Henry Gantt, Harrington Emerson, and Frank and Lillian Gilbreth, focused on the improvement of individual work performance. Based on his work experience at Bethlehem Steel, Taylor's research to improve work efficiency centered around four main principles (Filey & House 1969):

1. The development of the best method to perform a job. This procedure involved analyzing each task in detail. In modern organizations today, this principle is known as *work simplification.*
2. The selection and development of workers. Select the right worker using scientific methods and train him or her in the proper method of performing the job.
3. The bringing together of the proper method and properly selected and trained person.
4. The close cooperation of managers and workers.

Taylor's emphasis on breaking down components of the job and specialized training at the lower level as well as the managerial level were his greatest contribution to the scientific management theory.

Henry Gantt is noted for developing the *Gantt chart*, a device used to measure actual versus planned performance. The straight-line chart is used to measure the activity by the time it takes to perform it (George 1968). In addition, Gantt is known for his *task and bonus* plans for remunerating workers. According to his plan, a day's wages was paid for output less than standard, a bonus for achieving standard, and rewards for production above standard. His concern for efficiency was not at the expense of the human factors of management.

Harrington Emerson's work centered on efficiency, and he was the first to use the term *efficiency engineering* (George 1968). Emerson was an advocate of a strong staff, and of counsel as reflected in two of his 12 principles of management. For example, on the principle of common sense, he urged managers to strive for knowledge and seek advice from every quarter. On the principle of competent counsel, he states that managers should actively seek advice of competent individuals. He used the military as an example of strong staff and counsel. As one of the nation's first consultants, he served as the expert witness for Brandeis in 1910 and stated that the U.S. railroads could save a million dollars a day by adopting scientific management principles.

Frank and Lillian Gilbreth were also concerned with efficiency, as evidenced by studies centered on motion economy that laid the foundation for application of job simplification as we know it today. Gilbreth's interest was aroused during his work as an apprentice bricklayer, where he observed various work methods used by the bricklayers. His research led to the invention of a number of instruments and techniques relating to motion economy (George 1968).

1. Use of *motion picture film* to observe and analyze work motions.
2. The *microchronometer,* a clock with a sweeping hand, was used with the motion picture film to determine how long it took to perform various motions. The instrument was capable of recording time to $\frac{1}{2000}$ second.
3. The *cyclegraph,* which showed the motion patterns involved in performing a task, was made by placing a small lighted electric bulb near the employee's hand.
4. A *chronocyclegraph,* used to determine the acceleration, deceleration, and direction of movement, was added to the circuit in order to determine speed and direction of movement.
5. Used the technique of consolidating hand motions into 17 basic motions known as *therbligs.* (Gilbreth spelled backwards with the *th* transposed)
6. Invented the *process* chart and *flow diagram* to record patterns used in performing a task.

In their quest for the "one best method," the Gilbreths provided practical application of the science of management.

Human Relations

Early organization and management thought centered around efficiency, high productivity, and low labor cost. The feelings, needs, and attitudes of the worker were practically ignored. It was not until the middle 1930s that significant attention was given to the people in the organization. During this period, major contributions were made by Elton Mayo and his associates. These contributions are commonly referred to as the Hawthorne studies.

Hawthorne Studies

As reported by Henderson, Whitehead, and Mayo (1937), studies conducted at the Hawthorne plant of the Western Electric Company were initiated and influenced by two main factors: (1) There was interest in the problems of fatigue and monotony in factory work, and (2) the researchers were aware that there were no satisfactory criteria for dealing with people as compared with the carefully contrived experiments for materials and machines. The studies, conducted between 1927 and 1932, were in three phases.

RELAY ASSEMBLY TEST ROOM EXPERIMENT In this experiment, five women were transferred from their usual work surroundings to an experimental room where their work was supervised by an appointed observer. During the entire period of 5 years, continuous and accurate records were maintained on quantity of output, quality of output, room temperature, lighting, conversations, reasons for temporary stops, amount of sleep time, and number of developed human relationships. From time to time, experimental changes were arbitrarily introduced such as change in hours of work, introduction of rest periods, and change in illumination. The workers were informed about the nature of the experiments, and they agreed to cooperate. They were instructed to work at a comfortable pace and warned against attempts to increase output. Nevertheless, the rate of output increased throughout the study, regardless of changes in work conditions. The average increase in speed of about 30% was not attributed to skills development, since all of the women were experts at relay assembly. The increase in production can be attributed to changes in the social environment that is made up of sentiments and routine. The results also suggest that the achievements were largely due to an equilibrium between plant authority and the spontaneous social organization of the women.

THE BANK-WIRING ROOM EXPERIMENT This experiment consisted of two investigations simultaneously. One method was an indirect conversational interview; the other was by direct observation. Both the interviewers and the observers were studying the same group of workers. The interviewer conducted interviews by appointment, whereas the observer was placed with the group to record performance, conversations, and other significant events. The spontaneous social organization of this group centered on fear and mistrust because they were not sure of management's intentions. This was quite different from the previous experiment with women in the relay assembly room. The women were told about the experiment and they agreed to cooperate. This resulted in a high degree of accord between workers and management.

Employees in the bank-wiring experiment defeated the official plan of the company through formation of the informal organization. For example, individual differences in performance were related to the individual's position in the group rather than to his actual capacity. The employees established group norms for output levels, striking a medium between producing too much and producing too little.

The supervisory controls established by management failed. It was assumed that the worker was primarily moved by economic interests and that he or she would act to optimize the economic rewards.

Open System Theory

In the open system approach to organization, one of the key determinants is the degree of interaction with the environment. This approach is in direct contrast to bureaucracy theory, which considered the external environmental pressure as a threat, and to scientific and administrative management theories, which generally ignored the environment (Albanese 1975). During the period of classical theory, the organization was functioning in a more stable, predictable environment, in terms of economics, energy (personnel, materials, machines, and information), and uniformity of individual value system. Support for an open system theory is offered below by the succinct description of the milieu in which a complex organization must function:

> Today organizations are confronted with a magnitude and complexity of world change that strains the coping mechanism of bureaucracies. We face rapid technological advances, knowledge explosion, struggles of women and minorities for political and economic enfranchisement, limited raw materials, increasing environmental and social blight, inflation, shifted third world politics, and collisions of diverse values and philosophies (Mink, Shultz & Mink 1979).

Characteristics of an Open System

Organizations, as open systems, have common characteristics with other open systems such as input, process, and output, but they also have distinct characteristics. According to Mink, Shultz, and Mink (1979), an open organization is characterized as follows:

1. An *integrated whole.* In an open system, unity of organizational mission or purpose is fostered through the sharing of information, with credibility of leadership based on the ability to use a system-wide perspective for problem solving through persuasion rather than relying on legal authority.

2. *Interdependent components.* An open system discourages *empire building,* all parts of the system are responsive to each other. In the human body, for example, the various organs are interdependent subsystems that exchange nutrients, oxygen, nitrogen, and other biological elements. When the free flow or exchange of elements is blocked, disease results. In human organizations, blockage occurs with closed, belligerent members of defensive departments. In an open organization, internal responsiveness is fostered through collaboration of managers and staff rather than through authority.

3. *Interchange with the environment.* An open organization continually interfaces with the environment that it serves or on which it depends for survival. The interchange of activities, data, and energy with other systems in the environment that may affect decisions and goals of the organization makes for a proactive rather than a reactive relationship. An open organization anticipates new data and the possible change that may come with it. Thus it is prepared for decision making before a crisis develops.

4. *Interrelating individual, group, and organization.* Three characteristics (unity, internal responsiveness, and external responsiveness) are used to describe openness of the individual, group, and organization. Openness is increased on the individual level in terms of unity when there is positive self-concept. For internal responsiveness, an awareness of one's feelings, wants, and needs increases openness, and positive interaction with others increases openness in external responsiveness. On the group level, unity is fostered when one can identify with the team goals and objectives, realizing that group output is greater than the sum of individual outputs. For internal responsiveness, the group exhibits positive interpersonal skills, facilitating interaction among team members; and for external responsiveness, openness is increased when the group cooperates in gathering and relating external information relevant to task of the group. At the organization level, unity is increased when there is development of common goals of organization and the managerial process is in accord with purpose and mission. For internal responsiveness, unity is increased when there is positive reaction to and impact upon components within the organization. For external responsiveness, the organization is socially relevant and responsive to the larger community and is profitable and productive.

In addition to the foregoing, open systems share characteristic of negative entropy, feedback, homeostasis, differentiation, and equifinality (Katz & Kahn 1966). *Negative entrophy* means that the system must import more energy from the environment than it expends in order to survive and maintain internal order. *Feedback* refers to information input that describes the environmental condition, thus providing a signal to the system on its functioning in relation to the environment. The use of information input enables the system to correct malfunctions within the organization or adapt to changes in the environment, thus creating a steady state of *homeostasis.* Since organizations exist in a changing and demanding environment, they must be able to adapt to environmental demands as a means of survival. Open systems have a tendency toward *differentiation* or specialization among their subsystems, both because of dynamics and the relationship between growth and survival. Finally, the principle of *equifinality* suggests that there is no one best way to achieve an objective. Put another way, a system can use a variety of inputs and transform them in a number of ways, yet achieve the same final state. This principle suggests the flexibility associated with open system rather than the rigidity found in classical theory.

Open system theory is considered the most appropriate for organizations in today's environmental climate, but it also suffers from imperfection, as most other theories of organization. According to Albanese (1975), open system theory has two main problems: (1) lack of clearly defined boundaries, and (2) overemphasis on synergism. The boundary problem stems from the inability to establish defined limits, since all elements within a system are interrelated to some degree among themselves and with the environment. Establishing criteria to determine what is relevant as an entity into the system is somewhat arbitrary, and therefore different managers will define the system in different ways. The differences in system definition can be important in determining managerial effectiveness.

The second problem associated with the open system is that of synergism. The idea of synergism reflects the systems view in that the emphasis of the theory is on relationships and synthesis. Synergism means that the whole is greater than its parts. In terms of the organization, it means that the combined efforts of the various systems produce a greater total than would the individual systems acting independently. There is the possibility of de-emphasizing the importance of individual members and relying too much on relationships as a source of understanding systems parts.

Organization Design

An organization structure is analogous to the skeleton of the human body. Put another way, the structure provides a framework for the efficient flow of the many processes that are constantly going on. The structural design is static in nature and therefore cannot reflect all of the relationships and interrelations that exist. Although the formal organization is not realistic in some respects, it is a valuable tool for controlling and coordinating the network of activities.

Formal Organization

Formal organization is usually represented by a chart that is a graphic display of the organizational structure. The chart attempts to describe the formal relationships found in an organization in the performance of activities. A typical chart, with its lines and boxes, is designed to show some control over communication, authority, power, responsibility, and accountability (Hicks & Gullett 1975).

COMMUNICATION The chart depicts communication lines in all directions: downward, upward, and horizontal. For example, downward communication may take the form of management decision making, which flows down to systems and subsystems within the organization. Upward communication refers to reports to supervisors on results achieved, questions concerning policies, employee complaints, and other matters that need to be considered at a higher level. Horizontal communication is across departmental or unit lines such as the communication between the dietary and nursing departments.

AUTHORITY Authority may be viewed as the right to do something. It has also been referred to as institutional power, inasmuch as it is formally sanctioned by the organization of which the person who possesses the authority is a member. Authority typically gives an individual the right to issue instructions to others and to see that they are carried out. Authority may be centralized or decentralized. When authority is widely dispersed or delegated throughout the organization, *decentralization of authority* exists. When authority is in the hands of a few persons, *centralized authority* exists. Span of control, as discussed earlier, is also a form of authority and is typically depicted on organization charts. Line, staff, and functional authority are also defined through the organization chart, which shows that line personnel have the right to give orders, whereas staff personnel are limited to giving advice and consultation. For example, staff personnel may consult with the personnel director on matters of hiring, grievances, and other personnel activities. Functional authority allows a position holder to issue instructions in a limited area, such as requiring approval by the purchasing manager of expenditures over $100.

POWER The concept of power is broader than that of authority. Power can be defined as the ability to do something. An individual may possess power over activities or personnel without having legal or institutional authority. Power may stem from technical competence, seniority, and friendship with other powerful people inside or outside of the formal organization.

RESPONSIBILITY The obligation position holders feel for their actions is called responsibility. Unlike authority, responsibility cannot be delegated.

ACCOUNTABILITY When results are measured with predetermined standards, accountability is said to exist. Accountability may be thought of as flowing upward through the formal organization structure. Each level is accountable to the next.

Some problems associated with a formal organization are as follows:

1. Organizational status is associated with the placement of boxes.
2. The chart does not show the relationship of external influences.
3. Because the chart is static, it ignores dynamic interrelationships.
4. The chart does not depict the informal relationships that are present in all organizations.

Informal Organization

The informal organization operates outside of the formal organization. It arises out of the need for employees to interact socially, to establish cohesiveness with co-workers, and to satisfy individual motives. The informal organization facilitates communication in ways not open to the formal organization and therefore can foster the purpose of the formal organization or work against it.

The grapevine is a prime example of the informal organization that can be helpful, but can be detrimental if not used for organizational purposes. The manager has an excellent opportunity to use the grapevine to communicate information that will assist in the coordination of subordinate efforts. If recognized and used properly, the informal organization can supplement the formal organization in its goals and objectives.

Design of Medical Care Facilities

The level of care in medical facilities varies from *minimal care* in health-related facilities, to *acute care* found in hospitals. In between the two types, we find skilled nursing care in long-term care facilities and other facilities offering care for the mentally ill, homes for the aged, and homes for children and other adults that provide lodging, meals, social activities, and a minimum of health care. The organization design for the various facilities depends on the respective goals, objectives, and services rendered.

—— Long-Term Care Facilities ———————————

Long-term care is a broad term and includes a number of facilities that provide custodial, basic, and skilled nursing care. Confusion surrounding the nomenclature used to describe the various facilities is widespread, with most facilities lumped under the heading of nursing homes. Schneeweiss and Davis (1974) use the following classification for long-term care facilities:[1]

1. *Domiciliary care facilities.* This category includes homes for the aged, public and private homes for adults, and residence for adults.
    A. *Residency for adults.* A facility, that provides lodging, food, housekeeping services, and activity programs for adults who require such services on a continuous basis.
    B. *Proprietary home for adults.* A facility, operated for profit, that provides lodging, food, plus the services of attendants to ensure safety and comfort in bathing, dressing, feeding, and moving about. Medical and nursing services are not provided.
    C. *Public home.* A residence for adults, typically operated without an infirmary.
    D. *Home for the aged.* A proprietary or nonprofit facility with services similar to those for adult homes.
2. *Health-related facilities.* Intermediate care facilities providing lodging, food, social activities, social services, and minimal physical care. Nonambulatory patients are usually not admitted.
3. *Extended care facility or nursing home.* This facility provides 24-hour skilled nursing care, rehabilitative or restorative services, and other health services under the supervision of a physician.
4. *Senior citizen hotel.* A facility for the elderly who do not suffer from chronic illness.

The classification fails to delineate between the different types of nursing homes such as those providing skilled nursing care, intermediate care, and those providing minimal care. There are distinct differences, as noted in the Michigan Department of Public Health–Bureau of Health Care Facilities (1985). In Michigan, nursing homes are classified as follows:

1. An intermediate (or basic nursing) care facility (ICF).
2. A skilled nursing care facility (SNF).
3. An intermediate care facility for the mentally retarded (ICF/MR).
4. A nursing facility for the care of mentally ill patients.
5. A nursing facility for the care of mentally retarded patients.
6. A nursing facility for the care of tuberculosis patients.

This classification is based on the intensity of care provided, with the skilled nursing care facility providing the most intensive care. Because states may differ in their classification of care provided, the practitioner is advised to become familiar with local health codes.

---

[1]On February 2, 1989, the final rule was published for long-term care facilities participating in medicare and medicaid. The regulation removes the distinction between skilled nursing facilities (SNF) and intermediate care facilities (ICF). After October 1, 1990 both types of facilities will be known as "nursing facilities" and will operate under one set of requirements (USDHHS 1989). The regulations do not apply to ICFs for the mentally retarded.

The level of care in long-term care facilities improved considerably with passage of federal laws that governed both the physical facility and quality of care provided. Prior to 1935, care for the institutionalized elderly and the chronically ill individual was left entirely to the discretion of the various states, with different rules and regulations for licensure, level of care, and funding. The passage of federal legislation had a major impact on the growth and standards of operation for long-term care as follows (Moschetto 1981):

1. The *Social Security Act* (1935) provided monthly assistance to the disabled and to persons over 65 years of age. With the available funds, indigent individuals were able to pay for the improved quality of care.
2. The *Hill-Burton Act* (1946) contributed to improved facilities and care by providing grants and loans for the construction of and equipment for facilities.
3. *Amendments to the Social Security Act* (1950) marked the beginning of vendor payments to nursing home owners.
4. *The Small Business Act* and *Small Business Investment Act* (1958) made loans available to nursing homes.
5. *The National Housing Act* (1959) encouraged construction and renovation of nursing homes with the provision of mortgage insurance.
6. *The Kerr-Mill Program* (1960) encouraged expansion of medical care for the elderly by increasing federally matched funds to states using medical vendor payments.
7. *The Mental Health and Retardation Acts* (1963 and 1965) shifted the focus of care for mentally ill patients by promoting the transfer of mentally ill elderly from psychiatric hospitals to nursing homes.
8. *Medicare and Medicaid Amendments to the Social Security Act* (1965). Medicare provided medical insurance for persons 65 years and older; Medicaid provided a federal-state grant program for the indigent. Medicare is funded and administered by the federal government, whereas Medicaid is administered by the state with matching federal funds.

With the use of outside funding, long-term care facilities also had to comply with outside rules and regulations for licensure, certification, quality of care, and organization. In the state of Michigan, concerted effort has been made to unify standards of operation for foodservice with recommended standards formulated for all state-owned and -operated foodservice operations.

The organization of long-term care facilities depends on the intensity and nature of care provided. In an intermediate or basic nursing care facility, the organization may appear as shown in Figure 3-1.

The dietary department is usually supervised by a foodservice supervisor, with the advice and consultation of a Registered Dietitian. As a result of diagnosis-related groups (DRGs) with shorter lengths of stay in acute care facilities, patients are admitted to nursing homes in a more critical state of illness. In efforts to provide adequate nutritional care, Registered Dietitians are staffed on a full-time basis in large SNFs. As noted by the dotted lines, the consultant dietitian holds a staff position and reports directly to the nursing home administrator. The foodservice supervisor reports directly to the nursing home administrator and is responsible for production and service of food to both patients and personnel. The foodservice supervisor is a member of all mandated committees that concern patient foodservice, as required by the accrediting agency.

The skilled nursing care facility offers the most intensive care among the long-term care facilities. The facility, as all nursing home facilities in the state of

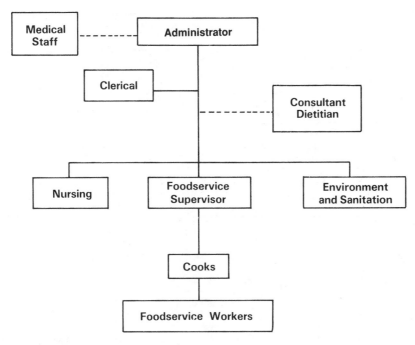

Figure 3-1. Organization chart for basic or intermediate nursing care facility. Broken lines indicate communication–not direct supervision.

Michigan, must be licensed. The facility may meet qualifications and request certification under guidelines for extended care facilities. Under these circumstances, the organization of skilled nursing care and extended care facilities are similar, as shown in Figure 3-2.

Nursing homes, along with other categories of medical care facilities became eligible for accreditation by the JCAH in 1967 as follows (American Medical Association 1967):

Category I: *Hospitals.*

Category II: *Extended care facilities. Established with medical staff and continuous nursing service to provide comprehensive post–acute hospital care for a relative short duration.*

Category II: *Nursing care facilities.* Establishments with medical staff or medical staff equivalent and continuous nursing care to provide long-term inpatient care (not necessarily posthospital) for a variety of medical conditions.

Category IV: *Resident care facilities.* Establishments which furnish regular and frequent, but not continuous medical and nursing service for the safe, hygienic, and sheltered living of residents not capable of or desiring independent living.

The extended care facility is an establishment or a designated part of an establishment that provides highly skilled nursing care and rehabilitative care to posthospital patients. Emphasis is on restorative care, such as physical, occupational, and speech therapy. The extended care may be provided in a facility separate from the hospital or it may occupy a *distinct* part of a hospital such as a designated floor or unit. In order to qualify as an extended care facility under the Medicare program, the provider of service must comply with the "conditions of participation" as specified in Public Law 89-97, amendment to the Social Security Act. (U.S. Department of Health and Human Services 1966).

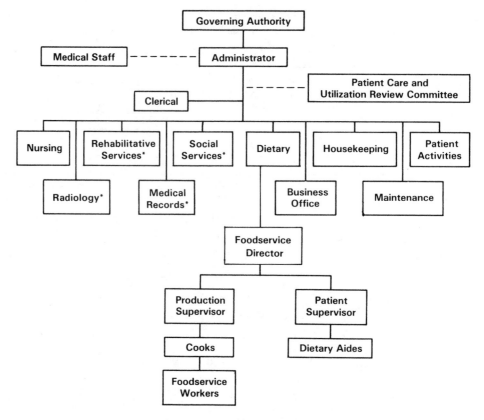

Figure 3-2. Organization chart for skilled nursing care and extended care facility. Starred entries may provide part-time or consultant services.

—Long-Term Care Survey —

The law and regulations governing conditions and standards of participation in Medicare–Medicaid for long-term care facilities have remained constant, but major changes have occurred in the process used to compile information on compliance. The purpose for implementing a new survey process is to ensure that the quality of care, intended by law and required by residents, is actually being provided in nursing homes.

The old survey process focused on structural requirements, such as written policies and procedures, staffing, and physical plant characteristics. The new Long Term Care Survey process (formerly referred to as Patient Care and Services, PACS) is patient outcome–oriented. For example, in ascertaining whether menus are planned and followed to meet the nutritional needs of each resident, surveyors will no longer routinely evaluate the written menu. Instead, surveyors will observe residents for physiological, psychological, and social factors that may affect food intake. In addition, surveyors will confirm through interviews with residents and staff that nutritional needs are met on a regular basis.

The Long Term Care Survey process was implemented nationwide in April 1986. Final procedural guidelines, as published in the Federal Register (June 1988) list the following components for a complete Skilled Nursing Facility (SNF)/Intermediate Care Facility (ICF) survey (USDHHS 1988):

- Life Safety Code requirements
- Administrative and structural requirements

- Direct resident care requirements, using the following worksheets:
  HCFA-520, Residents Selected for In-Depth Review
  HCFA-521, Tour Notes Worksheet
  HCFA-522, Drug Pass Worksheet
  HCFA-523, Dining Area and Eating Assistance Observation
  HCFA-524, Observation/Interview/Record Review

The above survey process is used for all surveys of SNF and ICF, whether freestanding, distinct parts, or dually certified. Advance notice to a facility that a survey is scheduled on a certain date is no longer provided. The surveyors may now enter an SNF/ICF unannounced. During the survey, the following tasks will be performed:

Task 1. Entrance conference
Task 2. Resident sample selection methodology
Task 3. Tour of the facility; resident needs; physical environment; meeting with resident council representative
Task 4. Observation/interview/medical record; review of each individual in the resident sample
Task 5. Drug pass observation
Task 6. Dining area and eating assistance observation
Task 7. Forming the deficiency statement (if necessary)
Task 8. Exit conference

The procedural guidelines provide surveyors with cross-references (conditions of participation) for the survey area; what to observe in patient outcome; suggested questions for interview with staff and residents; what to look for in the medical records; and how each factor is evaluated. (For details of the survey process relating directly to dietetic services see Appendix J.)

▬ Hospitals ▬▬▬▬▬▬▬▬▬▬▬▬▬▬▬▬▬▬▬▬▬▬▬▬▬▬▬▬▬▬▬

The acute care hospital provides the highest level of medical care and is the most complex of all medical facilities.

COMPLEX ORGANIZATION The complex organization found in hospitals is due to a number of factors (Rakich & Darr 1978):

1. There is a wide diversity of objectives and goals for the various personnel and subsystems within a complex facility. Conflict is likely to arise as subsystems carry out responsibilities involving complex medical and surgical cases, research, education, hotel-type accommodations, and other duties associated with patient care.
2. The diversity of personnel ranges from the most highly skilled and educated to the unskilled and uneducated. The task of the organization and management is to find ways to coordinate the efforts of the different groups so that they are able to work together.
3. The hospital is in continuous operation 7 days a week, 24 hours a day. The scheduling of personnel so that there will be adequate coverage is a monumental task.
4. In most hospital operations there are dual lines of authority. The duality refers to the board of governors, medical staff, and administrators, as discussed earlier. In addition, there is the legal authority of administrators and the functional authority of the medical staff, which often overlap and may create conflict.

5. Hospitals deal with problems of life and death. The nonroutine activities associated with complex hospitals often put undue psychological and physical stress on personnel at all levels. The consumer of hospital services cannot possibly understand the full thrust of ongoing activities and often becomes confused and hypercritical of the setting and results.

6. There is a problem in measuring the major product. Although there are accrediting agencies with mandated patient care policies, patient care has eluded precise measurement.

Because of the complexity of hospitals, it is evident that mechanistic, bureaucratic, formal authority principles of organization are not sufficient and cannot be applied across the board. Consideration must be given to the dynamics of sociopsychological forces at work within the organization. According to Georgopoulos (1972), organizational efficiency as well as high-level performance by members of the organization depends to a great extent on social efficiency. His theory is that social efficiency may be a more critical determinant of organization effectiveness than economic and technical efficiency since hospitals provide solutions to major problems. Considerations should center on the following.

1. *Organizational adaptation.* The ability for continuous adjustment to external conditions and the ability for successful response to relevant changes.
2. *Organizational allocation.* The ability to procure, deploy, allocate, and utilize human resources and materials; to resolve problems of access to and distribution of authority, rewards, and information; to apply work specialization and allocation of tasks; and to enact participative decision making.
3. *Organizational coordination.* The ability to articulate and interrelate the diverse roles and interdependent activities; to regulate and synchronize different functions so that all time and effort are expended toward solution of systems problems and goal attainment.
4. *Organizational integration.* The ability of the system to integrate all members into the organization in such a manner as to enhance cooperation and compliance in achieving overall sociopsychological unity and coherence.
5. *Organizational strain.* The ability to minimize tension as a result of friction and confrontation among key groups, unequal status participants, and highly independent groups and members of the organization.
6. *Organizational output.* The ability to maximize efficient and reliable performance by all departments and members; to maximize opportunities for personal growth and satisfaction in efforts to reach and maintain high levels of patient care or health services to the community.
7. *Organizational maintenance.* The ability to stabilize an organization's identity and integrity in the face of constant external changes and the potential disruptive and threatening situations that may develop internally.

An understanding of open system concepts, characteristics of complex human organizations, and the inherent problems associated with a dynamic, adaptive, and problem-solving social–technical system is a prerequisite for organizational design of a medical facility. The typical voluntary not-for-profit hospital is usually organized with the sharing of power in a triad: governing body, administrator, and medical staff. The trend, according to Rakich and Darr (1978), is changing to one of corporate structure in which the governing authority delegates power to a chief executive officer (CEO) who is responsible for all activities, including medical care. This type of structure is prevalent in hospitals where physicians are employed by the organization, such as Veterans Administration and military hospitals. Figure 3-3 is an example of an organization chart for a complex hospital. This teaching hospital prefers the title *pattern of administrative function* rather than the more traditional *organization chart*. The term implies a more flexible, less structured type of organization that encourages cooperative efforts of line and staff personnel. This is a 1000-bed hospital with extensive outpatient care at the main facility and at its various satellite units.

In this display, an executive committee, rather than an administrator or CEO, reports directly to the Board of Trustees. Of interest, also, is the lack of lines designating advisory relationships. According to White (1963), many companies omit dotted lines, which indicate communication, because they tend to clutter the chart. Furthermore, persons in a modern operation are free to communicate, for legitimate reasons, with almost anyone else in the organization. The direct lines are necessary to show relationships based on the power to discharge, discipline, issue orders, and communicate formal instructions and reports. Put another way, dotted lines may or may not be used at the discretion of the parties at either end of the chart, whereas solid lines must be used regardless of the interest or convenience of individuals involved.

The department of dietetics, as shown in Figure 3-3, is directly responsible to an associate administrator. Within the department (Fig. 3-4), three top administrators report to the director: (1) The assistant director of nutrition and education is responsible for in-service education, dietetic internship, and clinical services; (2) the associate director of production, service, and support services is responsible for unit kitchens, support services, and the executive chef; and (3) the assistant director is responsible for dining services, coffee shop, and special functions. Each major unit, as shown in Figure 3-4, is broken down into subunits. For example, Figure 3-5 depicts the three subunits in the production, service, and support unit. It is important for each individual to visualize how he or she fits into the organizational structure and why individual contributions are vital in accomplishing organizational objectives and goals. Further illustration of departmental breakdown is shown in Figures 3-6, 3-7, and 3-8, to include all levels of work distribution within the foodservice department.

The use of charts with vertical and horizontal lines is not universally accepted for all types of organizations. Two other modes frequently referred to are (1) the concentric and (2) the matrix organization.

CONCENTRIC ORGANIZATION The concentric organization chart has been used in business and industry for more than 30 years. The most distinguishing feature of the chart is the use of circles to indicate echelon levels. An illustration of organization charts for a hospital dietetics department, using both the traditional and concentric models, is shown in Figure 3-9.

According to Browne (1950), the concentric organization chart offers a more satisfactory presentation for the following reasons:

1. The chart improves representation of the dynamics of personal relationships because functions are centered around individuals, not below them. The schematic design, using circles rather than horizontal plane, surrounds the director with contracts, influences, and relationships that stimulate from all directions.

2. It eliminates the *above and below* concept. Various echelons of authority are represented by the distance of the circle from the center or focal point, thus avoiding the emotional concepts of above or below, higher or lower, superior or inferior, top or bottom.

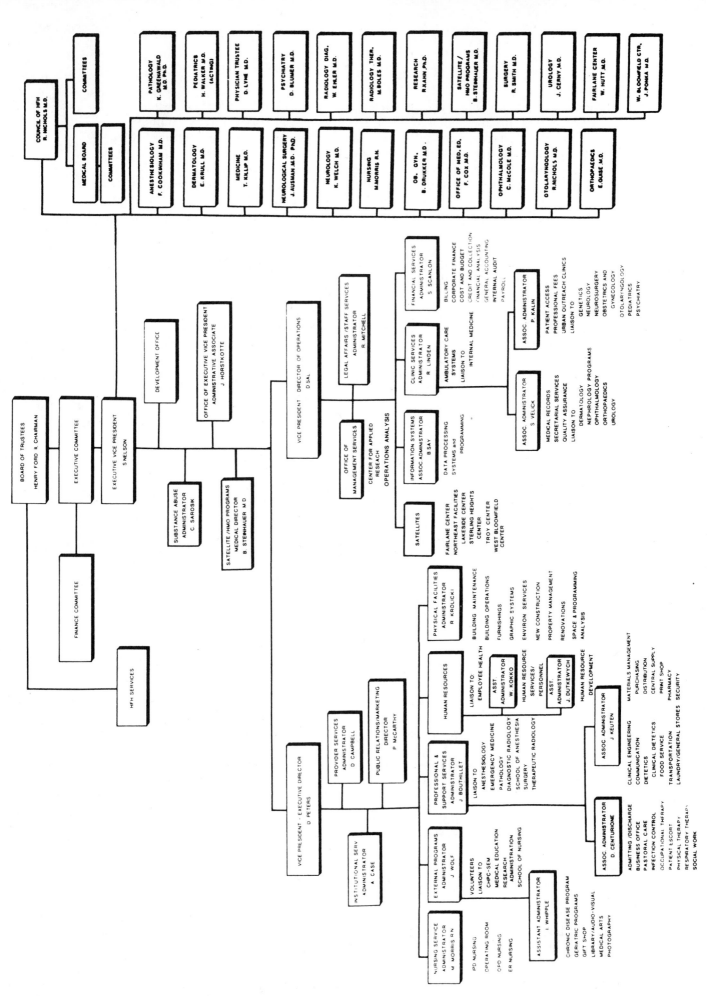

Figure 3-3. Organization chart for a large teaching hospital. *From Henry Ford Hospital, Detroit, Michigan*

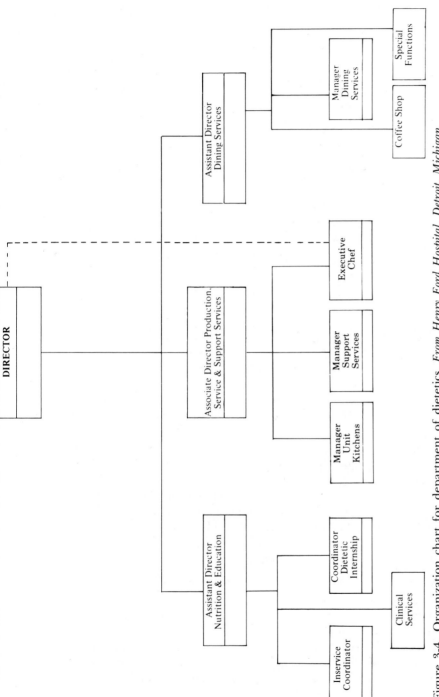

Figure 3-4. Organization chart for department of dietetics. *From Henry Ford Hospital, Detroit, Michigan*

35

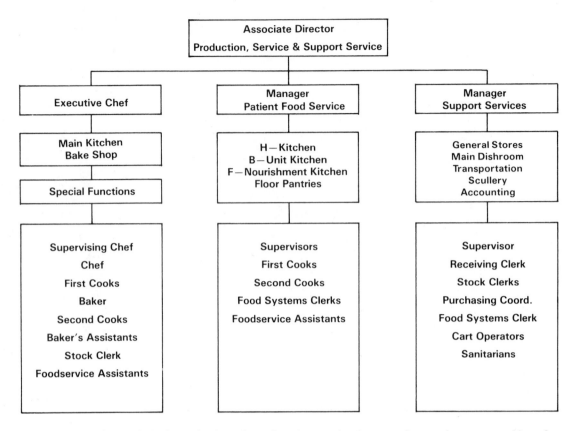

Figure 3-5. Organization chart for the production, service, and support units of a dietetics department. *From Henry Ford Hospital, Detroit, Michigan*

3. It presents an organization without loose ends. With the circular presentation, there is no left or right drop-off or vacuum of existing functions or relationships.

4. It eliminates the upside-down organizational structure since there is no top or bottom. The perspective is the same regardless of the angle or specific position from which the chart is viewed.

5. It simplifies designing and understanding. The problem associated with space in designing the traditional chart is eliminated with the use of circles. Using the traditional model, there are physical limitations to designing the fourth or fifth echelon level without decreasing the size of the boxes, thereby causing possible confusion in the interpretation of status.

MATRIX ORGANIZATION The concept of matrix organization, introduced more than two decades ago, was initially used for special projects only. Today, the matrix form of organizing is found in a variety of contexts: product management, task force management, production teams, and new business development teams. It is used by business and industry, government agencies, professional organizations, and hospitals. When the matrix form of management is introduced into an organization, there are changes in traditional management practices such as authority and responsibility, span of control, department specialization, resource allocation patterns, and personnel evaluation (Cleland 1981).

As shown in Figure 3-10, there is dual chain of command that departs from the traditional principle of reporting to only one supervisor. Since personnel in medical facilities frequently perform under dual lines of authority, the introduction of matrix management would not constitute a dramatic change in es-

MAIN KITCHEN

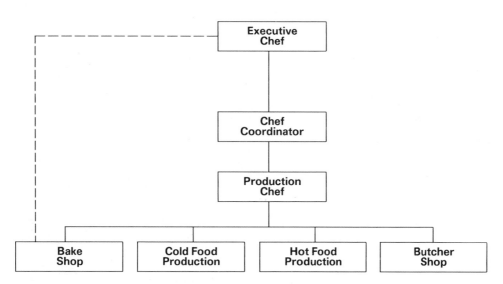

Figure 3-6. Organization chart for the main kitchen, a subunit of the production, service, and support unit of a dietetics department. *From Henry Ford Hospital, Detroit, Michigan*

tablished procedures. The essentials necessary for effective teamwork are also required for effective matrix management. In matrix management, as in the team approach to patient care, there must be integration and coordination of individual and group efforts as authority, responsibility, accountability, and power tend to shift and cut across functional lines. The matrix organization is used in hospitals to generate a number of reports to assist management in the decision-making process (Sinioris, Esmond, Glenesk, & Newman 1982). In hospitals, the matrix formation is centered on the patient as the product line and is closely related to physician specialty. In such cases, the specialty of programs form the horizontal lines (cardiology, obstetrics, and so on), whereas the vertical axis is represented by support services, such as nursing and physical therapy.

Matrix organization is complex and requires considerable attention to the organizational climate prior to implementation. Because matrix organization involves sharing of authority and responsibility, the struggle for power by individual managers can be one of the biggest problems. Other problems encountered with matrix organization, according to Davis and Lawrence (1978), include the following:

1. A tendency toward anarchy resulting from dual command, as people become confused over who is really the *boss*.
2. The misconception that matrix management is the same as group decision making, thus wasting an enormous amount of time.
3. During an economic crisis when business is slow, the matrix is used as a scapegoat for poor management practices and is discarded in favor or more direct action.
4. The fear that management cost will double because of the dual chain of command.
5. A tendency for the matrix to sink to lower levels in the corporate structure.
6. Fear of decision strangulation as a result of endless debate and the clearing of all decisions by higher administration.

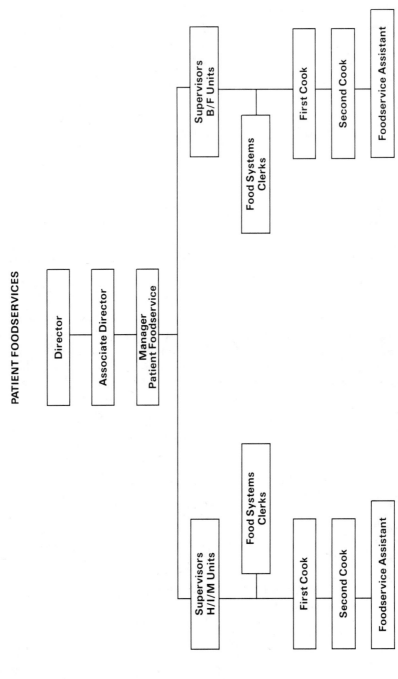

PATIENT FOODSERVICES

Director

Associate Director

Manager Patient Foodservice

Supervisors H/I/M Units

Food Systems Clerks

First Cook

Second Cook

Foodservice Assistant

Supervisors B/F Units

Food Systems Clerks

First Cook

Second Cook

Foodservice Assistant

Figure 3-7. Organization chart for patient foodservice, a subunit of the production, service, and support unit of a dietetics department. *From Henry Ford Hospital, Detroit, Michigan*

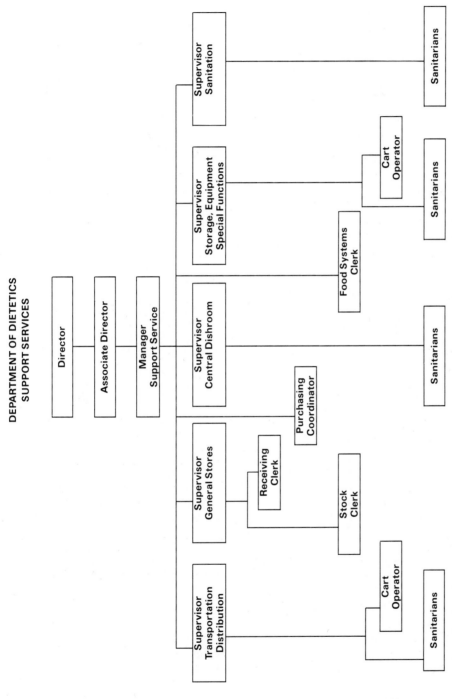

DEPARTMENT OF DIETETICS
SUPPORT SERVICES

Figure 3-8. Organization chart for support service, a subunit of the production, service, and support unit of a dietetics department. *From Henry Ford Hospital, Detroit, Michigan*

39

Organizational Chart: Traditional Model

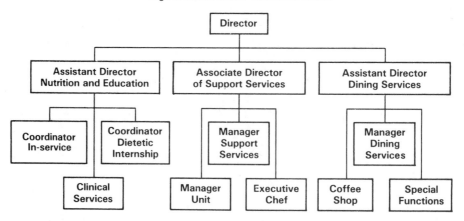

Organization Chart: Concentric Model

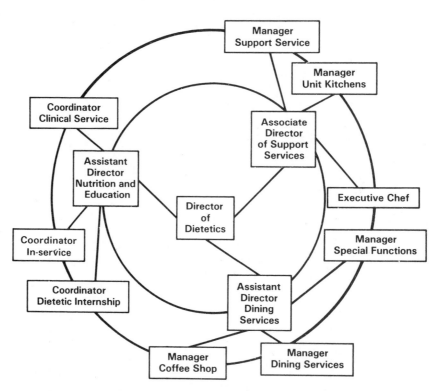

Figure 3-9. Two models of organization for dietary department.

The matrix organization will most likely be used to a greater extent by open organizations such as medical facilities simply because it lends legitimacy to what is now accomplished in an informal manner.

Multihospital Systems

A major trend in hospital organization is the advent of multihospital systems. The single hospital is gradually disappearing as hospitals ban together in efforts to maintain quality patient care during a period of adverse economic conditions. The major systems currently in use are as follows:

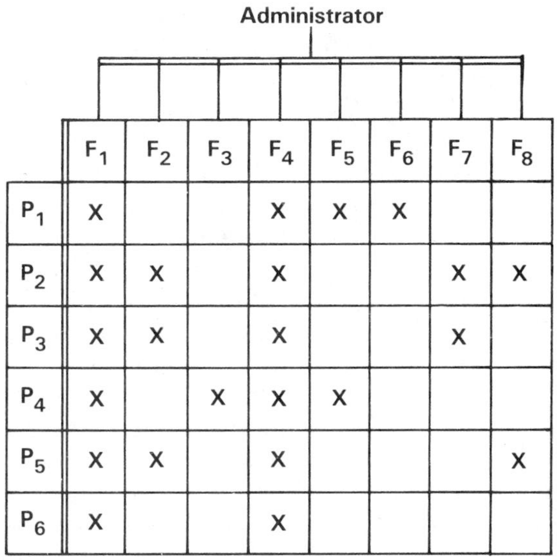

Administrator

	F$_1$	F$_2$	F$_3$	F$_4$	F$_5$	F$_6$	F$_7$	F$_8$
P$_1$	X			X	X	X		
P$_2$	X	X		X			X	X
P$_3$	X	X		X			X	
P$_4$	X		X	X	X			
P$_5$	X	X		X				X
P$_6$	X			X				

Figure 3-10. Conceptual model of matrix organiza
tion. P represents Patient–Project; F, Functional
Manager–Unit; and X, Patient–Function interface.

1. *Merger.* A merger takes place when the assets of two or more institutions are consolidated or when one institution acquires another (usually smaller) institution. When assets are consolidated, a new corporate structure is formed and may be housed in a new facility, or one facility may be closed and only one facility used. Legally, the merged hospitals must be under single ownership and have one governing body; one medical staff; one set of by-laws, rules, and regulations; and all mandated medical staff committees (Baydin & Sheldon 1978).

2. *Joint venture.* This system differs from the merger in how it is organized and controlled. The distinguishing feature is that each institution maintains its identity. This arrangement is possible when two or more institutions with powerful identities agree to combine resources in order to deliver improved patient care at lower cost. In a joint venture of hospitals in Boston (Baydin & Sheldon 1978), a new physical structure was built to house the three hospitals. The corporate structure, Affiliated Hospital Center, Inc., was organized with a vice president as Chief Operating Officer, with members from each institution constituting the Governing Board. Each hospital is responsible for its own financing, budget, medical staff appointments, teaching, research, and other components. Ambulatory care is to be run by all three. Cost of shared services is prorated to all three hospitals.

3. *Holding company.* A holding company owns and controls all stock of the other facilities and derives its income from interest and dividends. When facilities are nonprofit and without stock, all property, assets, and income as well as debts, liabilities and obligations of the facilities become those of the holding company (Baydin & Sheldon 1978). The holding company concept permits the small nonprofit hospital to maintain viable patient care by providing a broad economic base.

4. *Investor-owned system.* The system is owned and managed by national hospital chains that are proprietary and public. The largest of these national hospital companies is the Hospital Corporation of America (HCA). At the end of 1980, HCA operated 188 hospitals, with more than 80 new sites under development. Operating revenues increased 37% from 1979 to 1980 to more than $1.4

billion; income was up about 50% to approximately $81 million (Tinsley 1981). Ownership of facilities means total control, and the ability to provide unlimited managerial resources at the corporate level.

5. *Contract department management.* In this arrangement, there is a legal agreement between a health care facility and an outside management company for the management of a specified department. The degree of control granted to the management company is spelled out in the contract. During 1981, a total of 4951 departments in medical facilities were managed full-time by 138 outside contractors (Punch 1982A). Housekeeping, among 33 different departments managed by outside companies, is the most frequently contracted service. Food-service has the largest number of contract management providers, followed by housekeeping, respiratory therapy, and physical therapy.

6. *Contract Shared-Consultant Service.* This system provides services beyond departmental boundaries and is available to medical facilities in more than 50 different areas. One company, which limits its services to medical records abstracting, had the largest number of clients (2777) during 1981 (Punch 1982B). Other services offered by providers include financial consulting, management engineering, strategic planning, risk management, and others.

7. *Shared services.* These are cooperative ventures by two or more hospitals. Services can be classified as referred service, purchased service, multisponsored service, or regional service (AHA 1976). A *referred service* is maintained by one member of the group, and other institutions refer patients who need the service. Patients receive direct billing by the provider. A *purchased* service is a patient service provided by another institution. The institution requesting the service pays the provider directly and then bills the patient. A *multisponsored service* is jointly operated and controlled by a group of institutions. There is a legal arrangement, with controls established through mutual agreement or through a separate corporation to include board representation from each institution. A *regional service,* such as computerized information service, is sponsored by an association of institutions. The service is financed through association funds, assessment of members, direct charges to member institutions, or a combination of these. Shared food services include group purchasing, prepared food purchasing, sharing of preparation, and shared management and personnel.

All types of multihospital systems have proliferated during the past 5 years and are expected to continue in the same direction for years to come. The primary reason for the various types of networking is financial. A survey of 668 CEOs nationwide revealed that nearly as many hospitals are considering mergers as have already done so (Moore 1987). The survey also showed that hospitals in the Southwest have the highest level of merger activity (29.8%), whereas only 14.7% of hospitals in the Southeast have merged. A large percentage of hospitals have established referral networks instead of merging. Referral activity was highest in the Midwest (32.1%) compared with 17.6% in the Southeast. The same regions that displayed the most and least activity in mergers also displayed the most and least interest in managed care contracting. Three 10-year predictions affecting merger activity that may be of interest to the medical foodservice director are:

1. The industry will be downsized by 17.6% over the next 10 years as a result of decline in inpatient utilization.
2. There will be 479,000 fewer hospital full-time equivalents.
3. Managerial talents will be vigorously sought.

How is the increase in mergers affecting personnel? What thought is given to human resources, and when? How is administration assisting employees with the trauma involved when one or more facilities merge? According to Marks and Cutcliffe (1988), during the premerger phase, the CEOs are surrounded by bankers and lawyers until the deal is consummated. Little consideration is given to critical management components such as communication, integration, organizational design, and staffing until the merger is in place. In fact, key managers who will lead the postmerger and human resource personnel are usually absent from the initial planning.

A merger is a change. Employees approach change differently, depending on the nature and magnitude. When employees must rely on the "grapevine" for information, the result may be stress, anxiety, lower productivity, and even quitting the job in fear of what might happen. Fear and insecurity may have merit since downsizing is usually a consequence of merger. Steps that managers can take to alleviate the trauma associated with mergers are offered by Davy, Kinicki, Kilroy, and Scheck (1988) and Fink (1988):

1. *Communicate with employees in a timely manner.* If legally possible, make an announcement to the employees before the news media break the story. Maintain channels of communication throughout the transition period. Conduct honest, frequent meetings to enhance a feeling of security and to assist in reducing rumors.

2. *Reduce uncertainty and ambiguity.* Create transition committees to serve as information conduits between top management and the work force. Consider establishing a telephone merger hotline so that employees can anonymously express concerns and ask questions. Administer an open-ended survey to obtain information about employee expectations. Clarify any incorrect expectations.

3. *Address the issue of job security.* Provide honest information about the possibility of layoff. Consider providing an outplacement program. Provide an employee and family counseling program. Conduct seminars on how to cope with stress.

── Contract Food Management ─────────

The organization of a foodservice department can be affected in a number of ways when the medical facility decides to contract foodservice (Zaccarelli & Ninemeier 1982). Staffing becomes the number one concern for employees currently working at the facility. The food management company may bring in a completely new staff, or staffing may be divided—with some employees paid by the facility and others by the food management company. It is often the director of the dietary department and other members of the in-house management team who are in competition with the outside company. As shown by asterisks in Figure 3-11, managerial positions held by employees of the food management company are (1) director of dietetics, (2) foodservice director, and (3) cafeteria supervisor. The organizational structure is typical, with high-level managerial positions staffed by the food management company, and clinical service staffed by health care facility employees. In this structure, the director of dietetics is considered a department head and is responsible to both the health care facility administrator and the food management company. In some organizational structures, the director of clinical services reports directly to an administrator at the health care facility, rather than to the food management company director as indicated in Figure 3-11. This type of organization further emphasizes the need to understand concepts of the matrix organization.

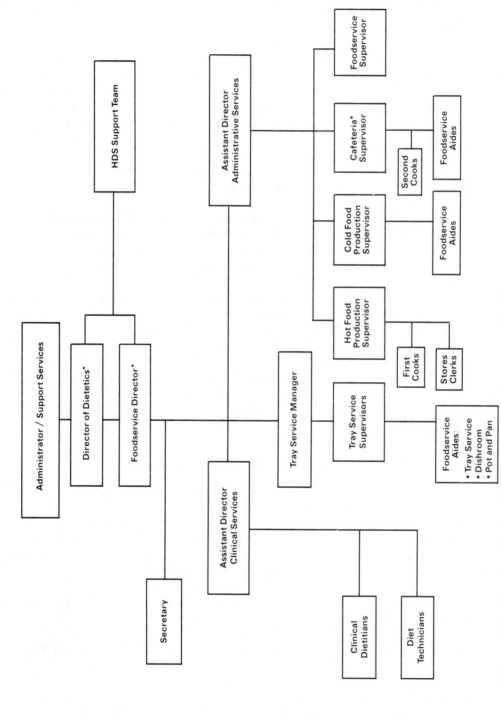

Figure 3-11. Organization chart for hospital foodservice operated by food management company. The starred employees are employed by the food management company. *From Detroit Receiving Hospital, Detroit, Michigan*

References

Albanese, R. (1975). *Management Toward Accountability for Performance.* Homewood, IL: Richard D. Irwin.

American Hospital Association. (1976). *Shared Food Services in Health Care Institutions.* Chicago: AHA.

American Medical Association. (1967). *The Extended Care Facility: A Handbook for the Medical Society.* Chicago: AMA.

Barnes, M. C., Fogg, A. H., Stephens, C. N., and Titman, L. G. (1970). *Company Organization: Theory and Practice.* Beverly Hills: Davlin Publishing.

Baydin, D., and Sheldon, A. (1978). Corporate Models in Health Care Delivery. In *Hospital Organization and Management,* J. S. Rakich and K. Darr, eds. New York: Halsted Press.

Browne, C. G. (1950). The Concentric Organization Chart. *J. Appl. Psych. 34*(6), 375–377.

Cleland, D. I. (1981). The Cultural Ambience of Matrix Organization. *Mgt. Rev. 70*(11), 25–39.

Davis, S. M., and Lawrence, P. R. (1978). Problems of Matrix Organizations. *Harvard Bus. Rev. 56*(3), 131–142.

Davy, J. A., Kinicki, A., Kilroy, J., and Scheck, C. (1988). After the Merger: Dealing with People's Uncertainty. *Training Devel. J. 42*(2), 56–61.

Filey, A. C., and House, R. J. (1969). *Managerial Process and Organizational Behavior.* Glenview, IL: Scott, Foresman.

Fink, C. A. (1988). The Impact of Mergers on Employees. *Health Care Supervisor 7*(1) 59–67.

Foyal, H. (1949). *Industrial and General Administration.* London: Pitman.

George, C. S. (1968). *The History of Management Thought.* Englewood Cliffs, NJ: Prentice-Hall.

Georgopoulos, B. S., ed. (1972). *Organization Research on Health Institutions.* Ann Arbor: The University of Michigan, Institute for Social Research.

Graicunas, V. A. (1937). Relationships in Organization. In *Papers on the Science of Administration,* L. Gulick and L. Urwick, eds. New York: Institute of Public Administration.

Gulick, L. (1937). Notes on the Theory of Organization. In *Papers on the Science of Administration,* L. Gulick and L. Urwick, eds. New York: Institute of Public Administration.

Hall, R. H. (1972). The Concept of Bureaucracy: An Empirical Assessment. *In Organizational Systems,* K. Azumi and J. Hage, eds. Lexington, MA: D. C. Heath.

Henderson, L. J., Whitehead, T. N., and Mayo, E. (1937). The Effects of Social Environment. In *Papers on the Science of Administration,* L. Gulick and L. Urwick, eds. New York: Institute of Public Administration.

Hicks, H. G., and Gullett, C. R. (1975). *Organization Theory and Behavior.* New York: McGraw-Hill.

Katz, D., and Kahn, R. L. (1966). *The Social Psychology of Organizations.* New York: Wiley.

Marks, M. L., and Cutcliffe, J. G. (1988). Making Mergers Work. *Training Devel. J. 42*(4), 30–36.

Michigan Department of Public Health–Bureau of Health Care Facilities. (1985). *Nursing Homes and Nursing Care Facilities.* Lansing: MDPH.

Mink, O. G., Shultz, J. M., and Mink, B. P. (1979). *Developing and Managing Open Organizations.* Austin, TX: Learning Concepts.

Mooney, J. D., and Reiley, A. C. (1939). *The Principles of Organization.* New York: Harper & Row.

Moore, B. (1987). What's Driving Upcoming Mergers? *Hospitals,* January 5.

Moschetto, C. A. (1981). Predictions about the Future of LTC (Long Term Care). *Nurs. Homes 30*(5), 42–50.

Punch, L. (1982A). Leading Firms Boost Contract Business 18.2%. *Mod. Healthcare 12*(7), 116–122.

Punch, L. (1982B). Shared Services Pacts Up 22%. *Mod. Healthcare 12*(7), 124–134.

Rakich, J. S., and Darr, K. (1978). *Hospital Organization and Management.* New York: Halsted Press.

Schneeweiss, S. M., and Davis, S. W. (1974). *Nursing Home Administration.* Baltimore: University Park Press.

Sinioris, M. E., Esmond, T. H., Glenesk, A. E., and Newman, R. S. (1982). Planning: Program Matrix Aids Planning Process. *Hospitals 56*(8), 75–77.

Tinsley, E. (1981). Health-Care Chains: Big Business' Niche in a $Billion Industry. *Restaur. Inst. 89*(10), 81–88.

Urwick, L. (1944). *The Elements of Administration.* New York: Harper & Row.

U.S. Department of Health and Human Services. (1966). *Conditions of Participation for Extended Care Facilities. Social Security Administration HIM-3.* Washington, DC: U.S. Government Printing Office.

U.S. Department of Health and Human Services, Health Care Financing Administration. (1988). *Medicare and Medicaid; Long Term Care Process; Final Rule.* Federal Register *53*(117), 22850–23100.

U.S. Department of Health and Human Services, Health Care Financing Administration. (1989). *Medicare and Medicaid; Requirements for Long Term Care Facilities.* Federal Register *54*(21), 5316–5373.

Weber, M. (1967). The Ideal Bureaucracy. In *Organization and Human Behavior,* G. D. Bell, ed. Englewood Cliffs, NJ: Prentice-Hall.

White, K. K. (1963). *Understanding the Company Organization Chart.* New York: American Management Association.

Zaccarelli, H., and Ninemeier, J. D. (1982). *Cost Effective Contract Food Service: An Institutional Guide.* Rockville, MD: Aspen Systems Corporation.

Chapter 4

Managerial Roles and Responsibilities

The concept of roles relates to the organizational expectations such as the work required, the tasks to be performed, and the situations and processes the individuals must deal with, as implicated by position, status, and relationships (Newman, 1973). All individuals within an organization have roles, either explicit or implicit. To avoid misunderstandings, the person in the role should be made aware of what he or she is expected to achieve and what objectives are involved, as well as what activities are required or permitted. A managerial role implies that the individual has other resources, including human resources, for which he or she is accountable.

Managerial Roles

In medical foodservice, the diverse, complex managerial roles and responsibilities are subject to both external and internal influences. In Michigan, the director of a medical foodservice must meet qualifications and guidelines established by the State Department of Health, federal guidelines for participation in Medicare and Medicaid programs, and standards of the Joint Commission on Accreditation of Hospitals (JCAH). Standard 1 of JCAH (1988) interprets the role for the director of dietetic services as follows:

> The dietetic department/service is directed on a full-time basis by an individual who, by education or specialized training and experience, is knowledgeable about foodservice management. The director is responsible to the chief executive officer or his designee. The director has the authority and responsibility for assuring that established policies are implemented; that overall coordination and integration of the therapeutic and administrative aspects of dietetic services are maintained; that the quality, safety, and appropriateness of the dietetic department/service functions are monitored and evaluated and that appropriate actions based on findings are taken.
>
> Dietetic services are provided by a sufficient number of qualified personnel under competent supervision. A qualified dietitian supervises the nutritional aspects of patient care and assures that quality nutritional care is provided to patients. Qualified dietitians or qualified designees participate in committee activities concerned with nutritional care. When the services of a qualified dietitian are used on a part-time basis, this individual provides such services on the premises on a regularly scheduled basis. The regularly scheduled visits are sufficient to provide for at least the following: Liaison with the hospital administration, medical staff, and nursing staff; Patient/family counseling as needed; Approval of menus, including modified diets; Any required nutritional assessments; Participation in the de-

velopment of policies and procedures; Participation in continuing education programs; and Evaluation of the dietetic services provided.

When a qualified dietitian serves only in a consultant status, this individual regularly submits written reports to the chief executive officer concerning the extent of services provided. When dietetic services are provided by an outside food-management company, the company compiles with all applicable requirements of this Manual, and the contract specifies the compliance requirements.

—— Director of Medical Foodservice ——————

The director of a medical foodservice operation affects nutritional care through the direction of all aspects of dietetic services, including the following responsibilities:

1. Organizes department as appropriate to the scope and complexity of services offered in meeting objectives of the organization.
2. Plans, organizes, controls, and evaluates components of foodservice systems (menu, equipment, food and materials, finances, and human resources).
3. Develops policies and procedures for the provision of optimal nutritional care in a safe and sanitary environment.
4. Adheres to established guidelines, both internal and external, in exercising managerial functions.
5. Participates in committee activities with reference to the nutritional care of patients.
6. Coordinates and integrates administrative and therapeutic services, inter- and intradepartmentally.
7. Develops, implements, and evaluates quality assurance standards for all aspects of the foodservice system.
8. Plans and controls fiscal resources through effective budget and cost measures.
9. Uses effective written and verbal communication techniques, inter- and intradepartmentally.
10. Maintains effective public relations, inter- and intradepartmentally.
11. Ensures adequate staffing for optimal level of nutritional care.
12. Plans, implements, and evaluates appropriate training and educational programs for personnel.
13. Utilizes current research on standards of practice relating to a medical foodservice operation.

The organization of a medical foodservice operation reflects both administrative and therapeutic duties, with personnel assigned according to level of care and complexity. The administrative and therapeutic services, in most instances, are assigned to Registered Dietitians (R.D.) To assist in the delineation of roles and responsibilities of dietitians, a position paper was issued by the American Dietetic Association (1981) with descriptions of the various classifications of dietitians, as detailed in the subsections that follow.

—— Administrative Dietitian, R.D. ——————

The administrative dietitian is a member of the management team and affects the nutritional care of groups through the management of foodservice systems that provide optimal nutrition and quality food. Responsibilities include the following:

1. Plans, develops, controls, and evaluates foodservice systems.
2. Develops short- and long-range department plans and programs consistent with departmental and organizational policies.
3. Manages and controls fiscal resources and recommends budget programs.
4. Utilizes human effort and facilitating resources efficiently and effectively.
5. Coordinates and integrates clinical and administrative aspects of dietetics to provide quality nutritional care.
6. Establishes and maintains standards of food production and service, sanitation, safety, and security.
7. Maintains effective written and verbal communications and public relations inter- and intradepartmentally.
8. Compiles and utilizes pertinent operational data to improve efficiency and quality of foodservice systems.
9. Plans, conducts, and evaluates orientation and in-service educational programs.
10. Interprets, evaluates, and utilizes pertinent current research relating to nutritional care.
11. Develops menu patterns and evaluates client acceptance.
12. Develops specifications for procurement of food, equipment, and supplies.
13. Plans or participates in the development of program proposals for funding.
14. Plans layout design and determines equipment requirements for foodservice facilities.
15. Administers personnel policies as established by department and organization.

Clinical Dietitian, R.D.

The clinical dietitian is a member of the health care team and affects the nutritional care of individuals and groups through the (1) assessment, (2) development, (3) implementation, and (4) evaluation of nutritional care plans. The clinical dietitian cooperates and coordinates activities with members of the management team. Responsibilities include the following:

1. Develops and implements a plan of care that is based on the assessment of nutritional needs and is correlated with other health care plans.
2. Counsels individuals and families in nutritional principles, dietary plans, food selection, and economics, adapting plans to the individual.
3. Utilizes appropriate tools in the provision of nutritional care.
4. Evaluates nutritional care and provides follow-up for continuity of care.
5. Communicates appropriate dietary and nutritional care data through record systems.
6. Participates in health team rounds and serves as a consultant on nutritional care.
7. Utilizes human effort and facilitating resources efficiently and effectively.
8. Evaluates food served for conformance to quality standards and dietary prescriptions.
9. Compiles and develops educational materials and uses them as aids in nutrition education.

10. Compiles and utilizes pertinent operational data to assure provision of quality nutrition care.
11. Interprets, evaluates, and utilizes pertinent current research related to nutritional care.
12. Provides nutrition education to students and personnel.
13. Plans and organizes resources to achieve effective nutritional care.
14. Plans or participates in the development of program proposals for funding.
15. Maintains effective written and verbal communications and public relations, inter- and intradepartmentally.
16. Administers personnel policies as established by the department and organization.

In large and/or teaching hospitals, managerial roles may include those in teaching and research.

Teaching Dietitian, R.D.

The teaching dietitian, with advanced preparation in dietetics or education, plans, conducts, and evaluates educational programs in one or more dietetic subject matter areas. Responsibilities include the following:

1. Develops curriculum, including courses to meet the needs of the students.
2. Plans, conducts, and evaluates the educational experiences for dietetic, medical, dental, nursing, and other allied health students and clients.
3. Guides and evaluates students' performance.
4. Plans and conducts orientation and in-service educational programs for the organization's personnel.
5. Prepares, evaluates, and utilizes current educational methodology and instructional media to enhance learning experiences of students.
6. Maintains accurate, detailed data records.
7. Contributes expertise as a member of the organization's teams for planning and evaluating and participates in committee and other organizational activities.

Research Dietitian, R.D.

The research dietitian, with advanced preparation in dietetics and research techniques, plans, investigates, interprets, evaluates, applies, and expands knowledge in phases of dietetics and communicates findings through reports and publications. Responsibilities include the following:

1. Plans, organizes, and conducts or participates in programs in nutrition, foods, or foodservice systems research.
2. Evaluates and utilizes appropriate methodology and tools to carry out program plans.
3. Maintains accurate and detailed records.
4. Evaluates and communicates findings.
5. Utilizes human and facilitating resources efficiently and effectively.
6. Interprets, evaluates, and utilizes pertinent current research related to program needs.
7. Maintains effective verbal and written communications and public relations, inter- and intradepartmentally.

8. Plans, conducts, and evaluates dietary studies and participates in epidemiological studies with a nutritional component.
9. Studies and analyzes recent scientific findings in dietetics for application in current research, for development of tools for future research, and for interpretation to the public.
10. Plans or participates in the development of program proposals for funding.

—— Consultant Dietitian, R.D. ——

The consultant dietitian, with experience in administrative and clinical dietetic practice, affects the management of human effort and facilitating resources by providing advice or services in nutritional care. The consultant does not assume responsibility for the day-to-day operation of the foodservice facility; that role is assigned to the dietetic service supervisor. The role of the consultant is to advise, observe, evaluate, instruct, and recommend. Responsibilities include the following:

1. Evaluates and monitors foodservice systems, making recommendations for a conformance level that will provide nutritionally adequate quality food.
2. Develops budget proposals and recommends procedures for cost controls.
3. Plans, organizes, and conducts orientation and in-service educational programs for foodservice personnel.
4. Plans layout design and determines equipment requirements for foodservice facilities.
5. Recommends and monitors standards for sanitation, safety, and security in foodservice.
6. Develops menu patterns.
7. Assesses, develops, implements, and evaluates nutritional care plans and provides for follow-up, including written reports.
8. Consults and counsels with clients regarding selection and procurement of food to meet optimal nutrition.
9. Develops, maintains, and uses pertinent record systems related to the needs of the organization.
10. Develops, uses, and evaluates educational materials related to services provided.
11. Consults with the health care team concerning the nutritional care of clients.
12. Provides guidance and evaluation of the job performance of dietetic personnel.
13. Interprets, evaluates, and utilizes pertinent current research relating to nutritional care.
14. Maintains effective verbal and written communications and public relations, inter- and intradepartmentally.

For optimal performance of the above tasks, the consultant should have a minimum of 3 years' experience with varied responsibilities such as therapeutic, administrative supervision, and staff education. In addition, the qualified consultant should be aware of pertinent legal codes to include (1) state nursing home licensing law; (2) federal regulations for Medicare and Medicaid; (3) Occupational Safety and Health Administration (OSHA) standards; (4) city and local codes, including fire, safety, and sanitation; and (5) labor laws such as compensation, unemployment, disability, and union contract (American Dietetic Association 1977A).

Federal guidelines specify that there must be a qualified dietitian as consultant but do not specify the frequency and time required. The amount of time spent by consultant dietitians vary from one visit every 6 months to 4 hours per week (Consultant Dietitians in Health Care Facilities 1987). The state of Maine requires 4 hours per week for a single unit (40 beds), plus an additional 2 hours per week for each additional unit. A survey of Illinois consultant dietitian's role and functions revealed that 74% of the 43 respondents reported insufficient time at nursing homes to perform in an efficient and effective manner (Welch, Oelrich, Endres, & Poon 1988).

The amount of time spent by consultant dietitians impacts on the outcome of resident care in a number of ways. In addition to direct resident care the consultant dietitians, with expertise in both management and clinical services, need ample time to monitor production and service; train staff, including nursing personnel; and promote interdepartmental communication.

Dietetic Technician–Dietary Manager

A dietetic technician is a technically skilled individual who has successfully completed an associate degree program in general, management, or clinical dietetics that meets the approval of The American Dietetic Association (ADA). A dietary manager is an individual who has completed a 90-hour classroom program plus 6 months of supervised work experience that meets certification standards of the Dietary Managers Association (DMA). Both the dietetic technician and the dietary manager may work in areas of administration or clinical, with appropriate responsibilities, and under the directions of a Registered Dietitian (R.D.). The dietary manager and dietetic technician are eligible for membership in the DMA. The dietetic technician is also eligible for associate membership in the ADA.

In long-term care facilities, the dietetic technician or dietary manager may have total responsibility of the foodservice operation, under the direction of a consultant dietitian. Depending on the level of services offered, duties and responsibilities may be as follows:

1. Plans menus on the basis of established guidelines.
2. Standardizes recipes and tests new products for use in the facility.
3. Procures and receives supplies and equipment following established procedures.
4. Supervises production and service.
5. Monitors foodservice for conformity with quality standards.
6. Maintains and improves standards of sanitation, safety, and security.
7. Selects, schedules, and conducts orientation and in-service educational programs for personnel.
8. Participates in determining staffing needs, in selecting personnel, and in on-the-job training.
9. Develops job specifications, job descriptions, and work schedules.
10. Plans master schedules for personnel.
11. Maintains a routine personnel evaluation system.
12. Understands and supports personnel policies and union contracts.
13. Assists in the implementation of established cost control procedures.
14. Gathers data according to prescribed methods for use in evaluating foodservice systems.

15. Makes recommendations that may be incorporated into policies and develops written procedures to conform with established policies.
16. Recommends improvements for the facility and for equipment.
17. Submits recommendations and information for use in budget development.
18. Compiles and uses operational data.
19. Obtains, evaluates, and utilizes dietary history information for planning nutritional care.
20. Guides individual and families in food selection, food preparation, and menu planning based on nutritional needs.
21. Calculates nutrient intakes and dietary patterns.
22. Assists in referrals for continuity of patient care.
23. Utilizes appropriate verbal and written communication and public relations, inter- and intradepartmentally.

A nursing care facility may recognize the role of a part-time or full-time dietitian, a dietetic technician, or a dietary manager. In the state of Michigan, rules and regulations for nursing homes (Michigan Department of Public Health 1985) specify the following qualifications for the supervisor of dietary or food-service:

1. Dietary or foodservice in a home shall be supervised by an individual who meets any of the following qualifications.
   a. Is registered by the Commission on Dietetic Registration of The American Dietetic Association.
   b. Is qualified to take the registration examination required for Registered Dietitian status.
   c. Is a graduate of a dietetic technician program approved by The American Dietetic Association.
   d. Is a graduate of an approved dietary managers training program that qualifies such person for certification by the Dietary Managers Association.
   e. Is a graduate of a dietary managers program granted approval status by the Michigan Department of Public Health before July 6, 1979.

In the state of Mississippi, regulations require that the dietary department *shall* be directed by a Registered Dietitian or a certified dietary manager with frequent and regularly scheduled consultations from an R.D., and must earn 15 hours of continuing education each year, approved by ADA or DMA (Consultant Dietitians in Health Care Facilities 1987). The functions and responsibilities of the consultant dietitian and the dietetic service supervisor in patient nutritional care for long-term care facilities have been defined by The American Dietetic Association (1977B) and are presented in Table 4-1.

Problems of Role Delineation

There are problems associated with listing tasks for managerial roles simply because no list is all-inclusive. The roles and responsibilities of health care professionals in dietetics are constantly under review. A study on how practitioners view future roles of the dietetic professional (Parks & Kris-Etherton 1982) concluded that the practitioner must have an awareness of (1) cost containment in the health care setting, (2) professional fees for dietary services, (3) shifts from

Table 4-1. Comparison of Duties of Consultant Dietitian and Dietetic Service Supervisor

Consultant Dietitian	Dietetic Service Supervisor
1. *Policy development*	
a. Reviews and participates in the development of the facility's patient care policies to insure the inclusion and support of nutritional care.	a. Provides operational information needed for determining patient care policies related to nutritional care.
b. Suggests revisions in these policies where necessary.	b. Understands policies and their impact on the daily operation of the dietetic service.
c. Consults with nursing, medical, dietetic, and other services on procedures to implement policies affecting nutritional care.	c. Assists in developing dietetic service procedures related to nutritional care.
d. Evaluates the effectiveness of nutritional care procedures and adjusts when necessary.	d. Provides feedback on the effectiveness of procedures.
2. *Setting priorities and goals*	
a. Evaluates the capability of dietetic service to deliver nutritional care, based on staffing, support systems and responsibilities of other services.	a. Provides operational information needed to determine priorities
b. Assists in setting realistic goals and priorities for establishing a system to assure that each patient has adequate daily intake.	b. Participates in the selection of priorities and goals affecting dietetic services.
c. Confers with the administrator, dietetic service supervisor, director of nursing and other appropriate heads of service to secure their concurrence in these priorities and goals.	
3. *Development of service to meet patient nutritional needs*	
A. *Nutritional assessment*	
a. Identifies the information needed for a nutritional assessment and the sources from which it can be obtained.	a. Participates in the development of forms and procedures for gathering information about the patients' food needs.
b. Assures that suitable forms are developed and that procedures are appropriate for collecting and recording information.	b. Collects information according to established methods and procedures. Some sources of information are (i) patient (foods liked and disliked); (ii) nurse (allergies, self-feeding ability, appetite and food intake, weight); (iii) patient's family; and (iv) observation of the patient at mealtimes.
c. Clarifies the responsibilities of the dietetic, nursing and social services in collection of assessment data. Offers training when necessary.	
d. Reviews information collected on individual patients to identify those needing further assessment by the dietitian. Identifies individual problems requiring nutritional intervention.	
B. *Nutritional planning and implementation*	
a. Develops the nutritional component of the patient's plan of care, including preparation for discharge.	a. Contributes nutritional assessment information to care planning conferences.

Table 4-1. (Continued)

Consultant Dietitian	Dietetic Service Supervisor

3. *Development of service to meet patient nutritional needs* (*continued*)

b. Reviews with dietetic supervisor, nursing service, physician and others as appropriate.	b. Assures that the menu served to the total population is nutritionally adequate and well received.
c. Participates in patient care planning conferences or shares information with the dietetic service supervisor to be taken to the planning conference.	c. Assures that each patient's menu is modified according to the plan of care.
d. Plans for periodic review.	d. Identifies and reports to the consultant dietitian any problems in the implementation of the plan of care.
e. Identifies responsibilities of the dietetic service in implementing nutritional care and provides appropriate guidance.	e. Reinforces diet counseling with patients and provides follow-up information to families.
f. Provides diet counseling to patients and families where necessary.	

C. *Evaluation*

a. Assures that there is a method for identifying patients who are not eating, not responding to the plan as anticipated, or whose condition has changed (e.g., food and fluid intake, weight survey, patient visitation).	a. Maintains the system to monitor the total facility population.
b. When a problem is identified, evaluates and changes plan when indicated.	b. Follows through on individual review of plans.
c. Suggests useful studies to the facility's committee on patient care evaluation.	c. Participates in the evaluation of the plan's effectiveness.

D. *Documentation*

a. Enters nutritional assessment and plan in the dietary and medical records and reports the patient's response, changes in plans and preparation for discharge.	a. After training, records information about each patient's food intake or implementation of plan of care in the appropriate records as designated by the policy of the facility.

4. *Staff training*

a. Develops a relevant plan for in-service training for all facility staff. Helps conduct some sessions. Reviews objectives and methods of nutritional care.	a. Assists in the development of a plan of in-service and participates in training sessions.
b. With the assistance of the dietetic service supervisor, provides appropriate training to the dietetic staff.	b. Conducts training sessions for the dietetic staff.
c. Assures the maintenance of records for orientation and training.	c. Keeps training attendance reports and updates personnel files as necessary.

5. *Provision of current information to facility staff*

a. Recommends suitable references on basic nutrition, therapeutic nutrition, medical terminology, food preparation, feeding techniques and aids, regulations, safety and sanitation, and others.	a. Refers to resources as necessary and identifies additional needs
b. Interprets current research findings.	

therapeutic to normal nutrition as the importance of preventive health care is recognized, (4) technological advances in health care, and (5) legislation that relates to the application of quality care. As reported by Neville and Tower (1988), the ADA Role Delineation Steering Committee has appointed members to five resource committees to participate in logical analysis to determine job responsibilities of entry-level dietitians, dietetic technicians, and R.D.s practicing beyond entry level. As noted in the following discussion of diagnosis-related groups, dietetic professionals have responded to future implications of cost containment, community outreach, and documentation of services rendered.

___ Diagnosis-Related Groups (DRGs) _____

The most recent federal law that impacts on the roles and responsibilities of medical foodservice personnel is the Social Security Amendment of 1983 (Public Law 98-21, 98th Congress, 1st Session); see USDHHS (1983). Changes have occurred in the method of payment for inpatient hospital services from a cost-based, retrospective reimbursement system to a prospective payment system (PPS), based on categories of 470 DRGs. The system is composed of major diagnostic categories, organized by organ systems and disease etiology, and 470 DRGs. In the September 1 Federal Register (1983), there is a complete listing of the DRGs, relative weighing factors, geometric mean length of stay, and length of stay outlier points used in the prospective payment system. The length of stay outlier points used in the prospective payment system refer to supplemental payment to hospitals for atypical cases. From 5% to 6% of the total DRG expenditure is used as a basis for calculating such additional payments. These cases include patients whose length of stay exceeds the average for the DRG.

To ease the transition, the PPS was phased in over a 3-year period. All Medicare payments were based on a combination of specific hospital rates and national and regional DRG rates, as shown in Table 4-2.

Rules governing DRG implementation are another form of accountability imposed on the hospital system in an effort to control costs of health care. As a subsystem of the hospital, the medical foodservice department is also affected. The degree to which DRGs impact on departmental functions and services depends on previous administrative practices, roles, and responsibilities, as well as involvement in professional activities such as Professional Standards Review Organization, Utilization Review, and other committees that demonstrate contributions to the health care team.

To counteract the financial effects of DRGs, the following activities have been initiated at the departmental level:

Table 4-2. Phase-In Periods for Diagnosis-Related Groups (DRG)[a]

Federal Fiscal Year Beginning	Hospital-Specific Rate Percentage	Federal Rate Percentage	
		National	Regional
October 1, 1983	75	—	25
October 1, 1984	50	12$\frac{1}{2}$	37$\frac{1}{2}$
October 1, 1985	25	37$\frac{1}{2}$	37$\frac{1}{2}$
October 1, 1986	—	100	—

[a] From *U.S. Department of Health and Human Services* (1984).

1. Communicating the possible roles and responsibilities of administrative and clinical personnel to top administration. Participating in hospital-based home health care. Supporting community outreach programs relating to follow-up patient care. Increasing outpatient services, such as diet clinics. Involving administrative and clinical staff in a corporate consulting program, with appropriate consultant fee schedules.

2. Documenting cost of service based on each of the DRGs. Conducting time studies. Emphasizing record keeping. Establishing fees for services.

3. Increasing marketing efforts with emphasis on revenue-generating activities. Enhancing food quality and customer satisfaction by balancing high- and low-cost foods on selective menus. Reducing menu cycle to correspond with length of patient stay. Expanding catering services to the larger community with carryout menus. Promoting competitive merchandising in the cafeteria. Reducing hours of operation. Increasing self-service. Participating in mobile home meal plans.

It has been 5 years since implementation of DRGs. Questions frequently asked are: (1) Did the new method of payment system for hospital inpatient care meet its objective to control cost? (2) How did the new method of payment impact on the financial status of hospitals? According to McCarthy (1988), the goals of the DRG system were met; however, there has been an increase in hospital closings, creating a fragile hospital system. In addition, the DRG system does not recognize new labor costs (salary raises), differences in costs based on severity of illness, differences in costs to hospitals for nonlabor resources, differences in the availability of nonacute care services, and new technology. McCarthy believes that reform of the payment system is essential, but the reform does not require abandoning the DRG system. One of the latest reforms (USDHHS 1987) is a rule that changes Medicare prospective payment regulation for inpatient hospital services in order to allow an adjustment for sole community hospitals that experience a significant increase in inpatient operating costs attributable to the addition of new inpatient services or facilities.

Multiple Roles

Another problem associated with the listing of tasks is that the role occupant frequently functions in multiple roles, with high dependence on other human resources. For example, as a specialist in administrative or therapeutic dietetics, the professional may also serve as consultant in nutritional care to other units within the organization or as a member of the health care team. Effective interaction as a member of the team will depend on the level of decision making and the amount of authority on the part of the individual professional.

The Health Care Team

The quality and effectiveness of care provided by an individual health care professional is limited by his or her own range of expertise. A team approach to health care combines the skills, knowledge, and experience of several professionals. Because the team approach emphasizes *multiple inputs,* a coordinated treatment plan for each patient may be achieved. The passage of federal legislation, with a primary objective of protecting invested funds, made the concept of health care teams a reality.

Professional Standards Review Organizations —— (PSROs) —————————————————————

Mandated under section 294F of Public Law 92-603 in 1972, PSROs are required to involve local practicing physicians in the review and evaluation of health care services provided by Medicare, Medicaid, and Title V (Maternal and Child Health) of the Social Security Act (American Dietetic Association 1976). The objective of the PSRO program is to assure quality of health care. The primary emphasis, as prescribed by law, is to determine whether health care services delivered to Medicare, Medicaid, and maternal and child health patients (1) are medically necessary, (2) meet professionally recognized standards of health care, and (3) are provided in the most appropriate setting to meet the patient's needs. The PSRO must specify its procedure for review of health care to include:

1. Concurrent review of the necessity of admission and continued stay in the hospital.
2. Medical care evaluation studies.
3. Retrospective analysis of health care practitioner, institutional, and patient profiles.

Screening criteria are established as part of the review process to determine whether (1) there is medical necessity for admission, (2) there is a need for continued hospitalization after a specified time period, (3) the services meet established standards, and (4) there is a discrepancy between the method of treatment and acceptable standards of treatment for a particular diagnostic category. The last condition would indicate the need for continuing-education programs for practitioners. Health care practitioners must develop norms, standards, and criteria to have an effective review and screening process. *Norms* are the numerical or statistical measures of observed performance. *Standards* refer to the range of acceptable variation from a norm or criterion. *Criteria* are predetermined elements against which the quality of services may be measured and developed and based on professional expertise and professional literature.

—— Role of the Registered Dietitian in PSROs ——————

The most appropriate level of involvement for the Registered Dietitian is in the form of peer review, as part of the Patient Care Audit Committee (American Dietetic Association 1976). This role is supported by laws governing PSROs, which require the involvement of nonphysician health care practitioners in the review of care provided by their peers. The director of the department of dietetics or a qualified dietitian designee must participate in the activities of one or more committees that must be established by the hospital as part of the review mechanism process. As a member of the committee, the Registered Dietitian should be involved as follows:

1. Provide dietary input by developing criteria, norms, and standards regarding the dietary management of problems or diagnoses chosen for review or audit.
2. Modify criteria, norms, and standards as new data and scientific evidence become available to ensure improved care as opposed to endorsing current practices.
3. Use the review process in the department of dietetics for the peer assessment of dietetic services alone.

4. Identify areas of deficit in dietary care and services and develop policies and/or educational programs to correct deficits.
5. Use the findings of the review system to plan continuing education for practicing dietitians and for input into the educational system for dietetic students.

There should be an effective working relationship between the patient care audit committee, the utilization review committee, and the continuing-education committee if quality assessment of patient care is to be accomplished. The findings of the Patient Care Audit Committee can assist the Utilization Review Committee in developing criteria for admission and continued-stay reviews, and assist the continuing-education program by defining educational needs of health care practitioners.

Developing a Nutrition Care Plan

The purpose of a nutrition care plan for patients is to return the individual to a state of wellness as soon as possible and in the most effective manner. Components of a patient care plan involve four basic steps: assessment, planning, implementation, and evaluation.

Nutritional assessment involves the screening process to collect facts and to identify problems and needs of the patients. The collection of data, based on both subjective and objective observations, should include the following:

1. Interviews with patients to determine food intake patterns, food restrictions and preferences based on cultural or religious factors, recent significant changes in weight or appetite, and observed emotional or physical limitations.
2. Reviews of medical histories from patients' medical records to include laboratory test results, anthropometric measures, and clinical findings from admitting examination.

Data collected during the assessment phase should be analyzed for nutritional deficiencies. If it is determined that a nutritional deficit exists, immediate steps should be planned to restore the patient to a state of well-being. The planning process includes:

1. Statements of short- and long-term goals for the patient in behavioral terms.
2. Development of specific dietary interventions, such as calculated diets, and supplements.
3. Outline of a system for communicating nutritional care plan to other members of the health care team, stating the required support for accomplishing goals. The system should be consistent with the format used by other team members in a particular facility.
4. Develop methods for checking response and or progress toward goals, such as diet acceptance and total intake.
5. Plans for discharge with consideration to such factors as ability or willingness to adhere to a dietary regimen, living conditions, and need for general assistance.

Implementation of a health care plan requires that the dietitian communicate with the health care team and with members of the production and service units within the dietary department. In order to ensure that patients will receive the nutritional care as planned, dietary personnel must be informed of special needs, including between-meal nourishments. Members of the health care team are informed through documentations in the patient's medical record. The recording of nutritional information in medical records may take the traditional form of entries in chronological sequence or a format of the problem-oriented medical record (POMR). Regardless of the method used, the documented information should support the dietary assessment, the care provided, and the results obtained (American Hospital Association 1976).

Using the POMR Method of Documentation

Nutritional care information based on the POMR is organized in three specific areas: data base, problem list, and progress notes. The data base includes information from physical examinations, complaints at admission, results of laboratory tests, dietary history, the patient's attitude toward and knowledge of food and nutrition, and home and family resources.

The list may include medical, physical, emotional, or religious problems— or any other problems affecting the patient that require additional information, treatment, or education. The list is maintained and updated as often as new problems arise. The advantage of having a problem list in the patient's medical record is that all team members can supervise and share in the solution.

Progress notes, recorded by the appropriate team member, indicate the actions taken on the particular problem. The progress notes may be recorded, using the subjective, objective, assessment, plan (SOAP) format:

S—*Subjective data.* Information derived from the patient during interviews.
O—*Objective data.* Clinical findings from initial physical examination, laboratory tests, and anthropometric measures.
A—*Assessment.* Interpretation and analysis of objective data, with emphasis on consistency.
P—*Planning.* Recommendations and plans to obtain more information, to treat, and to educate, including follow-up care.

Recording in Medical Records

The recording of information, consistent with policies of the organization, should be sufficient to (1) support the dietary assessment, (2) justify the nutritional care, and (3) document results accurately (American Hospital Association 1976). Progress notes should be brief, without sacrificing essential facts. Avoid professional jargon and any remarks that may be critical of treatment provided by other members of the team. Keep in mind that the patient has a right to see his medical record. Effective communication dictates that progress notes should be comprehensible by all members of the health care team.

AUTHORIZED PERSONNEL All entries in medical records should be signed and dated by the person making the entry. This person may be a dietitian, dietetic technician, or dietary manager, depending on the policies of the institution. In long-term care facilities where services of a full-time dietitian are not available, responsibilities for recording inpatient medical records may be assigned to the dietetic technician or dietary manager. The consultant dietitian is responsible for training the dietetic service supervisor and for determining whether the supervisor has the ability to document in medical records. In acute care facilities, where the nutritional care is more complex, Registered Dietitians should do the charting.

WHAT TO RECORD Guidelines for recording in the patient medical record by the qualified dietitian or authorized alternate is as follows (American Hospital Association 1976):

1. *Confirmation of diet order.* A notation that the prescribed diet is being fulfilled; it should be made within 24 hours of admission.
2. *Summary of dietary history.* Evaluation of the patient's daily pattern, nutrient deficiencies, food allergies, life-style, and socioeconomic resources; and an assessment of the diet–disease relationship.
3. *Nutritional care therapy.* Type of diet and restrictions, the patient's daily nutrient intake, diet acceptance, changes in diet order or diet instruction, and referral of the patient for assistance with the diet at home.
4. *Nutritional care discharge plan.* Description of the diet instruction given, with a copy placed in the patient's medical record, a description or copy of the diet forwarded to the referral agency or nursing home, and plans for nutritional care follow-up.
5. *Dietetic consultation.* Acknowledgment of the physician's written request for consultation. Consultation reports reflect assessment of the patient's dietary history, examination of the patient's medical record for previous dietary history, and recommendations for normal or modified diet. Subsequent counseling of patient or family should be recorded in the patient's medical record.

Committee Responsibilities

The role of the Registered Dietitian does not diminish the responsibilities of the foodservice director in assuring optimal nutritional care. To understand the diverse and complex nature of patient care the director must have an understanding of food and nutrition principles and the relationship to patient well-being. In addition, the director or an authorized designee must participate in the following committees concerned with patient care, as mandated by federal or state law.

INFECTION CONTROL COMMITTEE The purposes of the infection control committee are to establish preventive measures by developing policies and procedures for sanitation and aseptic techniques; to develop isolation procedures; to maintain records of all incidents of infection involving patients and personnel; to establish a system for evaluation and reporting infections; and to develop a system for in-service education on preventive and control measures.

ADMINISTRATIVE STAFF MEETINGS Regularly scheduled meetings are held in order to allow participation by department heads in the decision-making process; to provide for input and open communication; and to keep administrative personnel abreast of all changes affecting the organization and their respective departments.

BUDGET COMMITTEE The purposes of the budget committee are to include all department heads in the operational budget planning; to ensure appropriate input; and to ensure congruence with organizational goals and objectives.

QUALITY CONTROL COMMITTEE The primary purpose is to develop policies and procedures for optimal quality of patient care through ongoing quality assurance audits.

SAFETY COMMITTEE The safety committee is responsible for ensuring a safe environment for patients and a safe place of work for employees as mandated by OSHA and other regulations.

Effective teams within the health care setting, both administrative and clinical, are those that encourage and recognize contributions from members who possess various skills, knowledge, and experience. This cooperative effort is necessary for consistently high-quality nutritional care.

Professional Ethics

A health care professional needs a combination of both technical and ethical competence. Technical competence involves possession of adequate knowledge and skills to care for patients.

All professionals have a written and unwritten code of ethics to follow. To behave in an ethical manner is simply to do the *most good* and the *least harm* to others; to perform the proper professional dos and don'ts. Morality is a combination of judgment, actions, attitudes, and other behaviors of an individual that can be judged right or wrong (Tancredi 1974). In many situations, it is not always obvious which decision or approach is the morally or ethically correct one. Even when specific written ethical codes and guidelines exist, ethical dilemmas may emerge. An ethical dilemma exists when helping one patient may result in harm to another patient (Purtillo & Cassel 1981). A dietitian may be continually faced with the dilemma of how to delegate time spent with various patients. The health care professional must weigh alternatives to determine which option will be the most beneficial and the least harmful. Extreme examples of unethical conduct, which compromises patient well-being for personal gain, are situations in which the clinical dietitian accepts gifts or other favors from patients for services rendered or the director of foodservices accepts kickbacks from vendors. The practice of professional ethics in the health care environment requires that personal prejudices, preferences, and personal gains be set aside for the good of the patient.

A current ethical issue for dietetic professionals revolves around nutrition support for patients in varying states of illness. It joins the debate of medical support for use of artificial respirators, ventilators, kidney dialysis, and other forms of medical support. As societal values change with reference to death, dying, suffering, pain, and patient rights, dietetic professionals must face the ethical dilemma of whether to withhold or withdraw nutrition support. The question of who has the right to deny basic biological needs of nutrition and fluids has both legal and moral ramifications. According to Studebaker (1988), nutrition and hydration are different from other forms of medical therapy. All people, regardless of their state of health, require food and water. To deny them this is, de facto, a death sentence.

The position of The American Dietetic Association (1987) is that the dietitian should take an active role in developing criteria for feeding the terminally ill adult within the practice setting and collaborate with the health care team in making recommendations on each case. The position paper presents a comprehensive view of issues related to feeding the terminally ill from an ethical, legal, medical, and nutrition perspective, concluding with guidelines that dietitians can use in deciding the appropriateness of providing or withholding nutrition support.

In addition to the terminally ill adult, there are other situations that may be of ethical concern for the dietitian in the practice setting, such as malnourished patients, competent patients who refuse food, cancer patients, and incompetent patients in a permanent vegetative state (Schiller 1988). In addition to developing criteria through collaboration with health team members, Schiller recommends that the dietitian prepare for committee participation as follows:

1. Be familiar with basis legal and ethical principles.
2. Clarify personal values with reference to food and feeding, euthanasia, use of life-sustaining treatments, pain, Living Wills, artificial feeding, terminal disease, and prolongation of life.
3. Recognize the bases for conflicting legal judgments in nutrition support cases.
4. Review published guidelines, such as the ADA position paper, as a basis for decision making.

Since all health care professionals are individuals with various personal ethics and all patients have differing needs, it is crucial for professionals to be familiar with the Code of Ethics of their profession and ethical guidelines of the institution by which they are employed. General guidelines for dietitians (American Dietetic Association 1988) require a commitment from the dietitian to:

1. Provide professional services with objectivity and with respect for the unique needs of individuals.
2. Avoid discrimination against other individuals on the basis of race, creed, religion, sex, age, and national origin.
3. Fulfill professional commitments in good faith.
4. Conduct himself or herself with honesty, integrity, and fairness.
5. Remain free of conflict of interest while fulfilling the objectives and maintaining the integrity of the dietetic profession.
6. Maintain confidentiality of information.
7. Practice dietetics based on scientific principles and current information.
8. Assume responsibility and accountability for personal competence in practice.
9. Recognize and exercise professional judgment within the limits of his or her qualifications and seek counsel or make referrals as appropriate.
10. Provide sufficient information to enable clients to make their own informed decisions.
11. Inform the public and colleagues of his or her services by using factual information. Refrain from advertising in a false or misleading manner.
12. Promote and endorse products in a manner that is neither false nor misleading.
13. Permit use of his or her name for the purpose of certifying that dietetic services have been rendered only if he or she has provided or supervised the provision of those services.
14. Accurately presented professional qualifications and credentials.
    a. Use "R.D." or "registered dietitian" and "D.T.R." or "dietetic technician registered" only when registration is current and authorized by the Commission of Dietetic Registration.
    b. Provide accurate information and comply with all requirements of the Commission of Dietetic Registration program in which he or she is seeking initial or continued credentials from the Commission on Dietetic Registration.
    c. Refrain from aiding other persons in violation of any Commission on Dietetic Registration requirements or aiding other persons in

representing themselves as an R.D. or D.T.R. when they are not, thus avoiding disciplinary action.

15. Present substantiated information and interpret controversial information without personal bias, recognizing that legitimate differences of opinion exist.

16. Make all reasonable effort to avoid bias in any kind of professional evaluation. Provide objective evaluation of candidates for professional association memberships, awards, scholarship, and job advancements.

17. Voluntarily withdraw from professional practice if he or she:
    a. Has engaged in any substance abuse that could affect practice.
    b. Has been adjudged by a court to be mentally incompetent.
    c. Has an emotional or mental disability that affects practice in a manner that could harm the client.

18. Comply with all applicable laws and regulations concerning the profession and is subject to disciplinary action if he or she:
    a. Has been convicted of a crime under the laws of the United States that is a felony or a misdemeanor, an essential element of which is related to the practice of the profession.
    b. has been disciplined by a state and at least one of the grounds for the discipline is the same or substantially equivalent to these principles.
    c. Has committed an act of misfeasance or malfeasance that is directly related to the practice of the profession as determined by a court of competent jurisdiction, a licensing board, or an agency of a governmental body.

19. Accept the obligation to protect society and the profession by upholding the Code of Ethics for the Profession of Dietetics and by reporting alleged violations of the Code through the defined review process of the American Dietetic Association and its credentialing agency, the Commission on Dietetic Registration.

The American Dietetic Association has defined procedures for the review process when a member has allegedly violated the Code of Ethics for the Profession of Dietetics, as follows:

1. Complaint to Ethics Committee.
2. Preliminary review of complaint.
3. Response by person against whom the complaint is made.
4. Disposition of the complaint.
5. Remedial action.
6. Preparation for hearing and notice of hearing date.
7. Hearings—rights of concerned parties.
8. Cost responsibility.
9. Decision of Ethics Committee.
10. Appeals—rights of the respondent.
11. Notification of adverse action.

Rights and Responsibilities of Patients

All people are entitled to *conditional rights,* which include such basic goods as water, food, shelter, and medical care that facilitates a basic right to live (Purtilo & Cassel 1981). However, what a person feels morally entitled to may or may not be supported by legal rights. To clarify the responsibilities of the institution to ensure the individual rights of patients, as well as the responsibilities of patients, the Joint Commission on Accreditation of Hospitals (1988) issued the standards outlined in this section.

Patient Rights

Patients have the following rights:

Access to care. Individuals shall be accorded impartial access to treatment or accommodations that are available or medically indicated, regardless of race, creed, sex, national origin, or sources of payment of care.

Respect and dignity. Patients have the right to considerate, respectful care at all times and under all circumstances, with recognition of their personal dignity.

Privacy and confidentiality. Patients have the right, within the law, to personal and informational privacy as follows:

- To refuse to talk with or see anyone not officially connected with the hospital.
- To wear appropriate personal clothing, religious or other symbolic items, as long as they do not interfere with diagnostic procedures or treatment.
- To be interviewed and examined in surroundings designed to ensure visual and auditory privacy.
- To expect that any discussion or consultation involving their cases will be conducted discreetly and that individuals not directly involved will not be present without the patient's consent.
- To have their medical records read only by individuals directly involved in the treatment or in the monitoring of its quality only on the written authorization or that of the patient's legally authorized representative.
- To expect all communication and other records pertaining to their care, including source of payment for treatment, to be treated as confidential.
- To request a transfer to another room if another patient or a visitor in the room is unreasonably disturbing them by smoking or by other actions.
- To be placed in protective privacy when it is considered necessary for personal safety.

Personal safety. Patients have the right to expect reasonable safety insofar as the hospital practices and environment are concerned.

Identity. Patients have the right to know the identity and professional status of any individual providing service and to know which physician or other practitioner is primarily responsible for their care.

Information. Patients have the right to obtain, from the practitioner responsible for coordinating their care, complete and current information concerning diagnosis (to the degree known), treatment, and any know prognosis.

Communication. Patients have the right of access to people outside the hospital by means of visitors, and by written or verbal communication. The patient who does not speak or understand the predominant language of the community should have access to an interpreter.

Consent. Patients have the right to reasonable informed participation in decisions involving their health care. Patients should not be subjected to any procedure without their voluntary, competent, and understanding consent or that of a legally authorized representative. Patients have the right to know who is responsible for authorizing and performing the procedures or treatment. Patients shall be informed if the hospital proposes to engage in or perform human experimentation or other research or educational projects affecting their care or treatment, and the patients have the right to refuse to participate in any such activity.

Consultation. Patients, at their own request and expense, have the right to consult with a specialist.

Refusal of treatment. Patients may refuse treatment to the extent permitted by law. When refusal of treatment by the patient or legally authorized representative prevents the provision of appropriate care in accordance with professional standards, the relationship with the patient may be terminated upon reasonable notice.

Transfer and continuity of care. Patients may not be transferred to another facility unless they have received a complete explanation of the need for the transfer and of the alternatives to such a transfer and unless the transfer is acceptable to the other facility. Patients have the right to be informed by the practitioner responsible for their care, or the practitioner's delegate, of any continuing health care requirement following discharge from the hospital.

Hospital charges. Regardless of the source of payment for their care, patients have the right to request and receive an itemized and detailed explanation of the total bill for service rendered in the hospital. Patients have the right to timely notice prior to termination of eligibility for reimbursement by any third-party payer for the cost of their care.

Hospital rules and regulations. Patients should be informed of the hospital rules and regulations applicable to the conduct of patients. Patients are entitled to information about the hospital's mechanism for the initiation, review, and resolution of their complaints.

Patient Responsibilities

Along with rights, patients have certain responsibilities:

Provision of information. Patients have the responsibility to provide, to the best of their knowledge, accurate, and complete information about present complaints, past illnesses, hospitalizations, medications, and other matters relating to their health. They also have the responsibility to report unexpected changes in their condition to the responsible practitioner. Patients are responsible for reporting whether they clearly comprehend a contemplated course of action and what is expected of them.

Compliance with instructions. Patients are responsible for following the treatment plan recommended by the practitioner primarily responsible for their care. Patients are responsible for keeping appointments and, when unable to do so for any reason, for notifying the responsible practitioner or the hospital.

Refusal of treatment. Patients are responsible for their actions if they refuse treatment or do not follow the practitioner's instructions.

Hospital charges. Patients are responsible for ensuring that the financial obligations of their health care are fulfilled as promptly as possible.

Hospital rules and regulations. Patients are responsible for following hospital rules and regulations affecting patient care and conduct.

Respect and consideration. Patients are responsible for being considerate of the rights of other patients and of hospital personnel and visitors. Patients are responsible for being respectful of the property of other persons and of the hospital.

Foodservice personnel must be trained and made aware of the importance of treating all patients with human dignity and respect. Because of the length of stay for residents in skilled nursing facilities (SNFs) and intermediate care facilities (ICFs), resident rights cover additional topics, such as exercising rights, financial affairs, freedom from abuse and restraints, work, and personal possession. See Appendix K for a report on resident rights.

Malpractice

The director of a medical foodservice operation has total responsibility for the quality of nutritional care provided to patients. In small medical facilities, where only one dietitian is employed, the director of foodservice is responsible for providing both administrative and clinical nutritional care. In large facilities, the responsibility for nutritional care of patients is delegated to clinical dietitians. Since the patient is entitled to services from the dietitian, any dissatisfaction with the service provided may result in a malpractice suit (Baird & Jacobs 1981). Areas of obvious neglect would involve failure to carry out the diet order prescribed by the physician, incorrect assessment of the nutritional status of the patient, or incorrect or inadequate instructions to the patients. To protect against such liability, the dietitian should consider the following:

1. Follow the code of ethics of the ADA and the individual institution where he or she is employed.
2. Avoid statements that contradict the diagnosis given by the attending physician.
3. Explain all instructions carefully and clearly and support them with written literature, if possible.
4. Encourage the patient to contact the dietitian by phone in case of future questions or concerns regarding dietary regimen and instructions.
5. Assess, treat, and instruct patients only in a manner appropriate to his or her professional training and background.
6. Consult another dietitian or professional if in doubt regarding method of assessment, treatment, or instruction of any patient.

In addition to those general guidelines, a precise documentation by the dietitian in the patient's medical record is necessary. Besides being a tool for communication between health care professionals, the written record is the dietitian's best defense against potential malpractice suits.

Because of the current climate of changing moral and ethical thinking and patient rights, dietitians are joining physicians and other health care professionals in their concern with the legal aspects of their practices. As recommended in the discussion on ethics, the dietitian needs to review the full trial manuscripts of judicial decisions in order to gain a perspective of the arguments for and against the decision. A brief summary of four judicial decisions, involving nutrition and hydration, is as follows:

1. *Barber v. Superior Court (1983)*. Two physicians, charged with murder and conspiracy to commit murder, petitioned the California Court of Appeals for a writ of prohibition after a magistrate ordered the complaint dismissed and the trial court ordered it reinstated. The prosecution arose after life support measures were terminated in the case of a deeply comatose patient in accordance with the wishes of the patient's immediate family.

Clarence Herbert underwent surgery for closure of an ileostomy. Petitioner Robert Nejdl, M.D., was Mr. Herbert's surgeon and petitioner Neil Baber, M. D., was his attending internist. Shortly after the successful surgery, and while in the recovery room, Mr. Herbert suffered a cardiorespiratory arrest. He was revived and placed on life support equipment. Within the following 3 days, it was determined that Mr. Herbert was in a deeply comatose state from which he was not likely to recover. Tests and examinations indicated that Mr. Herbert had suffered severe brain damage, leaving him in a vegetative state, which was likely to be permanent. The physicians informed family members of his condition and chances for recovery. The family convened and drafted a written request to hospital personnel stating that they wanted "all machines taken off that are sustaining life." As a result, petitioners ordered the removal of a respirator and other life-sustaining equipment, but the patient showed no signs of change. After 2 more days and after consulting with the family, petitioners ordered removal of intravenous tubes that provided hydration and nutrition.

The court held that the cessation of heroic life support measures is not an affirmative act, but rather a withdrawal or omission of further treatment, and that the physicians' omission to continue life support measure, although intentional and with knowledge that the patient would die, was not an unlawful failure to perform a legal duty, given the fact that the patient had virtually no chance of recovery, and given the wishes of the family. The court further held that the failure to institute formal guardianship proceedings did not render the physicians' conduct unlawful, since there was no such statutory requirement, and that, under the circumstances, the wife was the proper person to act as surrogate for the patient. In addition, the court held that there was no legal requirement for prior judicial approval of a decision to withdraw treatment.

2. *In the Matter of Claire C. Conroy (1983).* The guardian of an 84-year-old nursing home patient, suffering from severe organic brain syndrome and a variety of other serious ailments, sought removal of a nasogastric tube from the patient, who was totally dependent on the tube for nutrients and fluids. The New Jersey Superior Court held that the nasogastric tube could be removed from the patient. The guardian ad litem of patient appealed. Conroy died while the appeal was pending.

From her teens until retirement at age 62 or 63, Ms. Conroy was employed by a cosmetics company. She was never married but was devoted to her three sisters. The last of her sisters died in 1975, leaving her nephew as her only living relative. In 1979, he petitioned for and was granted guardianship of Ms. Conroy, whom he then placed in a nursing home. Ms. Conroy was ambulatory upon admission but was somewhat confused due to her organic brain syndrome. In 1982, she developed necrotic ulcers on her left foot as a complication of diabetes. She was unable to maintain a conversation because of her extreme confusion, but was aware of and could respond to commands. It was observed that Conroy was not eating, and thus she was placed on a nasogastric tube. Except for a 2-week period, during which time she was fed pureed food but with poor results, this tube remained in place until her death. Her physician testified at trial that she was not brain dead, not comatose, and not in a chronic vegetative state. The physician who testified for the guardian described Conroy's mental state as "severely demented." Severe contractions of her lower legs kept her in a semifetal position. According to the physicians' testimony, if the nasogastric tube were removed, Ms. Conroy would have died of dehydration and starvation in about a week. Her physician described this as a painful death.

The Superior Court, Appellate Division, held that since the patient was not in a chronic vegetative state, but was simply very confused, the bodily invasion the patient suffered as result of her treatment was small and death by dehydration and starvation would be painful, the state's interest in preserving life outweighs the patient's privacy interest, and thus removal of nasogastric tube, upon which the patient was totally dependent for nutriment and fluids, would be improper.

3. *In the Matter of Shirley Dinnerstein (1979).* This Massachusetts case sought appeal on the question of whether a physician attending an incompetent, terminally ill patient may lawfully direct that resuscitation be withheld in the event of cardiac or respiratory arrest where such has not been approved in advance by a probate court.

The patient is a 67-year-old woman who suffers from a condition known as Alzheimer's disease, diagnosed in 1975. She suffered a stroke in 1978 that left her totally paralyzed on her left side. She is confined to a hospital bed, in an essentially vegetative state, immobile, speechless, unable to swallow without choking, and barely able to cough. She is fed through a nasogastric tube; intravenous feeding was discontinued because it caused her pain. She also suffers from high blood pressure, which is difficult to control. There is risk in lowering it because of a constriction in an artery leading to the kidney. She has a serious, life-threatening coronary artery disease as a result of arteriosclerosis. Her life expectancy is no more than a year, but she could go into cardiac or respiratory arrest at any time. In this situation her attending physician has recommended that if cardiac or respiratory arrest occurs, resuscitation efforts should not be undertaken.

The patient's family, consisting of a son who is a practicing physician, and a daughter, with whom the patient lived prior to her admission to a nursing home, concur in the doctor's recommendation. The family joined with the doctor and the hospital in bringing action for declaratory relief. The probate judge appointed a guardian ad litem, who opposed.

A judgment was entered in accordance with the prayers of the complaint for declaratory relief, declaring that on the findings the law does not prohibit a course of medical treatment that excludes attempts at resuscitation in the event of cardiac or respiratory arrest and that the validity of an order to that effect does not depend on prior judicial approval.

4. *In the Matter of Mary Hier (1984).* Prior to transfer to a nursing home, Mrs. Hier, 92 years old, spent 55 years at a psychiatric hospital. Both at the hospital and nursing home, she received thorazine to relieve her delusions and extreme agitation without suffering adverse side effects. Mrs. Hier resists administration of the medication because of an aversion to being injected with needles. She also suffered for many years from a hiatal hernia and a large cervical diverticulum in her esophagus. The combined effect impeded her ability to ingest food orally. In 1974 she received a gastronomy, but Mrs. Hier repeatedly pulled out the gastric feeding tube. Difficulty in replacing the tube at the nursing home prompted transfer to a hospital. Upon examination, the physician determined that the stoma was almost completely closed and that replacement of the tube would require surgery. Mrs. Hier refused to have any surgery performed. A petition was filed for appointment of a guardian with consent authority. The Massachusetts Probate Court ordered appointment of a temporary guardian with authority to consent to the administration of antipsychotic drugs but without authority to consent to surgical procedures necessary to provide her with adequate nutritional support. The guardian appealed. Physicians explored a number of alternative feeding methods, but decided that all were medically contraindicated because of the complexity of medical problems and lack of patient cooperation.

The judge, in applying the substitute judgment analysis, took into consideration the facts that the proposed operation is intrusive and burdensome; that Mrs. Hier has repeatedly and clearly opposed procedures necessary to introduce tube feeding (both gastric and nasogastric); that benefits of a gastronomy are diminished by her repeated history of dislodgement; that dislodgement cannot be prevented except by physical restraints; and that physicians who had evaluated her condition were making thoughtful recommendations that the surgery was inappropriate. *Judgment affirmed.*

Dietitians' activities in the institutions where they are employed are not the only possible places where they may be held accountable for dietary advice given. Talking at a group meeting or even talking to a friend can carry the possibility of a malpractice suit. It is crucial to avoid statements that may be interpreted as treatment, prescription, or diagnosis. Preventive measures instrumental for the dietitian include: choosing words carefully, provision of brief but clear documentation in patients' records, strict adherence to the code of ethics, and continual demonstration of high professional standards.

References

American Dietetic Association. (1976). *Professional Standards Review Procedure Manual.* Chicago: ADA.

American Dietetic Association. (1977A). *Guidelines for Consultant Dietitians in Long-Term Care Facilities.* Chicago: ADA.

American Dietetic Association. (1977B). *Patient Nutritional Care in Long-Term Care Facilities.* Chicago: ADA.

American Dietetic Association. (1981). Position Paper on Recommended Salaries and Employment Practices for Members of the American Dietetic Association. *J. Am. Diet. Assoc., 78*(1) 62–78.

American Dietetic Association. (1987). Position of the American Dietetic Association: Issues in Feeding the Terminally Ill Adult. *J. Am. Diet. Assoc. 87*(1) 78–85.

American Dietetic Association. (1988). Code of Ethics for the Profession of Dietetics. *J. Am. Diet. Assoc. 88*(12) 1592–1596.

American Hospital Association. (1976). *Recording Nutritional Information in Medical Records.* Chicago: AHA.

Baird, P. M., and Jacobs, B. (1981). Malpractice: Your Day in Court. *Food Management 16*(2), 41–43.

Barber v. Superior Court. 147 Cal. App. 3d 1006, 195 Cal. Rptr. 484 (1983).

Consultant Dietitians in Health Care Facilities (ADA Practice Group). (1987). *Dietary Regulations for Skilled Nursing Facilities: A Comparison of the State Regulations and the Federal Conditions of Participation.* Pensacola, FL: Ross Laboratories.

Joint Commission on Accreditation of Hospitals. (1988). Chicago: JCAH.

In the Matter of Claire C. Conroy. 464 A.2d 303 (N.J. Super. Ct. 1983).

In the Matter of Mary Hier. 464 N.E.2d 959 (Mass. Ct. App. 1984).

In the Matter of Shirley Dinnerstein. 380 N.E.2d 134 (Mass. Ct. App. 1979).

McCarthy, C. M. (1988). DRGs: Five Years Later. *New Eng. J. Med. 318*(25), 1683–1686.

Michigan Department of Public Health. (1985). *Rules and Regulations for Nursing Homes.* Lansing: MDPH.

Neville, J. N., and Tower, J. B. (1988). President's Page: Plans for Update of the Role Delineation Studies. *J. Am. Diet. Assoc. 88*(3), 356–357.

Newman, D. (1973). *Organization Design: An Analytical Approach to the Structuring of Organization.* London: Edward Arnold.

Parks, S. C., and Kris-Etherton, P. M. (1982). Practitioners View Dietetic Roles for the 1980s. *J. Am. Diet. Assoc. 80,* 574–576.

Purtilo, R. B., and Cassel, C. K. (1981). *Ethical Dimensions in the Health Care Profession.* Philadelphia: Saunders.

Schiller, M. R. (1988). Ethical Issues in Nutrition Care. *J. Am. Diet. Assoc. 88*(1), 13–15.

Studebaker, M. E. (1988). The Ethics of Artificial Feeding. *New Eng. J. Med. 319*(5), 306.

Tancredi, L. R. (1974). *Ethics of Health Care.* Washington, DC: National Academy of Sciences.

U.S. Department of Health and Human Services, Health Care Financing Administration. (1983). *Medicare Program: Prospective Payment for Medicare Inpatient Hospital Services.* Federal Register *48*(171), 39752–39886.

U.S. Department of Health and Human Services, Health Care Financing Administration. (1984). *Medicare program: Prospective Payment for Medicare Inpatient Hospital Services.* Federal Register *49*(1), 234–340.

U.S. Department of Health and Human Services, Health Care Financing Administration. (1987). *Medicare Program: Payment Adjustment for Sole Community Hospitals.* Federal Register *52*(157), 30362–30368.

Welch, P., Oelrich. E., Endres, J., and Poon, S. (1988). Consulting dietitians in nursing homes: Time in role functions and perceived problems. *J. Am. Diet. Assoc. 88*(1), 29–34.

Chapter 5

Management Functions

Managerial functions are discussed throughout the text as applied to specific areas in the management of a medical foodservice operation. The purpose of this chapter is to provide a sense of cohesiveness to what is conceptualized as the functions of management and to promote managerial responsibility for implementation of functions through leadership and employee motivation.

Classification of Managerial Functions

Managerial scholars have not reached agreement on what functions are fundamental to the management process. As illustrated in Figure 5-1, fundamental functions leading to goal achievement are classified into five categories (Terry 1978). Note in particular the four functions of management that are included in each of the five combinations: (1) planning, (2) organizing, (3) directing, and (4) controlling. Staffing, listed in two combinations, is considered a part of organizing as management allocates human resources. Actuating and coordinating are involved in carrying out the planning and organizing functions through the efforts of subordinates. Representing and motivating are accomplished through leadership as managerial practices impact on human behavior.

Planning

Planning involves identifying future activities that will promote the objectives and goals of the department. There are short-range and long-range goals. Plans for the next day, week, month, or year are considered short term. The foodservice manager should promote short-range planning to the lowest possible level. For example, the chef or head cook must plan for production and service (using a production worksheet) at least a day in advance. Long-range planning may involve periods of time up to 10 years or more. Plans should be in writing and reflected on the capital budget if large sums of funding are required. Long-range plans must be flexible enough to accommodate any technologic and economic changes and other external conditions that may develop over a period of time.

Organizing

Organizing is the dividing of work activity for the purpose of meeting objectives and goals of the department and organization. The result of organization is an orderly structuring of roles and responsibilities necessary to perform the various work activities. In order to perform the organizing function, the foodservice director must know what resources are available and the necessary in-

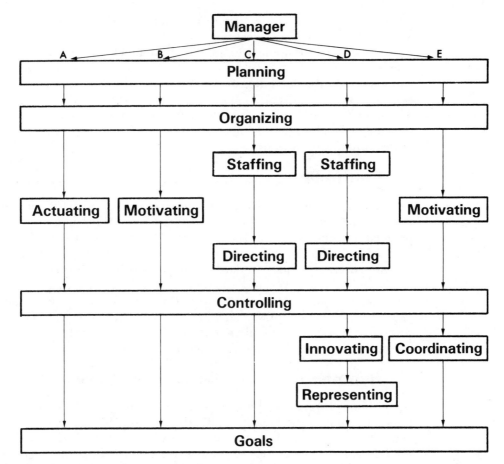

Figure 5-1. Five combinations of fundamental functions making up management process. From top to bottom, Category A consists of planning, organizing, actuating, and controlling; B: planning, organizing, motivating, and controlling; C: planning, organizing, staffing, directing, and controlling; D: planning, organizing, staffing, directing, controlling, innovating, and representing; E: planning, organizing, motivating, controlling, and coordinating.

terrelationships required in getting the job done. (See Chapter 3 for organization and design of foodservice departments.)

The most valuable resource, and the one requiring a large portion of the manager's attention, is the human resource. In organizing the various tasks and activities, consideration is given to the type of employee required to perform the function, based on experience, skills, and interest. Smooth organization depends on the relationship of the employee to the assigned job, the interrelationship of employees in a designated unit, and the relationship of one unit to another within the foodservice department.

As a result of organizing efforts, lines of communication, decision making, and authority emerge. Organization charts are used to provide visual displays of the levels within the department, divisions, units, section, and titles associated with each.

___ Directing _____

Directing is the coordinating, integrating, guiding, and initialing of subordinate's efforts in such a way that objectives and goals of both the department and employee are met. In carrying out the directing functions, the manager must assign tasks, give orders, train, and supervise work activity. In directing the work of others, the manager must provide all necessary information and the proper tools and equipment to get the job done effectively. Some of the managerial tools that are helpful in carrying out this function are job descriptions and job standards. Good direction is important if employees are to know what is expected of them. It is also important to realize that the work is done through human effort and that the methods used in directing may have a negative effect on employee morale. The manager must determine the most appropriate leadership approach to use.

Controlling

Controlling is a process of determining whether planned activities are carried out. In carrying out the control functions, a manager must know what was planned and the goals and standards that the plan must meet. To determine whether results are in line with plans, measurable standards must be in use. With established criteria (job standards), comparison of performance against standards can be made. Where a discrepancy is found between the expected and actual performance, it will be necessary to assess the significance of the differential. If the difference proves significant, corrective action must be taken. The corrective action taken should not be of a punitive nature but aimed at improving performance and promoting good human relations.

Hypothetical Example of Management Functions

Susan Doe is Director of Dietetics at a 350-bed hospital. In view of the current economic climate, the Hospital Administrator asked Susan to develop ideas for generating revenue. She conducted a feasibility study and submitted a proposal for operating a moderately expensive commercial restaurant, accessible to all visitors entering the hospital. The employee/visitor cafeteria, located in a remote area, would continue operation. The projected revenue and potential public relations were primary incentives for administrative approval. Susan used the four principles of management, discussed above, to carry out the project.

Planning. Susan used key personnel in the department to assist with details of planning and major decision making. Objectives and goals were clarified to ensure congruence with those of the department and hospital. Tasks to be completed prior to opening date were determined and assigned, such as remodeling of the proposed area, writing policies and procedures, purchasing equipment, and menu planning (the hub of the operation). Susan used the PERT technique (see Chapter 8) to ensure timely completion of the project.

Organizing. During this phase, Susan analyzed all functions to be performed, and divided work according to positions. She developed job specifications, job descriptions, and job standards. Staffing decisions were made regarding whether to hire new employees or train and use current staff. Salary scales were determined based on experience and skills required for each position. Lines of communication (in an organization chart) were established based on position and responsibility. The necessary equipment and tools to support functions were purchased, and printed menus were ordered.

Directing. The project was completed within the alloted time. Employees were hired or transferred from main production and service areas. Susan spent time coordinating all activities, such as orientation, training, and supervision of work. Restaurant opened for business.

Controlling. Susan used measurable Tools (job standards) to monitor quality and quantity of work. Susan remained flexible during initial phase and took corrective action when necessary, using the feedback loop (Chapter 1) to ensure customer satisfaction.

Leadership

Leading and managing are not synonymous, although the terms are used interchangeably. Simply being a manager, even a good manager, does not necessarily make someone a leader. The distinction, clearly drawn by Albanese (1975) infers that people follow managers because their job description requires them to follow; people follow leaders voluntarily and for reasons of their own choosing. The following discussion will attempt to distinguish the types of behavior exhibited by managers and leaders within organizations.

Management Defined

Management is the accountability to formulate and achieve the objectives of the organization. A manager has legal authority, within the organization, to plan, organize, direct, and control.

Leadership Defined

Leadership is the responsibility to represent the needs and goals of employees and to help them achieve what they want. A leader deals in emotions, excites camaraderie and unity, and guides vague notions into concrete actions. Leadership is generally recognized as the art of influencing and directing people in a manner that wins their obedience, confidence, respect, and enthusiastic cooperation in achieving a common objective. According to Lester (1981), leaders are self-starters, seeking out opportunity for making a change in the organization, rather than waiting for opportunity to come knocking at the office door.

The term *leader* is never found on the organization chart, except maybe as group leader. No one is officially known as the leader of one department or the other. But the term *manager* is frequently used to describe a position on an organization chart. The reason may be that there is more consensus of what a manager is or does, such as planning, organizing, directing, and controlling. A leader is not officially appointed by an organization; a leader asserts himself despite organizational constraints. One becomes a leader through recognition by superiors, peers, and subordinates.

Formal vs. Informal Leader

In every organization there is the formal manager, designated on the organization chart, with legal—that is, official—authority. Then there is the informal leader with no legal authority, but one who has a great deal of power and influence within the organization. A comparison of formal–informal leader characteristics are shown in Table 5-1. For the individual who wants to be effective as a manager and leader, one must be aware of where organization leaders are, both formal and informal. When support is needed for introducing change, one must make sure that the change is accepted by the informal leader, and he or she will persuade others to cooperate.

Characteristics of Managers and Leaders

Managers have the potential for becoming leaders. The degree to which an individual functions as both a manager and leader depends on the personal

Table 5-1. Characteristics of Formal and Informal Leaders [a]

Formal Leader	Informal Leader
Title is relevant to leadership position (Manager, Director).	Title is irrelevant, even misleading (Cook, Dishwasher, Union Steward).
Decision making tends to be through individual analysis and experience.	Decision making tends to be by consensus.
Frequently contacts others.	Frequently contacted by others. (Employees will check with informal leader on cooperation with changes.)
Almost always involved, regardless of issues.	Involvement is sporadic, depends on the issues.
Visible reminders of leadership position.	No visible *trappings* of leadership.

[a]From Weiss (1978).

attitudes toward goals, and the organizational climate. According to Zaleznik (1977), managers are basically different types of people and the work conditions favorable to the growth of one may be inimical to the other. Some of the major characteristics of managers and leaders are as follows:

1. *Attitude toward goals.* Managers tend to adopt impersonal, if not passive, attitudes toward goals. Leaders are active instead of reactive—shaping idea' rather than responding to them. In essence, leaders adopt a personal and acti e attitude toward goals.

2. *Conception of work.* Where managers act to limit choices, leaders devel p fresh approaches to long-standing problems and open issues for new o dous. Consequently, leaders create excitement in work. Leaders work from h n-risk positions, often seeking out danger, especially where opportunity and award appear high. In other words, they are not afraid to "rock the boat." For managers, the instinct for survival dominates their need for risk and their ability to tolerate mundane, practical work to assist in their survival.

3. *Relations with others.* Managers prefer to work with people; they avoid solitary work because it makes them anxious. The need to seek out others with whom to work and collaborate stands out as an important characteristic of managers. Often the manager communicates with his or her subordinates using signals instead of messages. One reason the manager does this is that signals are inclusive and subject to reinterpretation should people become angry or upset, whereas messages involve direct consequences that some people will not like. Messages are often referred to in less emotional terms, such as unscrupulous or detached. In contrast, leaders attract strong feelings of identity, such as love or hate.

The satisfaction of leadership comes from helping others get things done and changed, and not from getting personal credit for doing and changing things. Have you ever worked for someone who took credit for your creative and innovative ideas? Are you guilty of this kind of relationship with your subordinates? A positive answer to either question indicates poor leadership.

4. *Self-image.* Managers see themselves as conservators and regulators of the existing state of affairs within the organization. Perpetuating and strengthening the existing organization enhances a manager's sense of worth. Leaders tend to feel a separation from their environment. They may work in environments, but they never belong to them. Their sense of who they are does not depend on membership, work roles, or social indicators of identity.

The following discussion will examine some leadership styles and their effectiveness in the management of human resources.

Leadership Styles

The style of leadership has a direct influence on productivity and human relations, making the difference between an effective and ineffective organization.

THEORY X AND THEORY Y The theories developed by Douglas McGregor (1960) are basic assumptions to guide a manager's strategy in managing employees. Management practices that are consistent with theory X are commonly classified as those of an *autocratic leader;* those consistent with theory Y are classified as belonging to a *democratic leader.*

The autocratic leader uses force and position of authority to get others to do as he or she directs. The subordinate has no part or very little in influencing decisions. He or she often takes credit for accomplishments and puts blame for failure on others. This style of management tends to lose its effectiveness after the basic physiological needs of the employee have been met, because the manager is not concerned with the human elements involved.

The democratic leader seeks to lead mainly by persuasion and example, rather than by force, fear, or power. He or she encourages participation in decision making and seeks to fulfill the objectives of the worker as well as those of the organization. The style encourages the use of certain factors such as responsibility, delegation of work, and self-control in the work environment.

McGregor felt that the attitude of the manager was likely to have an effect on the attitudes and behavior of the employees. A manager with theory X assumptions believes that:

1. Work is inherently distasteful to most people.
2. Most people lack ambition, have little desire for responsibility, and thus prefer to be directed.
3. Most people have little capacity for creativity in solving work-related problems.
4. Most people must be closely controlled and often coerced to achieve organizational objectives.

In contrast, a manager with theory Y assumptions believes that:

1. Work is as natural as play, if conditions are favorable.
2. Self-control is often indispensable in achieving organizational goals.
3. The capacity for creativity in solving organizational problems is widely distributed in the population.
4. People can be self-directed and creative at work if properly motivated.

The manager with theory X assumptions generally ends up with theory X employees. Those same employees are likely to become theory Y employees when placed in an environment with theory Y asssumptions in practice. Put another way, employees generally live up to their expectations.

BOSS-CENTERED AND SUBORDINATE-CENTERED LEADERSHIP The autocratic–democratic dichotomy presents problems for managers who want to be democratic in their relations with subordinates and at the same time maintain the necessary authority and control in the organization. To assist managers faced with this dilemma, Tannenbaum and Schmidt (1973) developed a leadership pattern featuring a continuum of possible leadership behavior. Each type of action, as shown in Figure 5-2, is related to the degree of authority used by the boss and to the amount of freedom available to his subordinates in reaching decisions. The actions on the extreme left characterize the manager who maintains a high degree of control, whereas those seen on the extreme right

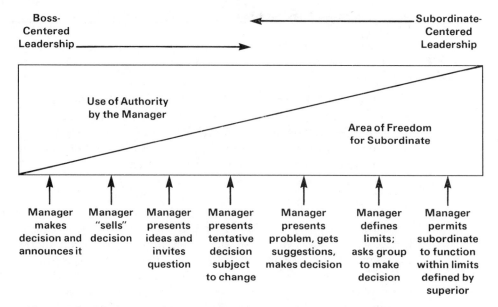

Figure 5-2. Continuum of leadership behavior. Reprinted by permission of the *Harvard Business Review*. An exhibit from "How to Choose a Leadership Pattern" by Robert Tannenbaum and Warren H. Schmidt (May/June 1973). Copyright © 1973 by the President and Fellows of Harvard College; all rights reserved.

characterize the manager who releases a high degree of control. Neither extreme is absolute; authority and freedom are never without their limitations.

The basic thesis is that the successful leader is one who is aware of those forces that are most relevant to his or her behavior at any one time and is able to behave accordingly. Regardless of the leadership style employed, it should be based on sensitivity and understanding for human relations and the tasks to be performed.

Motivation and the Employee

Motivation refers to the way external forces (managerial practices, organizational climate, and so on) affect human behavior on the job. Because motives are an internal state, motivation is inherent in the individual when he or she first enters the workplace. It is management's responsibility to elicit, rather than to instill motivation. An understanding of what motivated the individual to seek work is the first step to understanding employee motivation. Attempts are made during the selection process, by using sophisticated tools such as psychological tests, to screen individuals so that the employee fits the position. Yet employees of identical skills and abilities will perform at different levels of quantity and quality. The problem is not new, but the approaches to motivation have changed over the years.

Approaches to Motivation

TRADITIONAL THEORY OF MOTIVATION Frederick Taylor's approach to motivation, as discussed in Chapter 3, was that of the classic "economic man." He believed that wage incentives were enough to offset any other employee motives and that high productivity would continue as long as output was associated with the amount of earnings. The theory worked for a while because it met the needs of the employees at that time. However, the evaluation of management theory has shown that the economic theory is a less viable form of motivating employees than originally believed. For example, federal law now mandates a minimum wage for each employee, regardless of production level. As long as the employee remains on the job, a certain degree of economic security is guaranteed, In addition, the employee is further protected with worker's compensation should he or she be dismissed.

THE HAWTHORNE STUDIES The Hawthorne studies, discussed in Chapter 3, proved to be a major breakthrough in terms of employee motivation. It was concluded that productivity increased for the women in the relay assembly room due to the social relationships and improved work conditions. However, men in the test room established work norms to which they all conformed. In spite of wage incentives for piecework, productivity was not increased. The Hawthorne studies were the beginning of the human relations era in management. They proved that work incentives were not based primarily on economics.

MASLOW'S NEED HIERARCHY Maslow theorized that the needs of man exist in a hierarchical order and that one need must be met before another emerges. According to Maslow (1954), needs are classified (Fig. 5-3) from lowest to highest in the following order:

1. *Physiological.* This classification refers to basic survival needs such as food, drink, clothing, shelter, and sex.
2. *Safety.* This refers to both physical safety and job safety (job security).
3. *Belongingness and love.* As lower needs are met, the worker expresses concern for social relationships with other employees.
4. *Esteem.* This classification refers to self-respect, recognition, prestige, and other measures of esteem in the work environment.
5. *Self-actualization.* This is the highest classification of needs and is considered general in that the need varies with different individuals. It refers to the desire to become what one is capable of becoming. The need is rarely met.

Maslow's theory can help managers to understand employee motives, both the complexity and the importance. Since each employee may be at a different level of need, the manager must get to know employees on an individual basis in an effort to meet both personal and organizational goals. It is important to know what satisfies a worker and also the sources of dissatisfaction.

HERZBERG'S THEORY OF MOTIVATION The two-factor model on motivation is based on motivators (satisfiers) and hygiene factors (dissatisfiers). According to Herzberg (1974) there are especially satisfying and therefore potentially motivating job situations that differ from especially dissatisfying job situations (Table 5-2). Satisfying situations include opportunities to experience achievement, responsibility, recognition, and advancement in types of work that are interesting to the individual. Dissatisfying work situations include incompetent supervision, inadequate salary, poor working conditions, unfair company policies, inadequate employee benefits, and other such negative work-related factors. If hygiene factors are missing, dissatisfaction may develop; however the mere presence of hygiene factors will not guarantee satisfaction. It is not enough for the motivation factor to be fulfilled if the hygiene factor is lacking. Fulfillment of both factors is necessary for high employee job satisfaction.

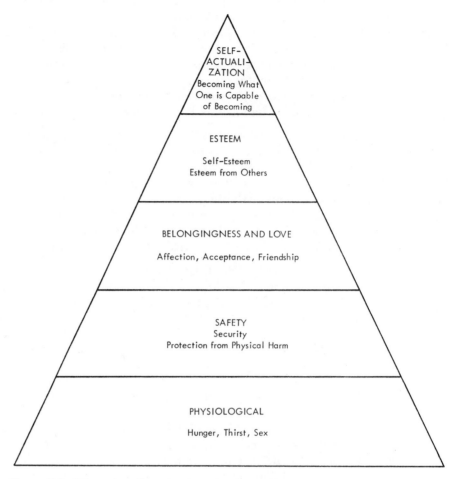

Figure 5-3. Hierarchy of needs. *From Maslow (1954)*

Table 5-2. Herzberg's Two-Factor Model on Motivation

Hygiene Factors	Motivators
Incompetent Supervision	Achievement
Inadequate Salary	Responsibility
Poor Work Conditions	Recognition
Inadquate Benefits	Advancement
Company Policies Unfair	Type of Work

Motivation and Work Values

Some of the traditional approaches, especially those relating to money or wage incentives, are no longer a major motivational factor. It requires more than the carrot-and-stick approach to motivate employees. The worker entering the work force today is seeking interesting, challenging work, with opportunities for advancement. The average worker seeks immediate gratification and is reluctant to work up the corporate ladder in the traditional manner.

MOTIVATING THE CONTEMPORARY EMPLOYEE One of the biggest managerial problems centers around contemporary employees and their differing work values. Motivating the employee to do more than put in 8 hours on the job requires that one understand people and the different values they hold regarding work. Equally important, managers must be aware of their own values. The questionnaire, as shown in Figure 5-4, can be used to make a quick assessment of a manager's orientation toward employee motivation. According to Howe and Mindell (1979), the instrument measures five major value dimensions:

Assessing Your Orientation Toward Employee Values

1. Organizational success is usually due more to chance than systematic planning.

    Strongly disagree   1   2   3   4   5   6   7   Strongly agree

2. When people advance in the company, it is often because of "who they know" rather than how well they perform.

    Strongly disagree   1   2   3   4   5   6   7   Strongly agree

3. There is little luck involved in running a department effectively.

    Strongly disagree   1   2   3   4   5   6   7   Strongly agree

4. I exercise a great deal of self-control in my position.

    Strongly disagree   1   2   3   4   5   6   7   Strongly agree

5. It is important to provide frequent feedback to employees on how well they are performing.

    Strongly disagree   1   2   3   4   5   6   7   Strongly agree

6. My ideas are rarely well understood by others in the company.

    Strongly disagree   1   2   3   4   5   6   7   Strongly agree

7. There is no such thing as "one right way" of doing things.

    Strongly disagree   1   2   3   4   5   6   7   Strongly agree

8. I often make decisions based upon insufficient information.

    Strongly disagree   1   2   3   4   5   6   7   Strongly agree

9. As a manager, I enjoy working in unclear situations.

    Strongly disagree   1   2   3   4   5   6   7   Strongly agree

10. Most people in an organization work because they have to, not because they want to.

    Strongly disagree   1   2   3   4   5   6   7   Strongly agree

11. It is often necessary to "step on some toes" in order to get the job done.

    Strongly disagree   1   2   3   4   5   6   7   Strongly agree

12. I try not to let my feelings get in the way of business.

    Strongly disagree   1   2   3   4   5   6   7   Strongly agree

13. I often worry about what my job will be in five years.

    Strongly disagree   1   2   3   4   5   6   7   Strongly agree

14. I have a strong degree of loyalty to my company.

    Strongly disagree   1   2   3   4   5   6   7   Strongly agree

15. Job security is very important to me.

    Strongly disagree   1   2   3   4   5   6   7   Strongly agree

---

Figure 5-4. Instruction for assessing managerial orientation toward employee values. *From Howe and Mindell (1979)*

1. *Locus or control.* Both the traditional and contemporary managers believe that they have control over events through their decisions; that success cannot be left to chance but must be planned; and that advancement of subordinates depends on achievement rather than politics, over which they have a great deal of control. Statements 1, 2, and 3 in Figure 5-4 represent three measures of locus of control. The *ideal manager*[1] of either type of employee (contemporary or traditional) would strongly disagree with 1 and 2, and strongly agree with 3.

2. *Self-esteem.* The ideal manager should recognize employee accomplishments by providing feedback as a measure to preserve and enhance individual self-esteem. Managers who exercise self-control, who feel that their ideas are creative, understood, and accepted, and who believe that feedback is important tend to have high self-esteem. Managers who have a mistrust of employees—who appear critical and are annoyed or irritated with those with different ideas or values—tend to score low in self-esteem. Items 3, 5, and 6 in Figure 5-4 are concerned with self-esteem. The ideal manager would score high and strongly agree with 4 and 5, and strongly disagree with 6.

3. *Tolerance of ambiguity.* Managers holding contemporary values can and often want to function in unstructured, ambiguous situations; believe that no problem is too complex to be solved; and strongly believe that there is more than one right way of doing things. Items 7, 8, and 9 relate to ambiguity. The ideal contemporary manager would strongly agree with each item. The ideal traditional manager would strongly disagree.

4. *Social judgment.* The contemporary manager is characterized by social perceptiveness, sensitivity, empathy, social intelligence, and social insight. Contemporary employees value good interpersonal relationships and personal recognition and therefore work best for managers with these values. The contemporary manager believes it possible to create an environment where people work because they want to, rather than need to; where worker feelings contribute to, rather than detract from, task accomplishment; and where rewards, rather than punishments, get the job done. Items 10, 11, and 12 refer to social judgment. The ideal contemporary manager would strongly disagree with each item. The more traditional manager would tend to agree with them, since he or she displays these characteristics only moderately.

5. *Risk taking.* Managers who seek excitement and changes and enjoy taking chances are more likely to have contemporary values than those who are cautious, consider matters very carefully, and are reluctant to take risk. The contemporary manager may be regarded by the traditional manager as impulsive and erratic. The contemporary manager has low dependency needs; is more concerned with the immediate future than with a long-term career; is loyal first to personal needs and desires over those of the organization; and is only moderately concerned with job security. Items 13, 14, and 15 measure risk taking. The ideal contemporary manager would generally disagree with all three. The converse is for the ideal traditional manager.

As more and more contemporary employees enter the work force, there will be an increased demand for managers who understand their values.

---

[1]Ideal manager is used as a frame of reference; the terms *contemporary* and *traditional* as dichotomy.

References

Albanese, R. (1975). *Management Toward Accountability for Performance.* Homewood, IL: Richard D. Irwin.

Herzberg, F. (1974). Motivation-Hygiene Profile: Pinpointing What Ails the Organization. *Organizat. Dynam. 3,* 18–29.

Howe, R. J., and Mindell, M. G. (1979). The Challenge of Changing Work Values: Motivating the Contemporary Employee. *Mgt. Rev. 68*(9), 51–55.

Lester, R. I. (1981). Leadership: Some Principles and Concepts. *Personnel J. 60*(11), 868–870.

Maslow, A. H. (1954). *Motivation and Personality.* New York: Harper & Row.

McGregor, D. (1960). *The Human Side of Enterprise.* New York: McGraw-Hill.

Tannenbaum, R. and Schmidt, W. H. (1973). How to Choose a Leadership Pattern. *Harvard Bus. Rev.* May–June.

Terry, G. (1978). *Principles of Management.* Homewood, IL: Learning Systems Company/ Richard D. Irwin.

Weiss, A. J. (1978). Surviving and Succeeding in the Political Organization: Becoming a Leader. *Supervis. Mgt. 23*(8), 27–35.

Zaleznik, A. (1977). Managers and Leaders: Are They Different? *Harvard Bus. Rev. 55*(3) 67–78.

Chapter 6

Effective Communication

Communication is the flow of information from a sender to a receiver. The purpose of communication is to convey meaning and promote understanding, and therefore the message should be clearly expressed in the appropriate language. However, the message may encounter a number of interferences during its travel. To reduce the number of "bottlenecks" a manager needs to understand possible causes and ways to overcome communication blocks.

Communication Channels

The three major channels used for communication are upward, downward, and horizontal.

___ Upward Communication ___

Upward communication is the flow of information from a subordinate to a superior. As a manager, you receive upward communication from your employees; and you communicate upwards to an administrator. In some organizations there is a free flow of information, whereas in other organizations blockage occurs. The difference is the organizational climate and how conducive it is to facilitating and encouraging the free exchange of ideas.

Based on past experience, employees may be reluctant to disclose information to superiors—especially if employees fear that disclosure may lead to punishment or retaliation in some way. The withholding of information, the failure to provide feedback, or the provision of distorted information can be costly for the superiors. How often has an employee been heard to remark, "I'm not sure I should tell you this"? Why do employees conceal their true feelings? Does the manager become angry, emotionally upset, or defensive? The attitude of the superior and the degree of openness exhibited with employees have a definite bearing on the amount of upward communication.

According to Gemmill (1970), if the superior's control over the personal goals of a subordinate were decreased, then their fear of receiving a penalty for disclosure would decrease. Given the organizational structure as it exists today, the superior has a high degree of control over subordinates in the form of firing, laying off, blocking promotions and salary increases, and holding back developmental assignments if the superior does not like what he or she hears. One way to elicit disclosure is through rewards. The more a superior rewards disclosure of feelings, opinions, and difficulties by subordinates, the more likely they will be to disclose them. Merely stating that there will be no punishment and that they should feel free to express their opinions is not enough. Words must be followed by action. For full disclosure, subordinates must know that they can express themselves without fear of reprisal and that they can look upon the superior as a source of help rather than as a powerful judge.

____ Downward Communication _____

Downward communication refers to information flow from the superior to the subordinate. Employees at the lowest level want to know what is going on in the workplace. The manager should make use of all available techniques to keep employees informed, including written memos, face-to-face contact, and regularly scheduled group meetings. According to Chase (1970), an element of good downward communication is the content of the message, to be transmitted as follows:

1. *The message must be accurate and true, whether it is good or bad news concerning the organization.* When employees realize that the information is only partly accurate, they will tend to ignore future messages.

2. *The message must be both definite and specific in meaning.* The message should state clearly why a certain position was taken. It must define all actions taken and what effects it will have on members of the organization.

3. *The message must be forceful.* A manager who does not agree or believe in a decision that has been made cannot expect his employees to believe in it.

4. *The message must be receiver-oriented.* Subordinates should not have any difficulty understanding how the message directly affects them.

5. *The message should not contain complexities.* It should be stated as simply as possible. An employee will spend 2 hours trying to compute the number of vacation days to which he is entitled, but will not give 5 minutes trying to figure out a management directive on how to reduce waste.

5. *The message should not contain hidden meanings.* To avoid misunderstanding, it is advisable to explain briefly the developments leading up to the message.

Employees can spend a great deal of nonproductive time discussing rumors that may or may not have any merit. Effective downward communication can reduce this waste of time and reduce any anxiety associated with distorted messages.

____ Horizontal Communication _____

Horizontal communication refers to information flow from one department to another. In complex, open organizations, direct horizontal communication is encouraged. Koontz and O'Donnell (1974) suggest that proper safeguards of horizontal communication rest in an understanding between superiors. Although interdepartmental relationships are encouraged, subordinates should refrain from making commitments beyond their authority and should keep their superiors informed on their activities.

In medical foodservice operations, upward, downward, and horizontal communication channels are necessary in order to coordinate patient care activities. For the foodservice director and other administrative personnel, information flow is most often between other department heads. For the clinical staff, information may flow to nurses, physicians, and other members of the health care team.

Feedback

Positive feedback lets an individual know that he is doing well; negative feedback identifies areas where improvement is necessary. Feedback is most helpful when it is provided as soon after the given situation as possible. However, negative feedback should not be given in public. In an organizational climate where feedback is encouraged, both the superior and the subordinate must be willing to accept criticism. It is up to the superior to convince subordinates that feedback is welcomed, and that management will not retaliate against an employee for the disclosure of information. Giving and receiving feedback is critical to effective communication since it lets individuals know how others view them.

—— Johari Window ——————————————————————

The process of giving and receiving information can be demonstrated by use of the Johari window (Fisher 1982). Looking at the four cells, as shown in Figure 6-1, the two vertical columns represent the *self* and the two horizontal rows represent the *others*. Column 1 contains "things I know about myself"; column 2 contains "things I do not know about myself"; Row 1 contains "things that others know about me"; row 2 contains "things that the others do not know about me." Cell information changes as the level of mutual trust and the exchange of feedback vary.

Information in the *arena cell* is public and is characterized by a free and open exchange of information. The *blind spot* contains information that a person does not know about himself, but that others know. A person communicates all kinds of information of which he or she is not aware but is picked up by others. The information may be communicated by what is said, the way it is said, or by management style. In the *facade* or *hidden area* there are things about a person that he or she knows but of which others are unaware. For one reason or another, this information is kept silent. One reason information is hidden may be fear of rejection if real feelings are known. The *unknown area* contains things that neither a person nor others know about the person. This material is below the surface and one may never become aware of it. However, the material can become public knowledge through an exchange of information. Internal boundaries in all cells can move backward and forward or up and down as a consequence of giving or receiving feedback.

ENLARGING THE ARENA To improve communication the arena must be made as large as possible. This is done by either reducing the blind spot

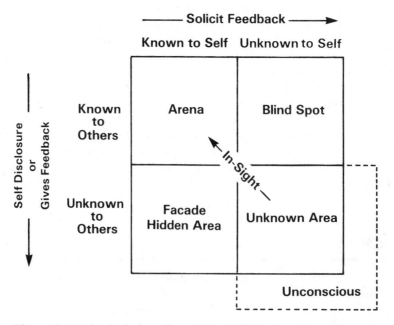

Figure 6-1. Johari window. *From Fisher (1982)*

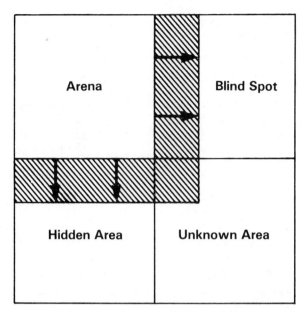

Figure 6-2. Johari window: Enlarging the arena. *From Fisher (1982)*

or the hidden area (Fig. 6-2). The blind spot is reduced by accepting feedback. The more self-disclosure and feedback one gives, the further down one pursues the horizontal line. The *ideal window,* in which there is a large arena, suggests that a person's behavior is open and aboveboard. Little questioning is needed to understand what the person is trying to do or say. A large facade or hidden area describes a person who asks for information but never volunteers any. Such a person eventually evokes feelings of distrust. When a person has a large blind spot, he or she gives feedback but cannot or will not accept it. A large unknown area reflects a person who does not know much about himself or herself and one about whom others do not know a great deal.

SUPERVISORY–EMPLOYEE RELATIONS The goal of soliciting or giving feedback is to move information from the blind spot or facade into the arena where it is available to everyone. As applied to relationships between a supervisor and an employee, the arena is composed of all activities performed by the employee and the supervisor (Fig. 6-3). The blind spot holds those activities that the supervisor expects the employee to perform but that the employee does not know he or she is expected to perform. The hidden area consists of activities performed by the employee. The supervisor does not know that the employee is performing these activities and does not expect them to be performed. The unknown area represents all activities that may be added or deleted from the employee's list of tasks and activities. The employee and the supervisor are both unaware of the activities to be added or deleted. The goal of using this model is to increase the arena of both the supervisor and the employee.

A climate of mutual trust is conducive to feedback and results in effective communication. The Johari window with the goal of increasing the size of the arena, is one way of promoting feedback and is objective and constructive.

Barriers to Communication

Effective communication is based on free flow of information. An understanding of why a message does not get through should be a major concern. Accord-

	Employee Knows	Employee Does Not Know
Supervisor Knows	**Arena** Actions performed by employee and known to employee and supervisor	**Blind Arena** Activities expected by supervisor but not known or performed by employee
Supervisor Does Not Know	**Hidden Area** Activities performed by employee but not known or expected by supervisor	**Unknown Area** Activities that may be added or deleted but unknown to employee or supervisor

Figure 6-3. Johari window: Supervisory-employee relations. *From Fisher (1982)*

ing to Strauss and Sayles (1960), reasons for communication breakdowns are as follows:

1. *We hear what we expect to hear.* What we hear is shaped by experience and background, and we reject messages that conflict.
2. *We have different perceptions.* Our perceptions depend on previous experience.
3. *We evaluate the source.* Not only do we evaluate the source in terms of our own background and experience, but also on how reliable we judge the source (sender) to be.
4. *Our emotional state conditions what we hear.* When we are insecure, worried, or fearful, we hear and view messages as more threatening.
5. *We ignore information that conflicts with what we already know.* Hearing that hard work leads to promotions conflicts with our knowledge that promotions are often based on favoritism.
6. *Words mean different things to different people.* The use of words allows for discretion in the interpretation.
7. *Words have symbolic meaning.* For some employees a particular word may have symbolic meaning that others overlook. For example, if the supervisor asks to see an employee in the office later in the day, one employee might feel important, whereas another employee might feel threatened.

Overcoming Barriers to Communication

Perfect communication may not be attainable, but there are techniques that the manager can utilize in the day-to-day superior–subordinate relationship.

1. *Feedback.* Provide both positive and negative feedback, when necessary. Observe nonverbal feedback such as a nod of the head, puzzlement, anger, and body movement. Check on reception of message with such questions as: "Do you understand? Is it clear? and Are there any questions?

2. *Face-to-face communication.* This provides immediate feedback. Certain parts of the message can be emphasized, questions can be answered, and further explanation provided. For important messages, both the spoken and written word may be used.

3. *Sensitivity to the world of the receiver.* Try to predict the impact of what is said on the receiver's feeling and attitudes.

4. *Awareness of symbolic meaning.* If an employee resists or objects to a certain procedure, find out if some symbolic meaning is attached.

5. *Careful timing of messages.* For example, employee conferences are often more effective at the end of the day.

6. *Reinforcing words with action.* Consistent reinforcement of words by action increases the likelihood that the message will be accepted.

7. *Direct, simple language.* Written communication, should be as intelligible and readable as possible. In face-to-face communication, use words understood by the receiver. Avoid double-talk and jargon that leaves the receiver with the feeling of "what did that mean?"

Developing good communication requires constant attention to channels of information flow, organizational climate, and day-to-day interpersonal behavior.

References

Chase, A. B. (1970). How to Make Downward Communication Work. *Personnel J.*, June, 478–483.

Fisher, D. W. (1982). A Model for Better Communication. *Supervis. Mgt. 27*(6), 24–29.

Gemmill, G. (1970). Managing Upward Communication. *Personnel J.*, Feb., 107–110.

Koontz, H., and O'Donnell, C. (1974). *Essentials of Management.* New York: McGraw-Hill.

Strauss, G., and Sayles, L. R. (1960). *Personnel: The Human Problems of Management.* Englewood Cliffs, NJ: Prentice-Hall.

Chapter 7

Decision Making

A decision is a choice among alternatives to act or not to act in a given situation. The alternatives provided the manager in a decision-making process may or may not be restrictive, depending on the nature and the urgency of the decision. To illustrate, Braverman (1980) classifies decisions as programmable and unprogrammable.

Types of Decisions

__ Programmable Decisions __

Programmable decisions occur with some frequency and are repetitive in nature. Because they occur over and over again, they can usually be solved without going through the decision-making process each time. As director of the foodservice operation, one is constantly faced with programmable decisions on a day-to-day basis. For example, when one decides to reduce the amount of food to prepare based on similar circumstances in the past, the decision maker is using past experience as the basis for decision making. However, as cautioned by Atchinson and Winston (1978), managers must take care to choose the appropriate programmed decision in situations that require new solutions. In the rush to make a decision, the situation confronted by a manager may resemble one for which there is an existing program. Other programmable decisions may be based on existing policies and procedures, requiring only minor changes based on environmental conditions.

__ Unprogrammable Decisions __

Unprogrammable decisions are more complex and difficult to resolve. They are one of a kind and will never recur in exactly the same manner. No common solution can be applied to unprogrammable decision making because of the uniqueness of the situation. However, general procedures can be formulated and used. Some examples of unprogrammable decisions are those related to the present economic conditions that may involve reorganization of the foodservice department as a result of reduced staffing, drastic changes in operating procedures, and embarking on a cooperative venture such as group food purchasing.

Decisions frequently result in a change of rules, policies, and procedures, or they may result in delay or inaction on the part of the decision maker. In both instances, a decision has been made because a decision to delay or not to act is as much a decision as the decision to act. Some managers use what is called *snap decision making,* based on judgment, intuition, and experience. Other managers make a choice among alternatives. One of the reasons for possible delay is a concern for the consequences of the decision. Some consequences are the acceptance or nonacceptance by those affected, the resulting social and psychological climate, and the profit or loss, if the decision involves monetary values.

Approaches to Decision Making

The manager, faced with a decision, will have to decide on the most appropriate method to use. Although a number of approaches are available, the following discussion is limited to intuitive versus scientific, and individual versus group decision-making processes.

Intuitive Decision Making

When a manager uses intuition in decision making, the decision is based on past experience. The correctness of the decision will depend on whether the current situation is similar to one that has happened in the past. In medical foodservice a manager is constantly involved in decision making. Most often the decision must be made immediately, thus limiting the time for deliberation or the use of time-consuming analytical procedures. The amount of experience a manager has in certain situations, and the degree of learning from these experiences, will form a basis for the intuition used in making the decision. In other words, it can be stated that intuition comes from experience. Problems arise when the manager's experience is limited, when a current problem is misjudged to be similar to a situation in the past, when the situation is viewed as a new or unique problem with no immediate solution, and when the situation involves uncertainty and risk. Since a manager's reputation, prestige, and even job security may be affected by the number of correct decisions made, it is advisable for managers to seek and use additional methods for decision making.

Scientific Decision Making

The scientific approach forces the manager to analyze all viable alternatives to the problem prior to making a decision. An experimental research type of format is used, such as (1) stating the problem, (2) establishing hypotheses, (3) experimentation, and (4) results and conclusions. The procedure may prove to be too costly to the organization in terms of carrying out the experiment. Also, the use of a strictly scientific approach will depend on the ability and skill level of the manager. A more practical approach is the use of problem solving. The problem-solving approach permits the analysis required in arriving at a decision, yet it does not involve the actual experimentation called for by the scientific approach.

PROBLEM SOLVING Problem solving and decision making are not the same. Problem solving is a part of the decision-making process and always leads to some decision (Braverman 1980). To solve a problem, one must realize that a problem exists. Problems are recognized in terms of the objectives and goals of the organization. When there is discrepancy between the current situation and the way it should be, a problem exists. Steps in problem solving (Fig. 7-1) are as follows:

1. *Define the problem.* Determine the nature of the problem. Get a clear understanding of cause—why there is a discrepancy between the actual and the expected outcome.

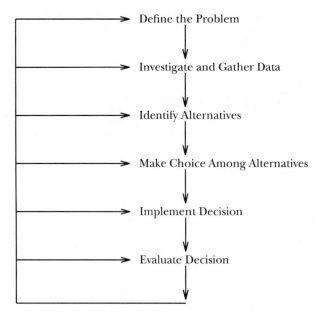

Figure 7-1. Steps in problem solving.

    2. *Investigate and gather data.* Conduct a thorough investigation to obtain all relevant data. Observe and talk to those involved. Gather reports, records, and other written documents.

    3. *Identify alternatives.* For each alternative, consider the impact on personnel in the involved department (e.g., determine the risks and benefits).

    4. *Make a choice among alternatives.* Select the most appropriate solution, with consideration to the impact, consequences, and probability of the outcome.

    5. *Implement the decision.* Avoid unnecessary delay in implementing the decision. Consider timing.

    6. *Evaluate the decision.* Monitor and follow up on the effects of implementation.

____ Individual vs. Group Decision Making ____

A manager is oriented toward making decisions independently, but at times it may be advantageous to share decision making with others. In addition to required sharing of decisions, such as in union matters, the manager may have other reasons for delegating decision making to a group or ad hoc committee. According to Massie (1971), a critical factor in the use of committees is to state in explicit terms what function the group is to perform. Managers tend to appoint committees to share in the decision-making process under the following conditions:

    1. When there is a need for consensus among different individuals, groups, or departments.

    2. When there is a need to gain acceptance by subordinates.

    3. When there is a need to minimize conflict among subordinates.

    4. When there is a need for creative ideas, suggestions, and alternatives.

    5. When there is a need for expert opinions in different areas.

    6. When there is a need to investigate and collect additional data.

7. When there is a need to train inexperienced personnel in decision making.
8. When there is a need to seek support for a decision that may prove unpopular.
9. When there is a need to make a final decision from among alternatives.
10. When there is a need to avoid the appearance of arbitrary decision making.

The previous conditions can be considered as advantages to group decision making. However, there are certain disadvantages to committee appointments. Committee decisions may result in *buck-passing*, by means of which no individual is held responsible for the decision. Further, committees are costly, considering the valuable time spent by individual members. Also, the group or committee decision-making process can become long and drawn out, resulting in compromise and indecision. Finally, committee decision making is not advisable if a decision must be made promptly.

Problem-Solving Tools

A number of sophisticated analytical tools are available to the manager for problem solving that may result in decision making, but most require high levels of mathematical skills. According to Koontz and O'Donnell (1974), there is a gap between the manager who is expected to use the models and the operations researcher who develops them. In essence, managers lack knowledge and appreciation of mathematics, and mathematicians lack an understanding of managerial problems. One technique, using systematic analysis has proved effective in the decision-making process—the decision tree.

The Decision Tree

The decision tree approach may be viewed as simple or complex, depending on the complexity of the decision to be made. The decision tree approach is most applicable when a decision must be made in an environment of uncertainty, and in high risk situations. A decision tree (Fig. 7-2) graphically illustrates all possible choices, risks, gains, and goals related to a decision. It also includes the likely payoff and the probability of success. Decision trees are normally drawn horizontally (Magee 1964), with the base at the left representing the current point. From the base, branches fork out to represent an alternate course of action. If the decision is a simple choice among alternatives, as shown in Figure 7-2, then the decision tree is reduced to a single-stage analysis. For more complicated decisions, more stages are necessary to reflect all possible alternatives.

The methodology used in establishing a decision tree is as follows (Carlisle 1976):

1. A decision is recognized (decision point).
2. Alternatives are identified (possible actions).
3. Possible future conditions or situations are identified (states of nature).
4. The likelihood of each state of nature is determined (probabilities).
5. Results of alternatives are determined (payoffs).
6. Outcomes of payoffs are calculated by multiplying the probabilities of the different states of nature (expected value).
7. Follow-up on sequential decisions are evaluated in the manner as the six previous steps.

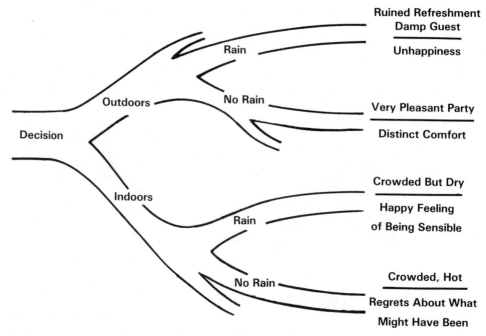

Figure 7-2. Sample decision tree. Reprinted by permission of the *Harvard Business Review*. An exhibit from "Decision Trees for Decision Making" by John F. Magee (July/August 1974). Copyright © 1974 by the President and Fellows of Harvard College; all rights reserved.

The major advantage of using a decision tree is that it helps decision makers to identify alternatives and clarify the nature of risks involved.

Brainstorming

Brainstorming is a creative method used in a group setting for generating ideas or alternatives in a problem-solving process. As developed by Osborn (1963), group brainstorming is not meant to be used as a substitute for problem solving but as a supplement, in these three ways:

1. *As a supplement to individual ideation* by generating a maximum number of potentially usable ideas in a minimum of time.
2. *As a supplement to conventional conferences* if and when creative thinking is the primary purpose.
3. *As a supplement to creative thinking* by including a more creative attitude and developing fluency of ideas.

The group is formed by appointing a chairperson to present the problem and promote a free exchange of ideas, and a recorder to write down all suggestions. The brainstorming environment encourages participants to talk freely by expressing any and all ideas, without criticism, judgment, or evaluation. The objective is to generate as many creative ideas as possible. At the end of the session, a compiled list is submitted to the decision maker for evaluation. The ideas may or may not be useful in providing a solution to the problem.

Synectics

Synectics is a group-oriented process for generating creative solutions to problems. It is similar to brainstorming except as follows:

1. The group is composed of a select group of experts on the particular problem.
2. The quantity of solutions offered is not of the essence.
3. Criticism is allowed as new and different viewpoints are formed.
4. The group is smaller.
5. Before solutions are offered, analogies are developed for a better understanding of the problem.
6. Every facet of the problem is analyzed in detail.

According to Braverman (1980), brainstorming attempts to promote new ideas by creating a climate conducive to generating a large quantity of suggestions. Synectics attempts to make the strange familiar and the familiar strange by looking at a problem in new and different ways.

The Delphi Method

The Delphi method is similar to brainstorming and synectics in that it is used to find solutions to problems. The method is used extensively by dietetic educators in arriving at competency statements for dietetic practitioners. Unlike other methods discussed, participants do not meet or communicate face-to-face. Generally, the procedure involves designing and sending a questionnaire to a large group of respondents, summarizing responses, analyzing results, and preparing and sending a new questionnaire based on results. The process is repeated, with feedback, to the respondents until an acceptable agreement is reached.

The use of problem-solving tools such as brainstorming, synectics, and Delphi can only assist the decision maker in making the best possible choice among alternatives; they cannot substitute for responsible judgment in making the final decision. An understanding of personal, organizational, and administrative factors that may affect decisions can be beneficial in the decision-making process.

Problems in Decision Making

There is a certain amount of risk involved in all decisions, in addition to other factors that have important bearings on the kind of decision made. The organization structure can be designed to facilitate and generate sound decisions and minimize forces that inhibit good decision making. The following administrative problems affect decision making (McFarland 1966).

1. *Correctness of decisions.* The probability that a particular decision will be correct depends on a number of factors, including the amount and accuracy of information gathered and the ability of the decision maker to analyze data correctly. Attempts are made to achieve the highest percentage of correct decisions possible and, if mistakes are made, to ensure that they are limited to minor decisions.

2. *The environment of decisions.* A manager may be reluctant to make decisions as a result of the organizational climate. Decisiveness on the part of top administrators will help promote decisiveness throughout the organization. However, if a manager is unclear as to the authority to decide or the responsibility to decide, decision making tends to be uncertain, erratic, or nonexistent. If decisions are rescinded over and over again, the manager will wait until he or she

can clear decisions with higher administration and thus will become too cautious and slow to make decisions.

3. *Psychological elements in decision making.* Decision making involves both personal and organizational factors. Personal factors that may influence an individual's organizational decision making include status, prestige, economic security, temperament, intelligence, energy, attitude, and emotions. The psychological view is that an individual's total personality must be considered in analyzing the decision-making process.

4. *Timing of decisions.* Those affected by a decision, including superiors, need to be informed in a timely manner. Supervisors should always be informed ahead of their subordinates so that the decision can be effectively communicated downward.

5. *Communicating decisions.* Timing is important in communicating a decision because undue delay may result in *leaks through the grapevine.* Leaks may be distorted, arousing antagonisms toward the decision before it is formally announced. Major decisions should be in writing. Because those affected by the decision should understand the logic or relevance; both the written and oral versions of communication should be clear and simple.

6. *Participation.* When individuals are allowed to participate in the decision-making process, there is a sense of belongingness on the part of employees, improved work efficiency, greater sense of responsibility, and a greater acceptance of change. To summarize, employees are more willing to carry out the demands of the decision if they had a part in the decision-making process.

References

Atchinson, T. J., and Winston, W. H. (1978). *Management Today.* New York: Harcourt Brace Jovanovich.

Braverman, J. D. (1980). *Management Decision Making.* New York: AMACOM.

Carlisle, H. M. (1976). *Management Concepts and Situations.* Chicago: Science Research Associates.

Koontz, H., and O'Donnell, C. (1974). *Essentials of Management.* New York: McGraw-Hill.

Magee, J. F. (1974). Decision Trees for Decision Making. *Harvard Bus. Rev.* July–Aug.

Massie, J. L. (1971). *Essentials of Management.* Englewood Cliffs, NJ: Prentice-Hall.

McFarland, D. E. (1966). *Management Principles and Practices.* New York: Macmillan.

Osborn, A. F. (1963). *Applied Imagination.* New York: Scribner.

Chapter 8

Time Management

Managerial personnel must be able to manage their own personal and organizational time. As work-related tasks increase in quantity and complexity, placing greater demands on one's time, a carefully organized and coordinated approach must be given to all aspects of the job. Such practices as working long overtime hours or taking work home to be accomplished on off-duty time should be scrutinized in terms of long-term solutions. The quality of time is more important than the quantity of time involved in completing a task.

Time Categories

According to a prescription for dynamic supervision in the hospital, published by the Bureau of Business Practice (1974), supervisors divide their time into four categories:

1. *Hospital time.* This is the time spent fulfilling obligations to other people in the organization. The time may include reports to higher management, meeting and discussions with associates and superiors, telephone calls, and progress reports.

2. *Investment time.* This is time spent directly on affairs that fall within the supervisor's immediate responsibility. Investment time means spending time now to make time in the future. An example of investment time is to train an employee who can eventually share the work load and help overcome the time pressure of the job. Other examples include time spent in planning the work of the department, making social contacts with people who may be able to help in some future activity, listening to complaints, and thinking creatively about the work.

3. *Immediate reward time.* This is time spent on activities that yield instant results. Delegation of activities fits into this category. When work is assigned to a subordinate, one can expect an immediate reward: one less thing to do. This category also includes helping an employee to solve on-the-job problems, dictating letters, writing interoffice memos, placing telephone calls, or any other activity that results in direct action or provides the information needed to take direct action.

4. *Wasted time.* This time represents work without beneficial results for the supervisor, the employees, or the department.

The first three categories may be classified as productive time; the fourth category may be classified as nonproductive time. It is important for managers to discuss the differences and make concerted efforts to reduce time wasters. It may involve changing or adjusting the daily routine, which may involve a break with tradition. Remember, it is necessary to invest time in order to save time.

Systems for Organizing Time

A systematic procedure for organizing and coordinating a time management program (Ashkenas & Schaffer 1982; Douglass & Douglass 1982; Ferderber 1981; Steffen 1982) is offered in the following subsections.

___ Assessing Use of Time

The following analysis and questions are helpful when one needs to assess how one's time is spent.

1. Analyze everything you do in terms of objectives. What needs to be done? When should it be done? Why should it be done? What are the consequences of not doing it? Maintain a time log of all activities on a daily, weekly, and monthly basis.

2. Analyze objectives and goals. Are goals clearly defined and measurable? Are goals realistic? Are goals essential for meeting objective?

3. Analyze planned versus spontaneous or interrupted time. How much time is lost through interruptions either by telephone or office drop-ins?

4. Analyze activities in terms of productivity. What activities that take more than 30 minutes per week can be eliminated? What activities taking an hour or more a week could be done in half the time? What activities taking more than 30 minutes could be delegated?

5. Analyze the number and types of meetings attended. Rate meetings according to effective use of time. Are meetings dull, unorganized, inefficient, and unproductive? Are meetings supportive of objectives and goals?

___ Planning Time

Objectives and goals must be considered when planning the use of time. The following should be considered.

1. Plan objectives and goals, both personal and organizational. Be realistic in planning what can be accomplished in a given amount of time. Consider relevancy of goals to objectives.

2. Plan ahead. Plan time on a daily basis to accomplish most important tasks first. Plan for upcoming meetings, conferences, and appointments. Be prepared with necessary supportive documents and data.

3. Plan to eliminate all nonessential, extraneous activities that are not supportive of objectives and goals.

___ Implementing Time Management

The use of time management practices can be very helpful and should include the following:

1. Clarify objectives and goals in writing. Focus on objectives, not activities. Set at least one goal that can be reached on a daily basis.

2. Set time limits for each task. Do not become a victim of Parkinson's law that says work expands to fill the time available. Implement a "quiet time" for blocks of uninterrupted time to work on major projects. Be realistic. Avoid overcommitting yourself. Learn how to say no.

3. Eliminate needless paperwork. Reduce the flow to your in-basket. Keep your desk clear of unnecessary paperwork by using the desk as a *temporary stopover*. Handle paperwork only once, decide if it should be filed or discarded.

4. Reduce telephone time. Make notes of essentials to cover before placing the call. Have your secretary obtain information on the nature of the calls

received while you are out of the office. When the call is returned, all files with necessary data can be available, thus eliminating additional calls.

5. Reduce interruption time. Set a certain time for appointments. For walk-ins, confer standing up; to sit down invites extended conversations.

6. Delegate. Give more of your own work to your secretary. Upgrade the job classification, if necessary. Assign tasks to subordinates with deadlines. Allow subordinate freedom to complete task independently without constant supervision. Make note of completion date on the calendar and follow up.

7. Conquer procrastination. Concentrate on priorities. Finish what you start. It is better to complete one project than to work on three or four and not complete any of them.

Evaluating the Effective Use of Time

The final step in organizing time is evaluation. The following processes are helpful in this phase.

1. Reflect on time usage. Use the last 15 minutes of the day to determine whether objectives and goals have been met.
2. Continually update priorities. Review at regular intervals, readjust, and make changes as necessary.

Program Evaluation and Review Technique

Time management is especially important in completing major projects that may appear difficult, complex, and ambiguous. The long-term effort required to complete such projects can be productive, if organized, carefully planned, and executed. One approach to time management that can be beneficial in completing major projects is the use of a Program Evaluation and Review Technique (PERT) network. PERT is a diagrammatic representation of a pattern of work assignments, consisting of activities and events (Anderholm, Gaertner, & Milani 1981). The PERT network is designed to allow the planner to organize and arrange the sequences of the subtasks in such a way that the project's final time limitations and constraints are met. PERT is also known as Critical Path Analysis (CPA), Critical Path Method (CPM), and Critical Path Planning (CPP). When time is chosen, the network analysis is referred to as PERT-time, and when cost is chosen, the network is referred to as PERT-cost (Taylor & Walting 1973).

The development of PERT is attributed to the U.S. Navy Special Projects Office. It was successfully used to develop the Polaris missile system. It is widely used in business management and government today.

In the following example, PERT is used to indicate PERT-time in terms of weeks required to plan a dietetic internship program.

Minisystem Task Analysis and Flowchart

A task analysis is recommended for all activities involved in the project. The minisystem task analysis permits one to *think through* all possible functions, elements, and components required for getting the work done for a single activity. For example, if the task were to formulate an advisory committee, functions might include the following:

Functions:

Determining type of input needed.
Determine optimum number of advisors.
Determine duties and responsibilities.
Listing first and alternate choices of advisors.
Submitting invitations to first choice.

Submit alternate if first choice declines.
Acknowledge positive responses.
Formulate committee.
Inform advisors of first meeting.

Elements and components might include:

Division faculty   Chalkboard
Place for meeting   Chalk
Chairs   Overhead projector
Desks, tables   Paper, (pads)
Printed hand outs   Pencils

After all activities and events have been identified, it is necessary to establish a time sequence (Fig. 8-1). PERT has proved to be an invaluable tool in the analysis of time, one of our most critical resources.

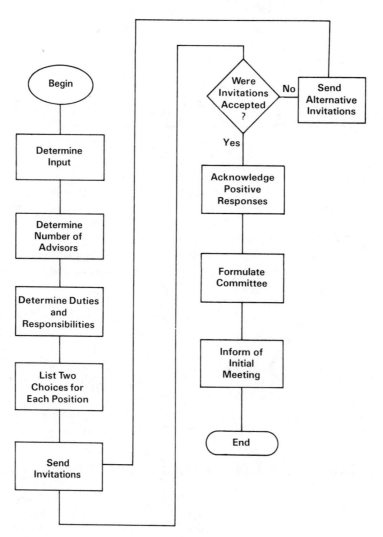

Figure 8-1. Flowchart for activity.

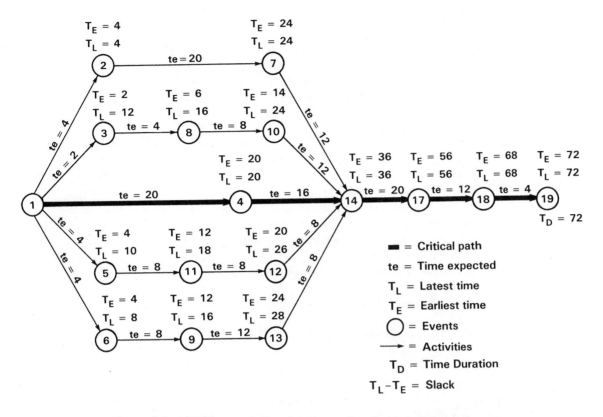

Figure 8-2. PERT network for planning a dietetic internship program.

PERT Network

The network diagram, as shown in Figure 8-2, represents the activities and events involved. An activity indicates work and is represented by an arrow. The length of the arrow has no significant meaning in the network; the main function is to indicate interrelationships and sequence of events. The events indicate accomplishments as a result of work or activity and are represented by a circle.

The critical path is the longest time path from the initial event and is determined by totaling the individual expected completion times (te). In the network, events 1–4–14–17–18–19 depict the critical path. $T\hat{E}$ represents the earliest time for completion of an event; $T\hat{L}$ represents the latest allowable completion time for an activity. To determine the amount of slack time for an event, subtract the event's earliest time from its latest time. In this PERT network, event number 14 is a critical point because all preceding events must be completed before the project can continue.

Gantt Chart

The Gantt chart is used to supplement the PERT network because graphically it illustrates when to begin each activity. It reflects the time element depicted in the PERT network in such a manner that the overlapping of activities can be readily viewed. For example, in the PERT network, activity 1→3 has a te = 2, but it does not tell when to start work on the activity.

Activities indicated on the Gantt chart (Fig. 8-3) are as follows:

1–2   Obtain program support (nonfinancial).
1–3   Develop program philosophy, objectives, goals.
1–4   Select internship program director.
1–5   Organize department to reflect internship program.
1–6   Formulate advisory committee.
2–7   Develop curriculum.
3–8   Designate clinical sites within hospital; select outside clinical sites.
4–14   Conduct clinical staff development.
5–11   Recruit and select additional clinical staff, if necessary.
6–9   Recruit and select clerical staff.
7–14   Purchase equipment and supplies.
8–10   Evaluate on-site and outside clinical facilities.
9–13   Determine criteria for program evaluation.
10–14   Formulate contracts with outside clinical facilities.
11–12   Develop clinical components.
12–14   Develop course outlines.
13–14   Plan for student services.
14–17   Apply for accreditation.
17–18   Select students.
18–19   Implement program.

PERT, used for planning comprehensive programs such as an internship program, offers the following advantages: (1) It permits participants to analyze all activities; (2) it serves to reduce the possibility of bottlenecks involved in massive organizational change, and (3) expedites the expenditure of time and energy on the part of the planning team during implementation.

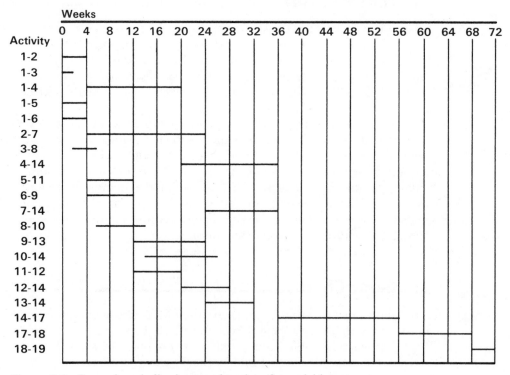

Figure 8-3. Gantt chart indicating starting time for activities.

References

Anderholm, F., Gaertner, J., and Milani, K. (1981). The Utilization of PERT in the Preparation of Marketing Budgets. *Managerial Planning 30*(1), 18–23.

Ashkenas, R. N., and Schaffer, R. H. (1982). Managers Can Avoid Wasting Time. *Harvard Bus. Rev. 60,* 98–104.

Bureau of Business Practice. (1974). *Dynamic Supervision in the Hospital: Solving Your Time Problems.* (Pamphlet No. 244, April 25). Waterford, CT: BBP. Bureau of Business Practice.

Douglass, M., and Douglass, D. (1982). It's About Time: Successful Time Habits. *Personnel Adminis. 27*(6), 19.

Ferderber, C. J. (1981). 10 Techniques for Managing Your Time More Effectively. *Practical Accountant 14*(8), 67–69.

Steffen, R. J. (1982). How to Stop Wasting Time. *Supervis. Mgt. 27*(5), 22–25.

Taylor, W. J., and Walting, T. F. (1973). *Practical Project Management.* New York: Wiley.

PART 2

FOODSERVICE SUBSYSTEMS

Chapter 9

Subsystem for Menu Planning

Menu planning is one of the most important parts of the foodservice systems. The menu dictates the need for and the utilization of other resources within the system. When the menu is viewed as the *hub* of the system, the concepts of dependency and interdependency can be readily visualized. If this conceptual view is accepted, the menu should be planned first; then consideration should be given to other subsystems, based on menu requirements.

The menu should reflect the philosophy, objectives, and goals of the organization since the menu represents and serves as a communication link with the larger environment. With this approach, it is expected that necessary resources (budget allocations for personnel, equipment, materials, and supplies) will be provided to meet stated objectives.

Menu Considerations

A basic objective of menu planning may be to serve nutritious, appetizing, and attractive food to meet the needs of patients and personnel. To this objective may be added the proviso *within budgetary allowances*. In order to meet this basic objective, the menu planner must have a knowledge of (1) the population to be served, which includes eating habits and resulting food preferences; (2) the nutritional needs of individuals and groups; and (3) a knowledge of a wide variety of foods, acceptable combinations, preparation, and service techniques.

Food Preferences

Food preferences are based on long-standing and traditional eating habits. When the patient enters the medical facility, he or she brings a group of traditional patterns of eating. Since food acceptance is important if the consumption of food is to meet therapeutic needs, an understanding of and a respect for diverse eating habits are major considerations. Traditional food preferences may be based on ethnic, cultural, regional, and/or environmental factors. Therefore, the menu planner needs to be sensitive to the reality that humans are omnivorous, capable of eating everything from sheep's eyes to old eggs. This sensitivity will make individuals aware of their own taboos as related to food (Gibson 1981). Personal preferences should not be the criteria for menu planning, nor should one attempt to apply the *melting pot* theory. Tables 9-1 to 9-9 depict some of the ethnic and culturally diverse eating habits of groups who may be part of the population served by a hospital foodservice.

Ethnic and cultural groups use a variety of ways to view foods in terms of what is appropriate to eat at mealtime, as between-meal snacks, on special occasions, and for various stages of growth, illness, and health.

In China food preferences vary, depending on the geographical location:

northern and western region (N), central region (C), and southern region (S). The styles of cooking are related to regional differences and are known as Mandarin (north), Shanghai (central), and Cantonese (south). A Chinese food pattern is given in Table 9-1. The eating habits are influenced by two main principles: (1) Fan-Ts'ai and (2) Yin-Yang. The *Fan-Ts'ai Principle* refers to the belief that the meal must be balanced with appropriate amounts of fan-ts'ai foods. Fan includes rice, wheat, millet, corn, flour, and noodles. Ts'ai includes any combination of meat and vegetables cooked in a variety of ways (boiled, steamed, stir-fried). The fan portion of the meal is considered indispensable and one cannot be full without it. The *Yin-Yang Principle* refers to the belief that there should be a balance of yin (hot) and yang (cold) foods. Fatty meats, fried, hot flavored, and oily plant foods are classified as yin. Yang foods include most water plants, crustaceans, and certain beans (mung). The classification is unrelated to temperature; it is based on beliefs of how food reacts within the body, and that an imbalance will result in improper bodily functions. This *hot–cold dichotomy* is widespread (Kirk & Eliason 1982). This principle is similar to practices observed by other Asian and Latin American groups. An Italian food pattern is presented in Table 9-2 and a Japanese food pattern in Table 9-3.

The Jewish food pattern (Table 9-4) encompasses religious considerations. The practice of *Kashruth*, the Jewish Dietary Laws, is observed in varying degrees by members of the Jewish faith. The three major religious groups are Orthodox, Conservative, and Reform. Orthodox Jews strictly observe the Dietary Laws by observing the Sabbath as a complete day of rest, study, and prayer. Conservative Jews are less strict in their observance of the Dietary Laws and believe that the Bible may be interpreted in many ways. Reform Jews consider the teachings of Judaism more important than the ritual; however, they do celebrate holidays as well as the Sabbath.

Milk and/or dairy products (milchig) and meat products (fleishig) may not

Table 9-1. Chinese Food Pattern[a]

Food Group	Characteristics of Food Habits
Milk	Limited use of milk or milk products. Cheese is rarely used except for a product made from goat or cow's milk which is eaten in Northern China.
Meat	Pork, fish, eggs, chicken, and shellfish are used in limited amounts, usually in mixed dishes.
Vegetables and Fruits	Widely used are spinach, broccoli, leeks, various greens, bok choy, carrots, pumpkins, mushrooms, sweet potatoes, soybeans, watercress, brussels sprouts, turnip, radish. Fruits are considered a delicacy. Regional additions: N[b]—corn, persimmon, peaches, pears, and large dates. C[c]—kohlrabi, white eggplant, apples, figs, winter melons. S[d]—yautia, eggplant, bamboo shoots, snowpeas, bananas, mango, tangerines, papaya, pineapple, orange, litchee nuts, figs, and small dates.
Bread and Cereal	Wheat products are preferred in northern region, including noodles, steamed bread. Millet and rice are used less extensively. Rice is the predominant product in the central region. In southern China, rice, rice flour, and *sticky* rice are used extensively.
Miscellaneous	Sweets include sugar, molasses, brown sugar, and preserves. Seasonings include salt, ginger, garlic, scallion, parsley, red and green pepper, sugar, and vinegar. The most highly seasoned foods are eaten in the northern region.

[a]Adapted from American Dietetic Association (1969), and Sanjur (1982).
[b]N—Northern and western region.
[c]C—Central region.
[d]S—Southern region.

Table 9-2. Italian Food Pattern[a]

Food Group	Characteristics of Food Habits
Milk	Consumption is limited by adults, except in coffee. Children may not consume recommended amounts. Cheese is eaten frequently and is used to prepare various dishes. Imported varieties are preferred, however, domestic types are used to a great extent.
Meat	A variety of meats are used, including veal, beef, pork, and chicken. Only small amounts of meat may be used in many dishes—often fried. Highly seasoned meats such as sausage and salami are used, as well as organ meats (liver, tripe, heart, and lungs). All kinds of seafood are eaten, including fresh, canned (sardines, anchovies, tuna), and dried. Fish is often fried in oil or used in stews or chowder. Eggs are widely used in omelets and other prepared dishes. A variety of dried beans and peas are used in soups, stews, with pasta, and in salads.
Vegetables and Fruits	Both cooked and raw green vegetables are used extensively. Escarole, Swiss chard, mustard greens, dandelion greens, and broccoli are very popular. Salads are eaten at most meals. Green vegetables are frequently boiled, then cooked in oil. Peppers and tomatoes are included in many of the prepared dishes. Pasta is preferred to potatoes. Eggplant and zucchini are favorite vegetables, as well as artichoke, mushrooms, and fava beans. All kinds of fruits are liked. Grapes, figs, and tangerines are favorites. Persimmons and pomegranates are holiday favorites, often served raw for dessert.
Bread and Cereal	Pasta is considered a staple food in the diet. Cornmeal (polenta) as well as rice are used in northern Italy. Italian bread is preferred and is usually eaten at each meal. Stale and day-old breads are used in prepared dishes. The consumption of whole grain and enriched cereals has increased.
Miscellaneous	Olive oil is preferred for cooking. Lard and salt pork may also be used in cooking. Butter is preferred for baking. Olives are well liked. Food may be highly seasoned. Cakes, pastries, and frozen delicacies are often used on festive occasions.

[a]Adapted from American Dietetic Association (1969).

Table 9-3. Japanese Food Pattern[a]

Food Group	Characteristics of Food Habits
Milk	Milk is used in small to moderate amounts. Tea is the most popular beverage. Milk is added to coffee and consumed in desserts such as ice cream. Cheese is used in small amounts.
Meat	An excellent variety of fresh fish is eaten as broiled, baked, boiled, and in soups. Raw fish is consumed occasionally. Smoked, dried, and canned fish are also eaten. Beef, pork, and poultry are preferred to lamb and veal. The main dish is often a combination of meat and vegetables, with soy sauce. Eggs are frequently eaten. Limited amount of beans and peas are consumed.
Vegetables and Fruits	An excellent variety of vegetables is eaten. Commonly used vegetables such as spinach, eggplant, peppers, broccoli, carrots, tomatoes, peas, cauliflower, and squash may be eaten separately or prepared with meat, poultry, or fish. Large variety of fresh fruit is consumed, especially oranges, tangerines, grapefruit, apples, pears, and melon.
Bread and Cereal	Polished rice is a staple food in the dietary pattern. The short grain, stick variety is preferred. Wheat products are consumed in breads and cereals.
Miscellaneous	Limited use of butter. Fat is used for deep-fat frying of fish, shellfish and vegetables (cooking method known as tempura). Simple cakes and cookies made from sugar and rice flour are eaten. Soy sauce is used in almost all dishes, including soups, meat, poultry, seafood, and vegetables. Pickles in great variety are used.

[a]Adapted from American Dietetic Association (1969).

Table 9-4. Jewish Food Pattern[a]

Food Group	Characteristics of Food Habits
Milk	Six hours must elapse after a meal before dairy foods may be eaten; half an hour must elapse after eating a dairy food before food may be eaten. Consumption may be adequate if used at both the breakfast and dairy meal. Cheese, such as American, Muenster, and Swiss, is well liked. Cottage cheese is eaten plain or in blintzes and noodle puddings.
	Low sodium milk from L. K. Baker and Co., Columbus, Ohio, may be used. Featherweight low sodium milk and Lonolac are also approved products.
Meat	Acceptable meat includes the flesh of all quadrupeds with a cloven hoof that chew cud such as cattle, sheep, goat, and deer. Orthodox Jews use only the forequarters (rib section forward).
	Meat of beef, lamb, goat, deer, chicken, turkey, goose, pheasant, and duck, is allowed. Liver and tongue are used liberally.
	Fish with fins and scales (fresh and as gefilte fish); smoked; lox (salmon); and caviar are eaten. Shellfish and scavenger fish such as sturgeon and catfish are not allowed.
	Eggs are eaten in abundance. An egg with a clot of blood must be discarded.
	Dried beans, peas, lentils are eaten, especially as soup.
Vegetables and Fruits	All fruits and vegetables may be used. Popular greens include spinach or sorrel leaves (used for schav, a popular soup), broccoli, and chicory. Carrots, sweet potatoes, green peppers are well liked. Green cabbage is often stuffed with ground beef and raisin mixture with tomato sauce. Fresh and canned tomatoes are used extensively. Root vegetables and potatoes are liberally used. Potato pancakes (latkes) and potato pudding prepared with egg are popular; as well as noodle pudding. Beets are used in soup (borscht).
	Orange or grapefruit or their juices are usually served for breakfast. Fresh or stewed fruits are often eaten as dessert with the meat meal.
Bread and Cereal	Bagel, rye bread, and pumpernickel are often used, as these do not have milk or milk solids and therefore can be eaten with meat or dairy meals. They are considered *pareve*. Matzoth is also considered *pareve* and is the only bread product allowed during Passover. Whole grains such as oatmeal, brown rice, buckwheat groats (kasha) are used.
	Ready baked products must have (U) or (K) certification (see under miscellaneous). Cooked cereals must be instant packets.
Miscellaneous	Sweet (unsalted) butter, usually whipped, is preferred to salted butter. Vegetable oils and shortenings are considered *pareve*. Fat of chicken is used to brown meat and fry potato pancakes.
	Danish pastries, coffee cakes, homemade cakes and cookies may be eaten in large quantities. Honey cakes are served for various holidays.
	Relishes such as pickled cucumbers and tomatoes, horseradish, and condiments are popular.
	Soup may be consumed at every meal. Chicken noodle and chicken rice soups are popular.
	Soft drinks are served with meat meals when milk beverages are forbidden.
	The following supplemental food products are approved for use: Sustagen, Sustacal, Ensure, Isomil, Vivonex 1000, Controlyte, Formula I, Meritene, Paygel–P, Nutramigen, Prosoybee, Isocal, and the fruit flavors of Precision LR, Flexical, and W–T Residue.
	Symbols used to indicate rabbinical supervision and certification are
	U The Union of Orthodox Jewish Congregations of America. Used for canned, boxed & bottled products
	VH or IVI Vaad Harabonim of Boston
	K Organized Kashrus Laboratories, not accepted by all observant Jews as rabbinical authority
	MK Montreal Vaad Ha-ir
	C.O.R. Council of Orthodox Rabbis of Toronto

[a]Adapted from American Dietetic Association (1969); Natow and Heslin (1982); Meador and Montalbano (1982).

Table 9-5. Muslim Food Pattern[a]

Food Group	Characteristics of Food Habits
Milk	Milk is encouraged and used extensively. Cream cheese is recommended. Aged cheese is prohibited.
Meat	Beef and lamb in limited amounts. Lamb is preferred. Young pigeons are allowed. Do not eat birds that are permitted to fly around and search for its own food. No ground meat allowed unless grinding process is observed. Chicken allowed if raised under controlled conditions. No wild game, except young pigeon. No pork or pork products allowed. Fish is allowed and should weigh less than 10 pounds. No halibut, carp, tuna, or scavenger seafood such as eel, catfish, oysters, crabs, clams, snails, and shrimp. No turtle or frog legs allowed. Portuguese sardines are recommended.
Vegetables and Fruits	Most green leafy vegetables are encouraged, except collards, turnip greens, kale, and green leaves of cabbage. Turnip roots, cabbage (white head only) and cauliflower are preferred. Rutabaga and spinach should be eaten sparingly. White potatoes and rice eaten only in cold climates. No sweet potatoes allowed. Fresh vegetables preferred to processed. Small navy beans allowed. Avoid use of all other types of beans, including soy or soy products. All fruits allowed and eaten extensively. Only sun-dried grapes allowed. Raw fruit is encouraged.
Bread and Cereal	Rye and whole wheat breads preferred (thoroughly cooked). Stale bread is better than fresh. No white flour or corn bread.
Miscellaneous	Butter is preferred to margarine. Vegetable oil is used (no soy). No fried foods. Brown sugar preferred. No white sugar. Bean pie (using navy beans) is a popular dessert. No nuts. Eat only one meal a day. No between meal snacks.

[a] Adapted from Muhammad (1967).

be prepared, cooked, or eaten together. Pareve (neutral) foods include eggs, vegetables, fruits, grains, and fish with scales and fins. Pareve foods may be eaten with either milchig or fleshig products.

Another group, the Muslims (Table 9-5), are also guided by religious considerations. The dietary pattern of the Muslims is based on the teachings of the Holy Quran. Strict guidelines on what to eat, as well as on the number of meals per day, are practiced by those observing the Muslim faith.

The Polish food pattern (Table 9-6) and the Puerto Rican food pattern (Table 9-7) are two more ethnic patterns that are important for today's medical foodservice director.

Regional differences also occur. The southern meal plan in Table 9-8 refers primarily to families living in rural areas. The food patterns of contemporary southern families living in an urban setting may be quite different. The differences may be attributed to changes in socioeconomic status and the degree of acculturation to urban living. The heavy meal is usually served midday (dinner); a lighter meal (supper) is served in the evening. Many of the foods listed can be classified by the more recent term "soul food." Soul food restaurants are popular eating places for those who have migrated to northern cities.

The southwestern part of the United States is a mixture of several cultural backgrounds. The food pattern given in Table 9-9 refers to the Spanish or Mexican cultures, although the Native American food pattern is similar.

Table 9-6. Polish Food Pattern[a]

Food Group	Characteristics of Food Habits
Milk	Children drink fresh milk; buttermilk is preferred by adults. Sour cream is used extensively in soups, salad dressings, with berries, and raw vegetables. Cheese is well liked.
Meat	Beef and pork are the most popular meats. Pigs' knuckles, sausage, smoked and cured pork, as well as chicken, goose, duck, and variety meats (liver, tripe, brains, tongue) are well liked. Fish—fresh, smoked, dried or pickled is used. Eggs are well liked and used in a variety of dishes (pancakes, noodles, dumplings, and soups). Legumes are used in soups. Cottage cheese is well liked and often served with sour cream.
Vegetables and Fruits	Potatoes are an important part of the Polish diet and are used in soups, stews, pancakes, and dumplings. Other favorites include carrots, beets, turnips, cauliflower, kohlrabi, peas, broccoli, sorrel, green pepper, spinach, and green beans. Citrus fruits used more liberally than in previous years.
Bread and Cereal	Bread eaten at most meals. Pumpernickel, sour rye, and white bread are well liked. Sweet buns are also popular. Oatmeal, rice, noodles, dumplings, cornmeal, porridge, and kasha are prominent in the diet.
Miscellaneous	A variety of fats and oils is used. Candy, sweet cakes, and honey are favorites. Coffee with cream and sugar is favorite beverage. Limited use of tea. Foods may be highly seasoned, especially with salt.

[a]Adapted from American Dietetic Association (1969).

Table 9-7. Puerto Rican Food Pattern[a]

Food Group	Characteristics of Food Habits
Milk	Milk is consumed more in cooking than as a beverage. Cereals are frequently cooked in milk. A cup of café con leche may contain 2–5 ounces of milk. Chocolate and cocoa are made with milk. Limited use of American cheese. Native white cheese (similar to farmer cheese, but firmer and saltier), is used.
Meat	Chicken and pork are eaten frequently, often in combination with other foods. Pork and beef are usually fried. Ham butts and sausage are used to flavor different dishes. Chitterlings are eaten fried (cuchifritos) or stewed with native vegetables (salcocho) and chick peas. Cod, tuna, salmon, and sardines are common fish choices. Crabmeat is a favorite. Fried and scrambled eggs are popular. Beans are eaten almost every day, often with rice. Pigeon and chick peas are popular. Red kidney beans are the preferred legume.
Vegetables and Fruits	Imported vegetables such as yautia (starchy root), apio, malanga, name (white yam), and plantain are used frequently. Pumpkin (used to thicken and flavor food), carrots, green pepper, tomatoes, sweet potatoes, cabbage, and onions are well liked. Lettuce is believed to be very nourishing. Potatoes are eaten in small amounts in stews, soups, or fried. Imported fruits are used often, especially acerola (the highest known food source of ascorbic acid). Oranges, bananas, and fresh pineapple are popular. Fruit cocktail, canned pears, and peaches are well liked. Peach, apricot, and pear nectar are commonly used.
Bread and Cereal	French bread, rolls, and crackers are the most frequent choices. Plantain is often eaten in place of bread. Breakfast cereals such as cornmeal, cornflakes, farina, and oatmeal are increasing in popularity. Cornmeal mush is popular.
Miscellaneous	Butter used in small amounts. Lard and salt pork used extensively. Olive oil is favorite on vegetables and salads. Sugar is liberally used in sweetening beverages and in prepared desserts. Black malt beer is a favorite beverage, often combined with beaten egg for convalescents and pregnant women. Canned soups, such as chicken and vegetables are often served as the main dish.

[a]Adapted from American Dietetic Association (1969), and Sanjur 1982.

Table 9-8. Southern United States Food Pattern[a]

Food Group	Charcteristics of Food Habits
Milk	Buttermilk is preferred. Fresh milk may be consumed in limited amounts. Cheese is well liked, especially aged cheese. Macaroni and cheese is a popular dish.
Meat	Chicken and pork are popular meats. Chicken is baked, stewed with dumplings, fried, and barbecued. Pigs' feet, hog jowls, ham hocks, cured ham and other variety meats (brains, liver, kidneys, and chitterlings) are eaten often. Chitterlings are steamed and served piping hot with seasoning and heat, or they may be steamed, breaded, and fried crisp. Beef is used, often as beef stew with vegetables. Cured tongue is also eaten. Fish (catfish and white buffalo) and shellfish are popular. Fried scallops, boiled shrimp, and fried, stewed, or raw oysters are popular in coastal areas. Rabbit, squirrel, opossum, and other small game are eaten. Eggs are usually fried. Black-eyed peas and beans, cooked with salt pork, are popular. Peanuts and peanut butter are consumed.
Vegetables and Fruits	Large amounts of leafy greens are consumed. Collards, turnip greens, mustard greens, green beans, and cabbage are cooked in water with bacon, ham hocks, or salt pork. The cooking liquid (pot liquor) may be eaten with cornbread. Tomatoes, fresh and canned, white and sweet potatoes are also favorites. Fruit is used; it may be eaten between meals rather than as part of a meal. Watermelon, cantaloupe, and lemonade are favorites in summer.
Bread and Cereal	Hominy grits with gravy, biscuits, polished rice with gravy, dumplings, pancakes, hoecakes, hush puppies, and cornbread are favorites.
Miscellaneous	Bacon and salt pork used in vegetables. Lard is used for frying. Butter is used for desserts. Gravies are used extensively. Sweets range from fried cookies and pies to layer cake—from soft gingerbread squares, skillet cake to pecan pies. Jams, jellies, and relishes are frequently eaten.

[a]Adapted from American Dietetic Association (1969); Jeffries (1969); Sanjur (1982).

Table 9-9. Spanish-Mexican American Food Pattern[a]

Food Group	Characteristics of Food Habits
Milk	Milk consumption may be limited. Limited amounts of cheese are used.
Meat	Chicken, pork chops, weiners, cold cuts, and hamburger are used predominantly but usually once or twice a week. Eggs are frequently used as fried, poached or scrambled with chili sauce and tortillas or as egg omelet. Beans are usually eaten with every meal, cooked, mashed, and refried with lard. Miscellaneous meats such as hog's head, tongue, tripe, brains, and kidney are well liked.
Vegetables and Fruits	Potatoes are a basic item, usually fried, and may be used three times a day. Chiles from green and red peppers are popular at each meal. Fresh tomatoes are purchased the year around and are a most popular vegetable. Occasionally canned tomatoes are used. Pumpkin, corn, greens, onions, green beans, green peas, squash, carrots, and chick peas (garbanzos) are frequently used. Bananas, melons, peaches, and canned fruit cocktail are the more popular fruits. Oranges and apples are used occasionally as snacks.
Bread and Cereal	Bread, purchased or homemade, is a popular item. Tortillas from enriched wheat flour are made daily. Sweet rolls are purchased. Breakfast cereal are usually the prepared type with emphasis on the sugar coated. Occasionally oatmeal is used.
Miscellaneous	Lard, salt pork, and bacon fat are used liberally. Most foods are fried. Soft drinks, popsicles, and sweet breads (pan dulce) or various kinds are used liberally.

[a]Adapted from American Dietetic Association (1969), and Sanjur (1982).

The *vegetarian diet* is gaining popularity and may require special attention by the menu planner. The diet can be divided into three categories (Endres & Rockwell 1980):

1. *Pure or strict vegetarian diet.* All foods of animal origin (meat, poultry, fish, eggs, and dairy products) are excluded from the diet. *Vegans* avoid one or more other food groups such as processed foods, cooked foods, legumes, cereals, grains, or fruits. *Fruitarians* limit food intake to raw and cooked fruits, nuts, honey, and oil.

2. *Lacto-vegetarian.* Meat, fish and eggs are excluded; however, dairy products and plant foods are permitted.

3. *Lacto-ovo-vegetarian.* The diet includes eggs, dairy products, and plant foods; meat, poultry, and fish are excluded.

With careful planning, basic nutrients can be provided in all categories except for the vegan and fruitarian patterns.

The effort expended to understand the patient profile can serve to maximize patient satisfaction. A knowledge of inhabitants for the geographical location is important. For example, Detroit, Michigan, has the largest Arabic-speaking population outside the Middle East; the largest concentration of Belgians, Chaldeans, and Maltese in the United States; and the second largest Polish population in the United States (Abonyi, Anderson, Horvath-Monnreal, & Travalini 1969).

___ Nutritional Adequacy _____

The nutritional adequacy of the menu is based on the general requirements as reported in publications such as the Recommended Dietary Allowances (RDA) (Food and Nutrition Board–National Research Council 1980), and the Daily Food Guide (U.S. Department of Agriculture 1980A). The RDA were first published in 1943 by a committee of the Food and Nutrition Board of the National Research Council, National Academy of Sciences.

Seventeen nutrient allowances are presented in quantitative units for 17 population groups based on age and sex; two groups (pregnancy and lactation) are based on conditions. (See Appendix Tables A-1 and A-2.)

The RDA, based on current nutrition research, is designed to provide nutritional maintenance for healthy persons in the United States. The RDA are not designed to assess individual nutritional needs, nor are they designed to meet abnormalities associated with various disease entities. For individual diet planning, requiring quantitative and qualitative nutrient modification, other tools are required. Since menu planning in an institutional setting is for a population group, the RDA serves as a frame of reference for meeting nutritional needs.

Daily food guides, as developed by the U.S. Department of Agriculture (1979, 1980A, 1980B) are recommended for the practical application of the RDA in group menu planning. The food guides, first developed in the 1920s, have evolved from the *Basic Four,* the *Basic Seven,* and currently to the *Five Food Groups.* According to Kinder and Green (1978), the *Basic Seven* is considered one of the better guides for menu planning because it puts emphasis on the consumption of fruits and vegetables. The most recent daily food groups are presented in Figures 9-1 to 9-5. It should be evident that there is a wide variation in the nutrient content of foods within a certain group. Therefore, it is wise to vary the kinds of food eaten within a group in order to ensure an adequate intake of all nutrients.

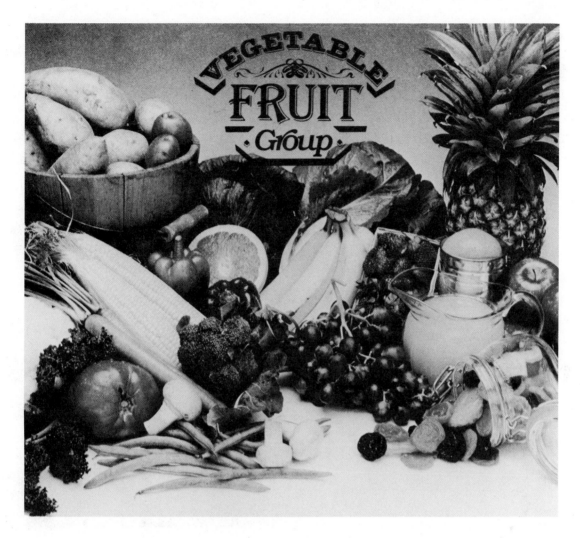

Figure 9-1. Food Group I—Vegetable and fruit.

After menus are planned, using Basic Four guidelines, they should be analyzed for nutritional adequacy and compared with Recommended Dietary Allowances (RDA). The menu shown in Table 9-10 was analyzed and compared to RDAs for 25- to 50-year-old males. The caloric level is 3% below the recommended range. The percentages by calorie are protein, 16%; carbohydrate, 48%; and fat, 38%. All nutrients exceed Recommended Dietary Allowances.

The menu was also compared with dietary guidelines published by the American Heart Association (AHA). The AHA guidelines (1988) are as follows:

1. Total fat should be less than 30% of calories.
2. Saturated fat should be less than 10% of calories.
3. Polyunsaturated fat should not exceed 10% of calories.
4. Cholesterol should not exceed 300 g/day.
5. Carbohydrate should constitute 50% or more of calories, with emphasis on complex carbohydrates.
6. Protein should provide the remainder of calories.
7. Sodium should not exceed 3 mg/day.

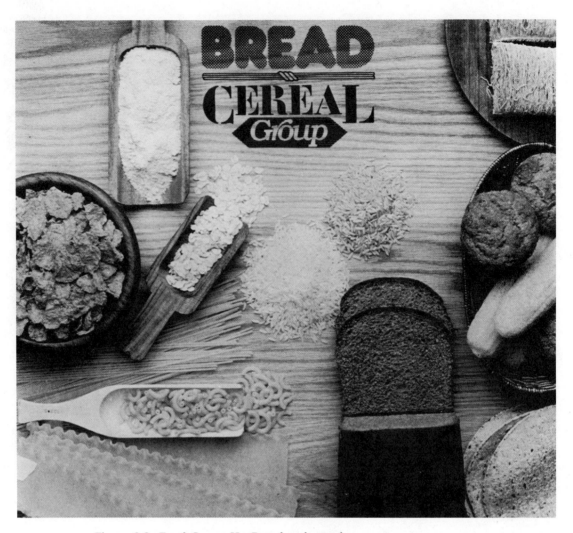

Figure 9-2. Food Group II—Bread and cereal.

8. Total calories should be adjusted to maintain recommended body weight.
9. Intake should include a wide variety of food.

The AHA comparison revealed that the menu is excessive in total fat by 8%, saturated fat by 4%, cholesterol by 220 mg, and sodium by 0.89 g. Polyunsaturated fat, protein, and carbohydrate were below recommended guidelines. Suggestions to correct nutrient and calorie imbalance are as follows:

1. To reduce saturated fat, change milk to 0.5% fat; use part of the milk in coffee and eliminate cream; remove skin from chicken before cooking; and check salad dressings to make sure polyunsaturated fats are used.
2. To increase calories, carbohydrate, and protein, increase carbohydrate such as grain and vegetables.
3. To reduce sodium, reduce milk to two servings per day; eliminate cream; and use salt-free crackers.

Knowledge of Food

Menu planning need not be limited to the imagination of the menu planner. Suggestions from a number of sources can serve the planner in using a wide

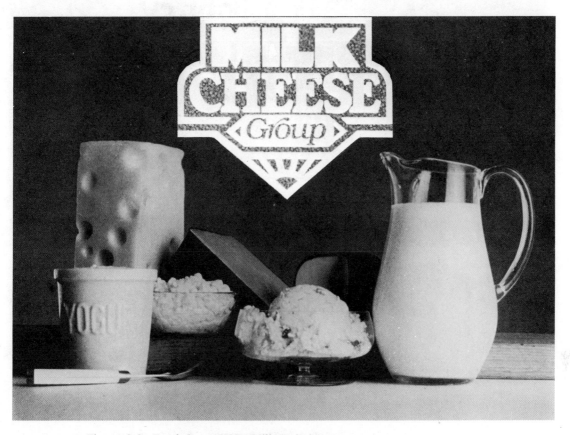

Figure 9-3. Food Group III—Milk and cheese.

variety of food choices. It is important to keep in mind that the process of menu planning is more involved than merely listing food as if one were making out a food purchasing list. The menu suggestions offered here reflect the distinction between the two processes. For example, *Braised Beef Cubes with Mushrooms* is a much more enticing menu item than simply Beef Cubes. As presented in Table 9-11, different menu names are offered in six categories. For maximum use of the menu suggestions, one may add or delete food items depending on client preferences, budgetary allowances, or other pertinent factors of menu planning.

Budgetary Allowances

In most instances the menu planner is given a prescribed budgetary allowance and must be able to provide nutritious, appetizing, and attractive meals within those allowances. In order to accomplish this task, the planner must know the cost of each food item placed on the menu, as well as the percentage of the food cost dollar allocated for each food category. (See Tables 15-1 and 15-2 for examples of food cost allowances and food category cost allowances.) When using precosted menus, it is necessary to update cost figures as often as significant price changes occur.

Equipment Needs

Equipment is one of the resources that should be available according to the planned menu. Frequently, the menu is planned around the equipment that has already been selected. In the latter instance, the menu planner must be aware of

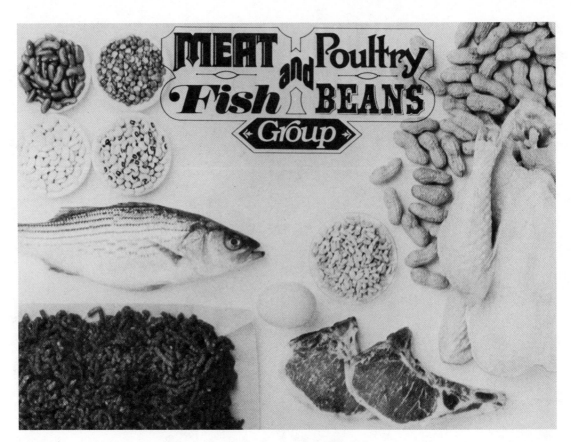

Figure 9-4. Food Group IV—Meat, poultry, fish, and beans.

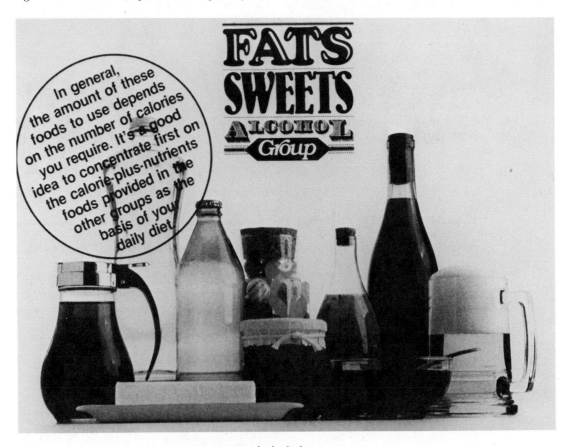

Figure 9-5. Food Group V—Fats, sweets, and alcohol.

Table 9-10. Sample Nutritional Analysis of One Day's Menu

Portion	Weight	Menu
½ cup	123 g	Chilled Orange Juice
½ cup	120 g	Oatmeal
1	50 g	Poached Egg on
1 slice	25 g	Whole Wheat Toast
1 tsp	5 g	Margarine
1 cup	245 g	Low Fat Milk
1 cup	240 g	Coffee
1 pkg.	6 g	Sugar
1 Tbsp	15 g	Light Cream
1 cup	250 g	Tomato Soup
4	11 g	with Crackers
¼	88 g	Baked Chicken
½ cup	87 g	Steamed Rice
½ cup	92 g	Broccoli
1 oz	33 g	Cranberry Sauce
1 cup		Tossed Salad, with
	34 g	Lettuce
	67 g	Tomato
	18 g	Green Pepper
	20 g	Onion
1 tsp	5 g	Margarine
1	50 g	Hard Roll
3-in square	63 g	Gingerbread
1 cup	245 g	Low Fat Milk
1 cup	240 g	Coffee
1 pkg	6 g	Sugar
1 Tbsp	15 g	Light Cream
1 Tbsp	15 g	Italian Dressing
½ cup	124 g	Apple Juice
3 oz	85 g	Braised Beef Cubes with
	8 g	Mushrooms
½ cup	80 g	Noodles
½ cup	91 g	Mixed Vegetables
⅛	17 g	Lettuce Wedge
1 Tbsp	16 g	French Dressing
1 slice	25 g	Whole Wheat Bread
1 tsp	5 g	Margarine
1 cup	245 g	Low Fat Milk
1 cup	240 g	Coffee
1 pkg	6 g	Sugar
1 Tbsp	15 g	Light Cream
½ cup	128 g	Cling Peaches

Nutritive Components

Calories	2633 cal	(97%)	Cholesterol	520	mg
Protein	107.8 g	(192%)	Carbohydrate	313.1	g
Calcium	1498.5 mg	(187%)	Potassium	3961	mg
Phosphorus	1956.1 mg	(244%)	Sodium	3868.7	mg
Iron	15.8 mg	(158%)	Fat	111.6	g
Vitamin A	12434.7 IU	(248%)	Saturated Fat	41.0	g
Thiamin	1.64 mg	(117%)	Oleic Fat	36.4	g
Riboflavin	2.76 mg	(172%)	Linoleic Fat	17.5	g
Niacin	22.4 mg	(124%)	Weight	3260	g
Vitamin C	185.5 mg	(309%)	Water	2243	g

Percentages by Calories

Protein: 16%	Carbohydrate: 48%	Fat: 38%

Table 9-11. Descriptive Menu Suggestions

Menu Item	Description
Entrees	
Beef Stew	Savory Beef Stew with Vegetables
Roast Beef	Roast Sirloin of Beef au Jus
Fried Chicken	Country Fried Chicken with Cream Gravy
Broiled Whitefish	Broiled Whitefish with Lemon–Garlic Butter
Pork Chops	Stuffed Pork Chop au Vin
Tenderloin of Beef	Savory Beef Strips
Appetizers	
Fantail Shrimp	Feathery Shrimp Cocktail
Apple Juice	Chilled Apple Juice
Cantaloupe	Fresh Melon Balls
Orange Juice	Tangy Orange Juice
Prunes	Sun Ripened Prunes
Soups	
Mushroom Soup	Fancy Cream of Mushroom Soup
Pea Soup	Zesty Split Pea Soup
Vegetable Soup	Home Style Vegetable Soup
Minestrone Soup	Hasty Minestrone Soup
Broth	Golden Chicken Broth
Vegetables	
Cauliflower	Parslied Crisp Cauliflower
Carrots	Tangy Glazed Carrots
Broccoli	Chopped Broccoli Cuts
Mixed Vegetables	Mixed Vegetables Medley
White Potatoes	Boiled New Potatoes
Green Beans	Green Bean Amandine
Salads	
Lettuce–Spinach	Fresh Garden Salad
Cranberry Mold	Jellied Cranberry Salad
Lettuce Heart	Crispy Lettuce Hearts
Coleslaw	Creamy Coleslaw
Celery Sticks	Crunchy Celery Sticks
Desserts	
Baked Alaska	Flaming Baked Alaska
Brownies	Chewy Fudge Brownies
Applesauce Cake	Spiced Applesauce Cake
Peach Slices	Yellow Cling Peach Slices
Lemon Cake	Lemon Ice-box Cake
Peach Halves	Peaches en Gelee

preparation techniques in order not to overload certain pieces of equipment. For example, the menu should not consist of all food items requiring roasting if only one oven is available.

Personnel Needs

Personnel should be selected based on menu planning. When personnel are in place prior to menu planning, the planner must be aware of skills, employee limitations, and the number of employees available to produce planned menu items. Although in-service training, with emphasis on work simplification and use of standardized recipes, can reduce the burden and frustrations of production workers, there are limits to the amount of quality food that can be produced in a specified time period.

Purchasing System

The menu planner will need to consider the form in which food is purchased, such as the amount of built-in convenience, the availability of certain food items, the frequency of deliveries, and the storage capacity.

Production System

The type of production system may pose limitations on the menu should menu planning take place after the system has been decided upon. For the total-convenience production system, menu planning may be limited because of the unavailability of prepared food items. In the cook-chill and ready-serve systems there may be problems with certain food items not suitable for the required holding and rethermalizing processes. In the commissary system, problems may occur with attempts to maintain quality while transporting large quantities of prepared foods. Finally, the factor of time to meet culinary schedules may present problems in the conventional system where all food for each meal is prepared as needed.

Meal Patterns

Meal patterns vary from the most common type of three meals a day to four or five meals. Traditionally, patients receive three full meals daily with between-meal nourishments. In the four-meal plan, patients receive three full meals daily with a substantial night nourishment. The five-meal pattern (Table 9-12) consists of two full meals and three small meals. Regardless of the meal pattern used, there should not be more than 14 hours between the serving of the evening meal and the next substantial meal for patients who are on oral intake and do not have specific dietary requirements.

The five-meal pattern gained popularity during the early sixties. In this pattern, meals are usually scheduled to begin at about 6:00 A.M., with three meals spaced between the first and the last meal, which is served about 8:00 P.M. The nutritional composition of the five-meal pattern can be as adequate as the traditional three-meal pattern. However, considerably more thought in the planning process is required in order to ensure that nutrients are spread out over the total day's diet. The balancing of nutritional components is especially important in instances where the patient is a poor eater or simply refuses to eat all five meals. One should be careful to avoid the tendency to increase calories and neglect other nutrients, such as protein. The continental breakfast of sweet rolls and coffee or a small meal of juice and coffee are examples of incomplete meals. It is believed that nutrients are utilized more efficiently by the body if each meal contains a balance of protein, fats, and carbohydrates.

Menu Format

Establishing a menu format ensures that food from each of the five groups is included in the daily meal pattern. When the menu is planned, there must be at

Table 9-12. Sample Selective Menu for Five-Meal Feeding Pattern[a]

6:00 A.M.	9:30 A.M.	1:00 P.M.	4:30 P.M.	8:00 P.M.
Orange Juice Pineapple Juice[b] *Fresh Grapefruit*[c]	Orange Juice Apple Juice *Fresh Banana*	*Vegetable Soup* Tomato Juice	*Beef Noodle Soup* Fresh Fruit Cup	*Chicken Broth* Grapefruit Juice

Shredded Wheat
Cornflakes
Hot Oatmeal
 	
White Toast
Whole Wheat Toast
Raisin Toast
 	
Whole Milk
Skim Milk
Chocolate Milk
Buttermilk
	Crisp Bacon
	Broiled Sausage
	Grilled Ham
	Corned Beef Hash
	Eggs, any style
	
	Hotcakes with syrup
	French Toast with
	  Honey
	Blueberry Muffin
	White Toast
	Whole Wheat Toast
		Cottage Cheese and Fruit
		  Plate
		Assorted Cold Cuts w/
		  Potato Salad
		Tuna Stuffed Tomato
		  with Chips and Relishes
		Maurice Salad Bowl
		
		Fresh Fruit in Season
		Baked Custard
		Assorted Jello
			Grilled Cubed Steak
			Baked Pork Chop
			Roast Chicken Breast
			Broiled Halibut Steak
			Roast Leg of Lamb
			
			Buttered Mashed
			  Potatoes
			Baked Potato
			Buttered Rice
			
			Buttered Green Beans
			Buttered Carrots
			Buttered Broccoli
				Submarine Sandwich
				Corned Beef on Rye
				Ham & Swiss Cheese
				  Sandwich
				Assorted Cheese & Crackers
				
				Fresh Fruit in Season
				Assorted Ice Cream
				Sugar Cookie

Coffee Tea Sanka Cocoa			Tossed Vegetable Salad Creamy Coleslaw *Lettuce & Tomato Salad*	
Butter Cream Sugar Jelly Salt Pepper			Cheesecake with Strawberries *Apple Pie* Chocolate Fudge Cake	

[a] From Flood (1968).
[b] Condiments and beverages listed under 6:00 A.M. meal are available at other meals.
[c] Italicized words indicate specials of the day.

least one food item offered for each category specified. As shown in Table 9-13, the three-meal menu format may be simple or elaborate. Terminology used to designate the type of meal may be breakfast, dinner, and supper, or breakfast, lunch, and dinner. When the supper meal appears in the menu format, it is usually a lighter meal consisting of combination dishes, meat substitutes, or entrees with meat extenders. In the elaborate-menu format, the lunch and dinner meals have the same number of food categories.

Nonselective vs. Selective Menus

The *nonselective menu* offers only one food item in each category of the menu format, thereby offering no choice. In contrast, the *selective menu* offers at least two choices of food items for each category. A comparison of the two is given in Table 9-14. The nonselective menu is more often used in nursing homes and small acute care facilities. Arguments by those who continue to use the nonselective menu are as follows:

1. The nonselective menu is less costly because fewer food items are offered.
2. Additional personnel are not required for production of menu items.
3. It is easier to control food intake with a nonselective menu.
4. It is not left to chance that a patient will select a balanced diet.
5. Purchasing is simplified.
6. It is easier to control portions and service.

Although the list supporting a nonselective menu is impressive, it does not address issues of optimal patient care. Many of the arguments for a nonselective

Table 9-13. Comparison of Simple and Elaborate Menu Formats

Simple Menu Format	Elaborate Menu Format
Breakfast	*Breakfast*
Fruit or Juice	Fruit or Juice
Cereal or Egg	Cereal
Toast	Entree (egg, sausage, etc.)
Butter or Margarine	Bread (Pancakes, Muffins, Biscuits, Toast, etc.)
Milk/Beverage	Butter or Margarine
	Milk/Beverage
Dinner	*Lunch*
Entree (meat, fish, poultry)	Appetizer (soup, juice, etc.)
Potato or Substitute	Entree
Vegetable	Potato or Substitute
Salad	Vegetable
Bread	Salad
Butter or Margarine	Bread
Dessert	Butter or Margarine
Milk/Beverage	Dessert
	Milk/Beverage
Supper	*Dinner*
Appetizer (soup, juice, etc.)	Appetizer
Protein Main Dish	Entree
Vegetable or Salad	Potato or Substitute
Bread	Vegetable
Butter or Margarine	Salad
Dessert	Bread
Milk/Beverage	Butter or Margarine
	Dessert
	Milk/Beverage

Table 9-14. Comparison of Nonselective and Selective Menus

	Nonselective Menu	Selective Menu
Soup or Appetizer	Cream of Asparagus Soup	Cream of Asparagus Soup or Chilled Tomato Juice
Entree	Broiled Beef Liver with Sauteed Onions	Broiled Beef Liver with Sauteed Onions or Roast Chicken with Giblet Gravy
Potato or Substitute	Buttered Mashed Potatoes	Buttered Mashed Potatoes or Candied Sweet Potatoes
Vegetable	Buttered Green Peas	Buttered Green Peas or Steamed Fresh Cauliflower with Almond Butter
Salad	Crisp Lettuce Wedge	Crisp Lettuce Wedge or Molded Cranberry Relish Salad
Bread	Hot Bran Muffin	Hot Bran Muffin or Hot Cloverleaf Roll
Dessert	Lemon Meringue Pie	Lemon Meringue Pie or Chilled Watermelon

menu are related to employee convenience rather than patient satisfaction. Some of the advantages cited by those who have used the selective menu are as follows:

1. The selective menu is often less expensive because the menu can be balanced with less expensive food choices (such as the use of liver, as shown in Table 9-14) that may be desired by some individuals.
2. There is increased food acceptance since patients are able to make their own selections.
3. Selective menus can be used as a training tool to encourage proper eating habits.
4. There are fewer leftovers since preparation is based on selections.
5. There is less plate waste since patients will usually eat what they select.
6. There is no increase in the quantity of portions produced, only in the variety of food items.

Use of the selective menu requires close monitoring to ensure that patients are receiving a balanced diet. After food selections are made by the patient, the individual menu should be checked by a qualified person to make sure that minimum daily requirements are met.

Steps in Menu Planning

Menu planning, whether done on a weekly basis or for an extended period, is a time-consuming process. The individual responsible for this task must be skilled in both production and service, as well as have a knowledge of other menu factors, if a balanced menu is to be produced. Menu planning can be made easier when an established menu format is used along with a suggested list of food items that have proved to be acceptable by patients and personnel. The suggested order of writing the menu is as follows:

1. Plan the lunch and dinner entrees for the entire week or extended period of time. When the entree is planned first, one is able to build the rest of the meal around the main dish by selecting foods that will enhance the appeal and attractiveness of the total meal.
2. Plan the vegetable and potato categories to accompany the entree. Give consideration to variety in color, texture, flavor, form or shape, and consistency.
3. Plan salads to accompany rest of meal. Use fruit or vegetables, rather than high-protein foods such as egg, cheese, and seafood. Consider variety and avoid using foods that already appear on the menu.
4. Plan bread category. The use of at least one hot bread a day will add variety and appeal.
5. Plan appetizer. If soup is used, do not repeat items, such as chicken noodle soup along with baked chicken as the entree. If fruit or juice is used, it should be different from the salad or dessert category.
6. Plan a dessert to complement the meal. Do not repeat items in other categories. Seek variety in texture, temperature, and other factors that will add interest. Limit *empty-calorie* desserts as much as possible.
7. Plan the breakfast entree. Offer eggs at least four times during the week.
8. Plan fruit or juice for breakfast meal. Consider a good source of vitamin C.
9. Plan cereal category. For selective menu, plan one hot and one cold cereal.

10. Plan breakfast bread. In addition to toast, plan for a hot bread, pancakes, or French toast for added interest.
11. Beverages such as coffee, tea, and milk are standard items, as well as condiments.
12. Plan a bedtime nourishment if it is served on a daily basis for all patients.

Modified Diet Menu Planning

The menu for modified diets should be based on the regular menu. This practice should be used for a number of reasons:

1. Patients on modified diets are more likely to eat their food if they receive the same food as those on regular diets. The primary differences may be modification of calories, nutrients, texture, seasoning, and method of preparation. For example, when fried chicken is planned for the regular diet, the preparation technique may be modified to baked chicken for patients on calorie-restricted diets.
2. Frequently, patients in the same room may be on different diets. When patients realize that they are all eating the same basic foods, the meal is more acceptable.
3. To modify the menu in this manner serves as training for patients when they leave the medical facility. The patient is taught that emphasis is not on the purchasing of "special diet food," but merely on adjusting the preparation technique.
4. Purchasing for the department is simplified when most patients can eat the same basic foods.
5. Production is simplified. Cooks can simply subtract the number of modified servings from the regular menu and prepare according to respective diet modifications.

As shown in Table 9-15, this system results in minimizing the use of different foods. When planning the modified diet menu, the menu should not be cluttered with portions and amounts for individual diets. The menu should be used as a guide for planning individual diets. When planned individually, each patient's diet can be adjusted for quantity, quality, and patient preferences as appropriate for the particular diet. Individual tray cards or individual menu selection sheets can be used to individualize the menu for each patient.

The use of arrows to indicate foods allowed on modified diets is not recommended. The procedure may be convenient for the typist, but is too easy for cooks and others responsible for production and service to make errors when they must follow arrows across the page instead of reading the written word for each diet.

An approved diet manual should be used as a basis for planning all modified diets. Depending on the nature of care, such as a nursing facility or an acute care facility, the manual may range from simplified (Iowa Dietetic Association 1984) to comprehensive (The American Dietetic Association 1988). According to the Joint Commission on Accreditation of Hospitals (1988), a qualified dietitian must develop or adopt a diet manual in cooperation with medical staff and other appropriate dietetic staff. The manual must meet standards for nutritional care in accordance with those of the Recommended Dietary Allowances (see Appendix Table A-1); must specify nutritional deficiencies; serve as a guide for ordering diets; be reviewed and revised as necessary; and be accessible for use in each patient care unit. In the states of Iowa and Texas, diet manuals

Table 9-15. Modified Diet Menu

Regular	Restricted Calorie	Restricted Fat	Restricted Fiber	Restricted Sodium	Full Liquid
Orange Juice	Unsweetened Orange Juice	Orange Juice	Orange Juice	Orange Juice	Orange Juice
Cream of Wheat	Cream of Wheat	Cream of Wheat	Cream of Wheat	SF Cream of Wheat	Cream of Wheat Gruel
Scrambled Eggs	FF[a] Scrambled Eggs	FF Scrambled Eggs	Scrambled Eggs	SF[b] Scrambled Eggs	
Buttered Toast	Dry Toast	Dry Toast	Buttered Toast	SF Toast	
Whole Milk	Skim Milk	Skim Milk	Whole Milk	Whole Milk	Whole Milk
Coffee/Tea	Coffee/Tea	Coffee/Tea	Coffee/Tea	Coffee/Tea	Coffee/Tea
Vegetable Soup	Vegetable Soup	FF Broth	Cream of Tomato	SF Vegetable Soup	Cream of Tomato Soup
Baked Honey Chicken	FF Baked Chicken	Baked Chicken (no skin)	Baked Chicken	SF Baked Chicken	
Buttered Noodles	FF Noodles	FF Noodles	Buttered Noodles	SF Buttered Noodles	Vanilla Pudding
Broccoli Spears	FF Broccoli Spears	FF Broccoli Spears	Asparagus Spears	SF Broccoli Spears	Grape Juice
Cranberry-Gelatin Mold Salad	Diet Gelatin Mold Salad	Cranberry-Gelatin Mold Salad	Cranberry-Gelatin Mold Salad	SF Cranberry-Gelatin Mold Salad	
Chocolate Fudge Cake	Diet Peaches	Cling Peaches	Cling Peaches	Cling Peaches	
Whole Milk	Skim Milk	Skim Milk	Whole Milk	Whole Milk	Whole Milk
Coffee/Tea	Coffee/Tea	Coffee/Tea	Coffee/Tea	Coffee/Tea	Coffee/Tea
Chilled Apple Juice	Unsweetened Apple Juice	Chilled Apple Juice	Chilled Apple Juice	Chilled Apple Juice	Chilled Apple Juice
Tenderloin Strips	Braised Tenderloin Strips	Braised Tenderloin Strips	Braised Tenderloin Strips	SF Tenderloin Strips	Cream of Mushroom Soup
Baked Potato with Sour Cream	Baked Potato	Baked Potato	Baked Potato (no skin)	Baked Potato	
Green Peas	Green Peas	Green Peas	Green Beans	SF Green Peas	Baked Custard
Fresh Garden Salad	Fresh Garden Salad	Fresh Garden Salad	Lettuce Wedge	Fresh Garden Salad	
Creamy Dressing	Lo-Cal Dressing	FF Dressing	Salad Dressing	SF Dressing	
Cherry Pie	Diet Cherries	Bing Cherries	Bing Cherries	Bing Cherries	
Whole Milk	Skim Milk	Skim Milk	Whole Milk	Whole Milk	Whole Milk
Coffee/Tea	Coffee/Tea	Coffee/Tea	Coffee/Tea	Coffee/Tea	Coffee/Tea

[a] FF indicates fat free
[b] SF indicates salt free

used in nursing homes must also be approved by the State Nutrition Consultant or by the Department of Health, Nutrition Section (Consultant Dietitians in Health Care Facilities 1987).

Cycle Menus

A cycle menu is one that is planned for a specified period of time such as 3, 4, 5, or 6 weeks. The menus are used for the specified period of time, then the cycle is repeated. The use of seasonal cycle menus are obsolete, for all practical purposes, since most foods are available throughout the year. Prohibitive use of certain foods may relate more to cost than availability.

The most current trend in cycle menu planning is to plan the menu for a number of days that is not a multiple of seven, such as 22, rather than for 21 days. Using this procedure, the same foods are not served on the same day of the week when the cycle is repeated. Therefore, when the menus are planned, they are not labeled as week no. 1, but as day no. 1, day no. 2, and so on. Another trend in cycle menu planning is to plan menus for special occasions to be inserted into the menu cycle as appropriate. Figure 9-6 presents a cycle menu rotation, using numbers instead of days of the week. The symbol H-4 represents the fourth holiday or special menu for the year.

Special menus are also planned for Friday meals since most patients prefer

MARCH 1988

Sunday	Monday	Tuesday	Wednesday	Thursday	Friday	Saturday
						1 No. 1
2 No. 2	3 No. 3	4 No. 4	5 No. 5	6 No. 6	7 F-1 Special	8 No. 7
9 No. 8	10 No. 9	11 No. 10	12 No. 11	13 No. 12	14 F-2 Special	15 No. 13
16 No. 14	17 H-4 Special	18 No. 15	19 No. 16	20 No. 17	21 F-3 Special	22 No. 18
23 No. 19	24 No. 20	25 No. 21	26 No. 22	27 No. 1	28 F-4 Special	29 No. 2
30 No. 3	31 No. 4					

Figure 9-6. Rotation for 22-day-cycle menu.

some type of seafood on those days. For a 22-day menu cycle, four Friday menus are sufficient.

The length of the cycle depends on the type of facility. In nursing homes, the cycle may need to be planned for at least a 4-week period since the length of stay for most patients is for an extended period of time. In acute care facilities, the cycle may be shorter since the average stay for patients is less than 10 days.

Cycle menus must be reviewed in order to take advantage of data collected during the previous cycle. The cycle also must be reviewed when new food items are added, when old items are deleted, or when substitutions must be made. In the review of menus, it is important that food choices at the end of the cycle (menu no. 22) are different from choices at the beginning of the menu cycle.

Advantages of planning and using a cycle menu are as follows:

1. *Reduces menu planning time.* After the menus have been planned and evaluated, the amount of time spent in menu review is minimal.
2. *Streamlines purchasing procedures.* Purchasing is somewhat repetitive, except for changes resulting from menu review.
3. *Aids in standardizing production.* Employees become more proficient as they prepare the same menu items over and over again.
4. *Serves as a training tool.* Repetitive production and service improves ability of supervisors and others in organizing activities.
5. *Aids forecasting techniques.* Data collected during previous menu cycle can be used to project future food needs.

The cycle menu, as planned for patients, may also be used for employees. It may be necessary to supplement the number and variety of foods offered in order to avoid menu boredom. The use of a "make your own salad bar," "items from the griddle or broiler," and "specials of the day" can add menu interest.

Menu Review Committee

The Review Committee is responsible for analyzing data collected during the previous menu cycle so as to make intelligent decisions relative to menu changes. For adequate representation, the committee may include the chef or head cook, purchasing personnel, production and service supervisors, and clinical dietitian, and be chaired by the foodservice director or a representative of administration.

Data collected may include census records, food acceptance results, plate waste studies, popular or unpopular food items, problems of quantity and/or quality control, and cost. The menu committee may recommend new recipes for testing or may add new items that have been tested with positive results. After all the changes have been made, the menu must be reevaluated. The following criteria are suggested for menu evaluation:

1. *Nutritional adequacy.* Does the menu adhere to daily food guidelines as listed in food groups?
2. *Food preferences.* Do menu items reflect the ethnic, cultural, and regional food preferences of patients and employees?
3. *Personnel.* Are employee skills adequate for preparation and service of planned menu items?
4. *Equipment.* Is there an overload on any one piece of equipment that would interfere with quality preparation and service?
5. *Flavor.* Is there a combination of mild and strong flavored foods?

6. *Consistency.* Is there a combination of soft and crisp food items?
7. *Texture.* Is there variety in ground and whole cuts of meat? Is there variation in texture?
8. *Color.* Are contrasting color combinations used? Will food items appear attractive and appetizing when plated together?
9. *Variety.* Is the same food item used more than once during the meal or during the day? For example, does the menu offer tomato juice for breakfast, lettuce and tomato salad for lunch, and veal cutlet with tomato sauce for dinner. Does the same food appear on the menu cycle for the previous day or the day after? Is the end of the menu cycle different from the beginning of the cycle?
10. *Cost.* Is the daily menu within prescribed budgetary allowances?

Quality assurance should begin with menu planning and prevail throughout the foodservice system. When effective menu evaluation techniques are used, one can be assured of quality control.

Standardized Recipes

Standardized recipes are mandated for use in medical foodservice operations by outside accrediting agencies. The primary purpose for this requirement is to ensure that all meals served to patients meet quality and quantity standards. The term "standardized recipe" does not mean that recipes are developed by outside agencies and used by all foodservice facilities. Rather, a standardized recipe is defined as one that has been tested and adopted for use in a particular facility. In some respects, a standardized recipe is analogous to an organization chart; each must reflect the objectives and goals of the particular operation. A standardized recipe system involves recipe development and serves as a basis for menu pricing.

To develop, maintain, and use a standardized recipe system requires time, effort, and full cooperation of both management and employees. The task is compounded when there are a number of cooks on staff who prepare their own special dish and are unwilling to share their *secret* recipe. The importance of seeking and gaining participation in all aspects of the developmental process cannot be overemphasized.

Recipe Development

It is not an easy task to develop recipes. The initial step is to decide on the format for the recipe card. As shown in Table 9-16, the card should include adequate information necessary for product uniformity in both quality and quantity. The recipe card should provide the user with:

1. Recipe number
2. Name of product
3. Number of servings
4. Size of servings
5. Ingredients (listed in order of use; ingredient first and the form later—i.e., onions, chopped; fully described, i.e., flour, pastry, or bread). Group ingredients that are to be combined or mixed together.
6. Measurements (listed by weight, where possible)
7. Yield increments (allow 2–3 columns for different yields on each card)

Table 9-16. Sample Recipe Card

PLAIN MUFFIN   Recipe No. _____
Total servings: 100
Serving size: 2 muffins each

Ingredients	200 Muffins Weight	Muffins Weight	Muffins Weight	Procedure
Flour, all purpose	10 lb			1. Mix flour, baking powder, sugar, and salt
Baking Powder	9 oz			
Sugar, granulated	2 lb, 10 oz			
Salt	3½ oz			
Eggs, beaten	2 lb, 4 oz			2. Mix eggs, oil, and milk. Stir into flour mixture…stirring only until flour mixture is moistened; batter will be lumpy.
Oil	3 lb			
Milk, whole	10 lb			3. Using No. 20 scoop (3⅕ Tbsp), portion into greased muffin tins.
				4. Bake at 400°F for 20 minutes or until lightly browned.

Cost Data

	Cost per Recipe	*Cost per Serving*
Labor		
Food		
Energy		

   8. Procedure (listed opposite ingredients)
   9. Cooking temperature and time or cooling temperature and time
   10. Pan size and number of servings per pan or amount of mixture per pan
   11. Type and size of serving utensils (ladle, scoop, weight, volume)

The recipe card should be large enough so that it can be easily read from a standing position with the card placed on a tabletop or clipped to a board. A suggested size is 5 × 8-inch index cards or 8½ × 11-inch sheets with bold, heavy type. For protection against soils as a result of employee handling, the card or sheet may be laminated or covered with plastic. A notebook, with plastic sheet covers, can be used for each set of menus (e.g., soups, entrees, desserts). List the source of the original recipe for future reference. Additional information on the recipe card may include cost data for food, labor, and energy.

To minimize the possibility of errors, use standard terminology in describing ingredients, volumes, and weights. The employee responsible for preparation of a food product should not have to guess whether the ingredient amount is "as purchased" (A.P.) or "edible portion" (E.P.).

After the format has been established, start with some of the more popular food items currently prepared in the facility. Do not pressure the employees by attempting to standardize too many recipes at the very beginning. It may be advisable to gain the cooperation of the informal leader among the cooks and have this employee share and adjust the initial recipes. Other employees are more likely to cooperate when the project is approved by the informal leader. For recipes that have proved to be acceptable, the following suggestions are offered.

   1. Have the cook record the ingredients, amounts, and procedures, using the suggested recipe format. Convert all measurements to weights if possible.

2. Observe preparation of food item. Check to determine whether steps have been omitted in procedures or extra ingredients are added. Observe mixing or other manipulations and record time required; for example, mix for 3 minutes at high speed.
3. Weigh and record weight of raw product.
4. Observe cooking temperature, time, type, and size of cooking utensils.
5. Weigh and record weight of cooked product.
6. Determine net yield, number of servings, and serving size. Indicate serving utensils required.
7. If necessary, adjust the recipe as a result of observations.
8. Have another employee prepare the same food item, using the adjusted recipe.
9. Repeat steps 2–6.
10. If product quality and quantity are consistent, record the recipe in the permanent recipe file.

— Developing New Recipes ——————————

In standardizing new recipes, such as those found in newspapers, magazines, and food company brochures, it is suggested that the initial preparation should be in the smallest yield possible. Analyze the new recipe for answers to the following:

1. Does the recipe contain foods that are acceptable to patients and personnel?
2. Are ingredients readily available?
3. Is the cost per serving within budgetary allowances?
4. Is the preparation time reasonable for assigned personnel?
5. Are personnel skills adequate for required preparation and service?
6. Are utensils and equipment available for preparation and service in large quantity?

If answers to the above questions are positive, continue with the following steps:

1. Record all pertinent information from the new recipe on a recipe card. For accuracy, convert all measurements to weights. If procedures for preparation are incomplete or unclear, leave space on the recipe card so that information can be recorded during trail preparation.
2. Discuss original recipe with the cook responsible for preparation. Emphasize the importance of accuracy in recording information. Accuracy will be particularly helpful if a decision is made to adjust recipe to a larger quantity.
3. Develop a recipe evaluation sheet to assess quality and quantity—that is, appearance, aroma, taste, tenderness, serving temperature, total yield, number of servings, and serving size.
4. Modify the recipe, if acceptable, for larger quantities. Calculate ingredients according to the charts in Appendixes C and D, or use the factor method as illustrated in Table 9-17. Adjust procedures to allow for additional mixing, cooking, or cooling time.
5. Conduct a second testing of the recipe. Follow steps 1 through 3 above. Evaluate product.
6. Repeat testing of recipe for the third and fourth trials, using different employees.
7. If product quality and quantity are acceptable, record the recipe in permanent file.

___Adjusting the Recipe _____

Errors in adjusting volume and weights in a recipe can be expensive in terms of both labor and food costs. Adjusting a recipe is a time-consuming task. One should be familiar with the procedures and allow ample time for the calculations. It is considered poor management to request a cook to double a recipe at the last minute. Frequently used methods for recipe adjustment include (1) direct-reading weight tables, (2) direct-reading measurement tables, and (3) the factor method (Aldrich & Miller 1967).

The use of direct-reading tables requires a minimum amount of calculation (see Appendixes C and D). To obtain the desired yield in adjusting recipes, observe the following steps:

1. Locate the column that corresponds to the original yield of the recipe to be adjusted.
2. Move a ruler down the column until you find the ingredient amount you wish to adjust.
3. With the ruler in place, read across the line to the column that corresponds to the desired yield.
4. Record this figure as the amount of the ingredient required for the adjusted yield. Repeat steps 1, 2, and 3 for each ingredient in the original recipe to increase or decrease yield.
5. If it is necessary to combine two columns to obtain the desired yield, follow the above procedures and add together the amounts given in the two columns for the adjusted yield.
6. Amounts are given in exact weights, including fractional ounces. After yield adjustment has been made for each ingredient, refer to Appendix F for rounding off fractional amounts that are not of sufficient proportion to change product quality.

The values for rounding are within the limits of error normally introduced in handling of ingredients. The primary purpose of Appendix F is to aid in rounding fractions and complex weights and measurements to ensure product quality control.

Since the original recipe may list ingredients in either weights or measures, it may be necessary to use both direct-reading tables together. To arrive at ingredient amounts, using measurement tables, follow the same procedures as outlined above for weights. The limiting factor in using direct-reading tables is that they can only be used when both the yield of the original recipe and of the adjusted recipe can be divided by 25.

At times it may be necessary to adjust a recipe with an original yield of more or less than 25, especially when developing recipes for modified diets and for special activities. In such cases, the use of the factor method is suggested. The factor method can be used to decrease or increase any recipe, regardless of original yield. For example, to increase the original yield of the plain muffin recipe from 100 to 300 portions, one should follow the steps as follows:

1. Divide the desired yield by the known yield of the recipe ($350 \div 100 = 3.5$) to obtain the basic factor. When increasing a recipe yield, the factor will be greater than 1.0; when decreasing a recipe yield, the factor will be less than 1.0.
2. Convert to weight all amounts of ingredients given in other units (Appendix B). Add weights of all ingredients to get total weight of the original recipe. See Table 9-17 for the factor method of recipe adjustment.

Table 9-17. Illustration of the Factor Method for Recipe Adjustment

(1) Original Recipe[a]		(2) Change Measures to Weight	(3) Change Weight to Ounces	(4) Multiply by Factor	(5) New Recipe (ounces)	(6) New Recipe[b] (weight)
Flour	10 lb	Not	160	3.5	560	35 lb
Baking Powder	9 oz	necessary	9	3.5	31.50	1 lb, 15½ oz
Sugar, granulated	2 lb, 10 oz	for	42	3.5	147	9 lb, 3 oz
Salt	3½ oz	this	3.50	3.5	12.25	12¼ oz
Egg, beaten	2 lb, 4 oz	recipe	36	3.5	126	7 lb, 14 oz
Oil	3 lb		48	3.5	168	10 lb, 8 oz
Milk, whole	10 lb		160	3.5	560	35 lb
Total			458.50		1604.75	100.29
			(28.656 or 28 lb, 10½ oz)		(100 lb, 4 oz)	(100 lb, 4 oz)

[a] Original recipe calls for 100 servings. Servings to be increased from 100 to 350. Factor is 350÷100 = 3.5.
[b] Check for calculation accuracy. Original recipe × Factor = New recipe (28.656 × 3.5 = 100.29 or 100 lb, 4 oz).

3. Change all weights to ounces. This procedure makes the calculation easier. If you prefer to work with decimal parts of a pound instead of ounces for the multiplication, use Appendix G.
4. Multiply the amount of each ingredient in the original recipe by the factor.
5. Add together the new weights (ounces or decimals) of all ingredients for adjusted recipe.
6. Convert ingredient weights back to pounds and ounces for ease of weighing by cooks. Use Appendix F for rounding off unnecessary fractions. The totals for steps 5 and 6 should be the same. If not, check calculations for mistakes made in arithmetic.

Adapting Recipes to Metric System

In adapting recipes to the metric system, change all ingredient amounts in original recipe to weights, then convert to metric. All recipes should be tested in the same manner as suggested for enlarging a recipe. For recipes such as stews and soups a soft or approximate conversion is adequate. For cakes, pastries, and other baked products, where minor deviations may result in failure, exact conversions are suggested. (See Appendix H for soft and exact metric conversions.)

A recipe with both English and metric units may be confusing for employees responsible for preparation. In Table 9-18 only the metric units are used.

Recipe Costing

It is good management practice to know what is being served (standardized recipe), how much is being served (portion control), and how much each portion costs (recipe costing).

To determine recipe cost, add the cost of each ingredient in the recipe. Total all ingredient costs and divide by the number of servings or portions to find *portion cost*.

Table 9-18. Illustration of Adapting a Recipe Using Metric System

(1) Original Recipe[a]		(2) Change Measures to Weight	(3) Change Weight to Grams	(4) Multiply by Factor	(5) New Recipe (grams)	(6) New Recipe (weight)
Flour	4.536 kg	Not	4536	3.5	15876	15.876 kg
Baking Powder	255 g	necessary	225.15	3.5	788.02	788 g
Sugar, granulated	1.190 kg	for	1190.7	3.5	4167.45	4.167 kg
Salt	99 g	this	99.22	3.5	347.27	347 g
Egg, beaten	1.020 kg	recipe	1020.6	3.5	3572.1	3.572 kg
Oil	1.360 kg		1360.8	3.5	4762.8	4.763 kg
Milk, whole	4.536 kg		4536	3.5	15876	15.876 kg
Total			12968.47		45389.64	
			(12.968 kg)		(45.389 kg)	(45.389 kg)

[a] Metric weights are conversions of weights in original recipe (see Table 9-17). Servings to be increased from 100 to 350. Factor is 350 ÷ 100 = 3.5.
[b] Accuracy check: 45389.64 ÷ 12968.47 = 3.5.

$$\frac{\text{Total recipe cost}}{\text{Number of portions}} = \text{Cost per portion}$$

To determine the *food cost percentage,* divide the portion cost by the selling price. For example, if the portion cost is $0.26 and the portion sells for $0.55, then the food cost percentage is 0.47 or 47%.

$$\frac{\$0.26}{\$0.55} = 0.47 \text{ or } 47\%$$

If the objective is to maintain a minimum of 47% food cost, then divide the portion cost by the food cost percentage to obtain the *selling price.*

$$\frac{\$0.26}{0.47} = \$0.55$$

For more accuracy in computing the selling price of a food item, a *prime cost method* is used. The prime cost method includes both the food and labor costs, to which a percentage is added for profit and other costs. As shown in Table 9-19, the selling price of each food item can be standardized if basic information, such as portion size, recipe cost, and labor computations, is provided. To determine the labor cost involved in the preparation of a food item, it is necessary to monitor the time it takes for an employee to prepare an item, and then multiply the time by the hourly rate paid to the employee. For example, if it takes one employee (at the rate of $4.50 per hour) 1 hour to prepare 350 portions of plain muffins, the labor cost of each portion is $0.013 (i.e., $4.50 ÷ 350 = $0.013). The labor cost includes only the preparation time. Cooking time is included in the labor cost only when attention is required during the cooking process, such as constant stirring, turning of foods, and other similar techniques.

The mark-up percentage is related to ingredient cost. In this example, the food cost of two muffins is $0.08 and the labor cost is $0.013 for a total of 100%. To this cost (0.08 + 0.013 = 0.093) is added another 150% (1.5 times) to

Table 9-19. Illustration of Prime Cost Method for Determining Selling Price

Food Item	Serving Size	Food Cost per Serving	Labor Cost per Serving	Prime Cost	Markup	Selling Price
Plain Muffin	2 muffins	$0.08	$0.012	$0.092	250%	$0.23

determine the selling price of $0.23. Note that in order to derive at a 150% increase, the prime cost must be multiplied by 2.5 (100% + 150%) since the basic cost represents 100%.

References

Abonyi, D., Anderson, J. M., Horvath-Monnreal, M. and Travalini, P. (1969). *Ethni-City: A Guide to Ethnic Detroit.* Detroit: Wayne State University, Michigan Ethnic Heritage Studies Center and Center for Urban Studies.

Aldrich, P. J. and Miller, G. A. (1967). *Standardized Recipes for Institutional Use.* Chicago: ADA.

American Dietetic Association. (1969). *Understanding Food Patterns in the U.S.A.* Chicago: ADA.

American Dietetic Association. (1988). *Handbook of Clinical Dietetics.* Chicago: ADA.

American Heart Association. (1988). *Dietary Guidelines for Healthy American Adults.* Position Statement. Circulation No. 70-1003.

Consultant Dietitians in Health Care Facilities (ADA Practice Group). (1987). *Dietary Regulations for Skilled Nursing Facilities: A Comparison of State Regulations and the Federal Conditions of Participation.* Pensacola, FL: Ross Laboratories.

Endres, J. B., and Rockwell, R. E. (1980). *Food, Nutrition, and the Young Child.* St. Louis: Mosby.

Flood, C. (1968). *Proposals for Implementing Change in Hospital Feeding.* Detroit: Wayne State University.

Food and Nutrition Board–National Research Council. (1980). *Recommended Dietary Allowances.* Washington, DC: National Academy of Sciences.

Gibson, L. D. (1981). The Psychology of Food: Why We Eat What We Eat When We Eat It. *Food Technol. 35*(2), 54–56.

Iowa Dietetic Association. (1984). *Simplified Diet Manual.* Ames: Iowa State University Press.

Jeffries, B. (1969). *Soul Food Cook Book.* New York: Bobbs-Merrill.

Joint Commission on Accreditation of Hospitals. (1988). Chicago: JCAH.

Kinder, F., and Green, N. R. (1978). *Meal Management.* New York: Macmillan.

Kirk, D., and Eliason, E. K. (1982). *Food and People.* San Francisco: Boyd and Fraser.

Meador, R., and Montalbano, B. (1982). Practical Applications of Kosher Food Service in a Nonkosher Residential Health Care Facility. *J. Nutr. Elderly 2*(1), 61–69.

Muhammad, E. (1967). *How to Live to Eat.* Chicago: Muhammad's Temple of Islam, No. 2.

Natow, A. B. and Heslin, J. (1982). Understanding the Cultural Food Practices of Elderly Observant Jews. *J. Nutr. Elderly 2*(1), 49–59.

Sanjur, D. (1982). *Social and Cultural Perspectives in Nutrition.* Englewood Cliffs, NJ: Prentice-Hall.

U.S. Department of Agriculture. (1980A). *The Hassle-free Guide to a Better Diet* (Science and Education Leaflet No. 567). Washington, DC: U.S. Government Printing Office.

U.S. Department of Agriculture. (1980B). *Food* (Science and Education Administration Home and Garden Bull. No. 228). Washington, D.C.: USDA.

U.S. Department of Agriculture, Food and Nutrition Service. (1979). *Building a Better Diet* (Program Aid No. 1241). Washington, D.C.: USDA.

Chapter 10

Subsystem for Equipment Planning, Use, and Care

Most department heads have been involved in equipment selection, layout, and design. The involvement may have been the selection of a single piece of equipment or the complex responsibilities for planning a new or renovated facility. Foodservice directors are not expected to be experts in the area of equipment, but it is a costly resource that must be managed. Therefore, it is important to understand basic equipment principles and to possess sufficient knowledge necessary to convey departmental needs to the appropriate authority.

Managerial Responsibility

Since equipment does not last forever, one is expected to plan and submit an annual budget (capital expenditures) for the replacement of old or nonfunctioning equipment. To plan for capital expenditures with some degree of proficiency, the foodservice director must be knowledgeable about the condition of the equipment so that he or she can write a strong justification to the budget committee. The foodservice director should consider the following factors:

1. *Know equipment and keep appropriate records.*
    A. Keep an up-to-date library of books (include expense in annual budget) and review current literature.
    B. Learn to read manufacturer's brochures for an understanding of terminology. This knowledge will aid in communicating departmental needs to equipment companies, to the internal budget review committee, and assist in comparing features of different equipment models.
    C. Organize and maintain a working file of equipment catalogs and brochures.
    D. Keep in contact with equipment companies and their sales representatives. Make contacts at conventions and food shows. Be familiar with the latest equipment, whether you are currently in the market for new equipment or not.
2. *Analyze the foodservice department and set up a long-range equipment program.*
    A. Take an inventory of all major equipment in the department. List age and condition of each piece of equipment along with other pertinent data, as shown in Figure 15-19. The accumulated information can be used for justifying new equipment. It is not

enough to say that you are tired of equipment breakdowns; you must have support in the form of records to justify the need.
   B. Determine replacement cost or time and new items needed. Life expectancy is approximately 10 years for most major equipment.
   C. Be aware of equipment costs and analyze each requirement with the view of saving money in the long run. The savings may be in repair costs or in food or labor costs. Good records will assist in calculating the payback period.
3. *Budget for equipment.*
   A. Include equipment requirements in annual budget (See Figure 15-18 for a sample of a capital equipment budget request.)
4. *Establish priorities.*
   A. List equipment as absolutely necessary or as desirable. This task is important in case it is necessary to eliminate certain equipment requests because of budget constraints.
5. *Coordinate requirements.*
   A. Get to know the purchasing agent in the organization.
   B. Know the procedures and requirements for equipment requests.
   C. Be aware of budget meeting dates and deadlines for submitting requisitions. Know when requests should be submitted and make sure that your requirements are included.
6. *Be knowledgeable concerning equipment meetings.*
   A. Know when the equipment review committee meets so that you are there to defend your request, if necessary. Be aware that foodservice will have competition from other departments within the facility for dollars spent on equipment.
7. *Write effective justifications.*
   A. Provide complete description, including manufacturer's name, model, type, size, shape, color, and electrical or plumbing characteristics. If required, list more than one source.
   B. If request is for replacement, state whether the present equipment is obsolete or is functionally inadequate.
   C. If request is for an initial purchase, state how the function was performed in the past.
   D. If there has been a change in departmental function or basic objective, refer to workload increase.
   E. State estimated initial cost, plus installation and maintenance costs.
   F. State how nonapproval or request will affect departmental goals, employee morale, efficiency, or aesthetic value as related to patient care.

The above responsibilities should be performed whether the foodservice director is involved in selecting one piece of equipment, remodeling, or planning for a new facility.

Facility Planning

In planning for renovations or for a new facility, the foodservice director will or should be part of the planning team, along with the administrator, architect, contractor, and foodservice consultant. The foodservice director is sometimes not included as a member of the planning team for a number of reasons. It may be that the individual has not impressed administration with an interest or knowledge of equipment selection, layout, and design. The contract for a foodservice consultant should be based on how much can be contributed by the foodservice director. For effective contributions, the foodservice director should be included as a member of the planning team during the very early stages. After plans have been finalized, little impact can be made.

Foodservice Consultant

The foodservice consultant serves as the communicating link between the foodservice director and other members of the planning team. There are two organizations of foodservice consultants from which names of potential candidates may be obtained: (1) Food Facilities Consultant Society; and (2) International Society of Foodservice Consultants. Qualified consultants may or may not belong to one of the above organizations. One of the best methods to use in selecting a qualified consultant is through personal interview and information based on reputation. The foodservice consultant may be involved in the following duties (American Hospital Association 1977):

- Help to determine and select equipment.
- Prepare drawings of equipment layout.
- Prepare work flow for architect.
- Write specifications for specially fabricated equipment.
- Prepare equipment portfolio.
- Advise on ventilation, lighting, floors, walls, and other physical features.
- Check preliminary architectural drawings.
- Develop appropriate cost estimates.
- Advise on bids.
- Inspect fabricated equipment in plant before delivery.
- Assist in inspecting installation of equipment.
- Train personnel in use of equipment.
- Perform other services as required.

Factors for Preliminary Planning

The foodservice consultant works within limitations and guidelines established by the administrator and foodservice director. For realistic planning, the consultant must know the (1) objectives, goals, and basic functions of the department, (2) menu and menu pattern, (3) purchasing system, (4) production and service systems, (5) work load and personnel data, and (6) quality standards. Answers to the following questions will assist the foodservice consultant in formulating layout and design concepts:

1. What will be the bed capacity?
2. What will be the patient profile? Adults only _____. Females only _____. Children only _____. Adults and children _____.
3. How many floors for patient care? _____ Number of patient care units on each floor _____. Number of beds in each patient care unit _____.
4. How many buildings to be served? Main building only _____. Satellite units _____. Estimated capacity of each satellite unit _____. Distance of satellite units from main building _____.
5. In addition to patient service, what other services will be provided? Employee cafeteria _____. Vending _____. Coffee shop _____. Executive dining _____. Catering _____. Restaurant _____.

6. What is the estimated number of meals to be served daily? Patients _____. Personnel _____. Guests and others _____.
7. What will be the operating hours? _____.
8. What will be the meal schedule? Patients _____. Personnel _____. Guest and others _____.
9. What type of menu system used? Selective _____. Nonselective _____. Cyclical (length) _____.
10. Will the same menu be used for patients and personnel? _____.
11. What will be the purchasing form for meat? Frozen _____. Chilled _____. Preportioned _____. Quarters _____. Wholesale _____.
12. What will be the purchasing form for fruits and vegetables? Frozen _____. Fresh _____. Canned _____. Dried _____.
13. What will be the purchasing form for baked products? Bread _____. Rolls, buns _____. Pies, cakes, cookies _____.
14. What will be the purchasing cycle?

	Daily	Weekly	Monthly
Meat	____	____	____
Poultry	____	____	____
Seafood	____	____	____
Produce	____	____	____
Groceries	____	____	____
Dairy Products	____	____	____
Bread and Baked Products	____	____	____

15. What type of production system? Cook-serve _____. Cook-freeze _____. Cook-chill _____. Convenience _____.
16. What type of service system for patient trays? Centralized _____. Decentralized _____.
17. What type of distribution for patient service? _____.
18. What type of serviceware? China _____. Plastic _____. Disposables _____.

All decisions related to planning must have administrative approval to receive adequate funding. This initial planning stage provides an excellent opportunity for input by the foodservice director. The initiative taken by the foodservice director at this time will have a tremendous effect on the outcome of the final plans.

Space Allocation

The amount of space required by a foodservice department is directly related to the functions that must be performed and the various systems used to carry out those functions. For example, the dining space for a commercial restaurant may take priority over the production space because the operation is profit-oriented, with emphasis placed on seat turnover for volume sales. The production system, for the most part, is designed for individual orders rather than for preparing food in quantity. In contrast, most medical foodservice operations are nonprofit, with cafeteria seating used by a limited number of employees and guests. Furthermore, the production is designed to produce food for both employees and patients, with a large amount of space allotted to patient tray setup.

___ Dining Space ___

Most authorities begin calculation of foodservice space with the dining area. The amount of space allotted is based on the following factors:

1. *Heaviest customer load at any one time.* This factor is minimal for medical foodservice operations since most employees eat meals on a staggered basis so as to provide adequate coverage of patient units. Also, most employees are willing to adjust their meal hours to eat at a less busy time, if necessary.

2. *Speed of service.* An average of five persons per minute can be served with a straight-line system. Less time per customer is involved with the scatter system, but a bottleneck may develop at the cash register unless an adequate number of cashiers are scheduled for peak periods.

3. *Menu variety, preparation, and service techniques.* A large number of food items to choose from tends to slow down the selection process. Most cafeteria menus include a mixture of ready prepared food items and foods cooked to order, such as grilled sandwiches. The promptness of selection by the customer for self-serve items and the speed of the server for controlled items may speed or delay the rate of customer flow.

4. *Seat turnover.* The term *seat turnover* refers to the number of customers occupying a seat during the hour. For example, if the seat is occupied on an average of 20 minutes, the turnover rate is three (60 minutes $\div$ 20 = 3). For employees in medical foodservice, the average time allotted for meals is 30 minutes. Therefore the turnover rate is two.

5. *Length of serving period.* The longer the serving period, the fewer seats required to accommodate customers. As shown in Table 10-1, the number of seats required for 1000 customers, at a turnover rate of two, varies from 200 to 500.

6. *Space allocation per seat.* Space allocation for one seat ranges from 12 to 15 ft^2 (Kotschevar & Terrell 1977). Requirements vary from state to state; therefore, one should check local and state codes before a final decision is made on seat space allocations. To calculate the total cafeteria space required, multiply the space required for one seat times the number of seats required for one turnover, as shown in Table 10-2. When using the above allowance for cafeteria space, additional space must be added to the total square footage for seating. The estimated width of the service area should be approximately 14 ft. This allows for 4 ft as customer line-up space, 1 ft tray slide, 2 ft counter width, 4½ ft for workers behind counter, and 2½ ft for back bar (Kotschevar & Terrell 1977). The area allotted for the back bar may be reduced if reach-through refrigerators and warming units are used. The average length of a cafeteria counter in hospital foodservice operations is 30–32 ft.

___ Production and Service Space ___

Space allocations for production and service include pre-preparation, cooking, baking, salad-sandwich, tray setup, and nourishment, as well as office space and dishwashing and potwashing space. During the planning stage, preliminary estimates of space needs for production and service can be based on the number of beds. Depending on the type of systems used, an allowance of 20 to 30 ft^2 per bed is suggested (Kotschevar & Terrell 1977). More space is needed where full production is done, such as with the cook-serve system. Less space is required in production and service areas for a convenience system. As shown in Table 10-3, the need for space is reduced as the number of beds increases. The allowances do not include storage areas for dry, chilled, or frozen foods, nor do they include cafeteria, special dining rooms, employee facilities, or floor pantries.

Table 10-1. Seats Required for 1000 Customers Based on Length of Serving Period and Time Allotted for Meals

Time Allotted	Length of Serving Period		
for Meals	1 Hour	2 Hours	2½ Hours
30 minutes	500	250	200

Table 10-2. Cafeteria Space Requirements Based on Seat Space and Seat Turnover

Space per Seat (ft²)		Number of Seats		Total Space Required (ft²)
12	×	500	=	6000
12	×	250	=	3000
12	×	200	=	2400

Table 10-3. Variations in Space Needs in Relation to Number Served[a]

Meal Load	Areas per Meal (ft²)	Variations in Total Area (ft²)
0–100	5.00	500–1000
200–400	4.00	800–1600
400–800	3.50	1400–2800
800–1300	3.00	2400–3900
1300–2000	2.50	3250–5000
2000–3000	2.00	4000–6000
3000–5000	1.85	5500–9250

[a]From Kotschevar and Terrell (1977).

A more precise calculation of space for production and service needs can be made later as consideration is given to factors related to the planning of menu, purchasing, production, and service systems. It is suggested that space for each work center be calculated according to equipment needs, and then the space for all work centers totaled to provide space needs for the entire area (Avery 1979). See Table 10-4 for a guide to equipment selection, based on menu.

Space required for patient service and setup, which is located in the production area, depends on the following:

1. *Type of tray service.* A tray service system using carts to deliver trays to the patient units will require storage space for carts plus space for cart cleaning.
2. *Number of patients served.* For high volume patient service, more carts are required for distribution, thus requiring more space.
3. *Menu variety for regular and modified diets.* The number of different food items, each requiring serving space, will affect the amount of setup space needed.

The percentage of floor space required for production and service depends on the system used and the type of equipment associated with each system. According to Kotschevar and Terrell (1977), the space for equipment

Table 10-4. Menu Analysis for Equipment Needs

Menu Item	Purchased Form, Preparation Technique	Major Equipment Needs
Appetizers		
Chilled Cranberry Juice	Canned, bulk	Dry storage
Cream of Celery Soup	Fresh, scratch	Dry storage, refrigerator, kettle
Vegetable Soup	Fresh, canned, scratch	Dry storage, refrigerator, kettle
Entrees (hot)		
Roast Beef au Jus	Fresh	Refrigerator, convection oven
Breaded Veal Cutlet with	Frozen	Freezer, fryer
Mushroom Sauce	Fresh	Refrigerator, tilting kettle
Grilled Cheese Sandwich	Scratch	Dry storage, refrigerator, slicer, griddle
Char-Broiled Hamburger on a Bun	Fresh, scratch	Dry storage, refrigerator, broiler
Entrees (cold)		
Deluxe Club Sandwich	Scratch	Dry storage, refrigerator, slicer
Cottage Cheese–Fruit Plate	Fresh, scratch	Refrigerator
Maurice Salad	Fresh, scratch, precooked meat	Refrigerator, slicer, steamer
Vegetables		
Parslied Potatoes	Fresh, prepeeled	Refrigerator, steamer
Baked Potatoes	Fresh	Convection oven
Buttered Broccoli	Frozen	Freezer, steamer
Green Beans with Pearl Onions	Frozen	Freezer, steamer
Salads		
Tossed Vegetable Salad	Fresh, scratch	Refrigerator, vertical cutter-mixer (VCM)
Creamy Cole Slaw	Fresh, scratch	Dry storage, refrigerator, VCM
Molded Peach on Lettuce	Fresh, canned, scratch	Dry storage, refrigerator
Breads		
Hot Rolls	Scratch	Dry storage, mixer, proofer, oven
White, Wheat, Rye	Commercial	Dry storage
Desserts		
Lemon Cake with Lemon Icing	Scratch	Dry storage, refrigerator, mixer, oven
Cherry Pie	Canned, scratch	Dry storage, kettle, mixer, oven
Chocolate Chip Cookies	Scratch	Dry storage, refrigerator, mixer, oven
Assorted Ice Cream	Commercial	
Beverages		
Coffee	Scratch, bulk	Dry storage, urn
Tea	Bag, individuals	Hot water dispenser
Milk	Carton, individuals	Refrigerator

may comprise only 30% of the total space with 70% or more used for work areas, traffic aisles, and space around equipment for ease of operation and cleaning.

Space for storage includes dry storage, refrigerated, and low temperature frozen food storage. Depending on the type of production system, space for a blast freezer may be needed. In addition to the above, space must be provided for the receiving and inspecting of deliveries.

Table 10-5. Type and Dimensions of Scales Used in Receiving Area[a]

Type	Capacity (lb)	Gradation	Platform Dimensions (in.)
Bench-type counter scale	30	1 oz	10½ × 13½
	50	2 oz	10½ × 13½
	100	8 oz	10½ × 13½
Platform scale—36 in. high	60	2 oz	10½ × 14½
	100	1 lb	10½ × 14½
	100	2 oz	10½ × 14½
	200	4 oz	10½ × 14½
	300	1 lb	10½ × 14½
	50	1 oz	13 × 19
	100	2 oz	13 × 19
	200	4 oz	13 × 19
	300	1 lb	13 × 19

[a]From Wilkinson (1969).

In the receiving area, space is required for scales and for some means of conveying goods received to their proper location (such as flatbed trucks, two-wheeled hand trucks, conveyor belts); space is also required for the receiving office. Floor space required by the types of scales usually found in the receiving area is shown in Table 10-5.

Provision should be made for the storage and removal of trash near the receiving area. A separate room should be provided with enough space for a compactor and equipment for cleaning trash cans. Depending on how garbage is disposed of and the frequency of pickup, it may be necessary to provide for refrigerated storage in the trash area.

Space required for dry storage depends on the following:

1. *Menu.* The variety and type of food items.
2. *Stock level required.* The minimum and maximum amounts of food to be kept on hand.
3. *Frequency of delivery.* The size of deliveries is related to how often deliveries are made. Space is needed for the largest amount to be stored at one time.

Dry storage includes space for food items (canned, bottled, bagged), paper supplies and other disposables, and a separate area for cleaning supplies. According to Avery (1979), it is best to compute dry stores for 1 day, multiply this by the number of days food is to be stored plus 10%, and then double the amount to allow for aisles and waste space. Table 10-6 offers guidelines for estimating dry storage needs for a 100-bed hospital.

Space for refrigerated and low-temperature storage includes both the large walk-in refrigerators and freezers and the smaller units located throughout the production and service areas. Factors related to the amount of space needed for chilled and frozen food are the same as those associated with dry storage. Guidelines, such as those listed in Table 10-7, are suggested for refrigerated and low-temperature storage during preliminary planning.

The importance given to space utilization cannot be overemphasized. Each square foot of space represents an enormous outlay of capital. The previous discussion on space allocation is considered preliminary. As work proceeds to equipment selection and layout, more exact calculations can be made, with possible revisions in space allocation.

Table 10-6. Guidelines for Dry Storage Space[a]

Type of Facility—Hospital (ft³)	Criteria
2.4	Per bed
0.025–0.050	Per meal served
500	Per 500 meals served
262	For 100 bed hospital feeding, 480 meals per day and storing food for 30 days

[a]From Avery (1979).

Table 10-7. Suggested Guidelines for Refrigerated and Low-Temperature Storage[a]

Food Category	Percentage[b]
Meats[c]	20–35
Fruits and Vegetables	30–35
Dairy Products	20–25
Frozen Food	10–25
Leftovers and other prepared foods	5–10

[a]From Kotschevar and Terrell (1977).
[b]Percentage of total space. Allowance may be calculated on basis of 15–20 ft³ of refrigeration per 100 complete meals or 1–1½ ft³ for every three meals served.
[c]Portion cuts require ½ to ⅓ less space than carcass or wholesale.

Equipment Selection

The menu is the basis for determining equipment needs. Based on menu items served, other factors such as the form of purchase, storage, preparation, and service techniques combine to indicate specific equipment needs. For example, the kitchen range, loaded with big pots and pans, is practically obsolete in medical foodservice operations. Most foods are prepared with the use of steam equipment and ovens. If the menu does not require certain kinds of equipment, then it is a waste to spend money to purchase it. In addition, it uses valuable space. The complete menu cycle must be analyzed before decisions are made. An analysis of equipment needs based on one meal for a typical day is shown in Table 10-4.

The analysis, such as listed in Table 10-4, will only provide the type of equipment needed, it will not give information on the capacity needed or how many pieces of each type. To arrive at specifics in terms of size and number, one needs to calculate the portion size, total amount of food needed, batch size, and at what interval the food item is needed during the meal hour. For example, to cook 500 (4-oz) servings of roast beef (rolled and tied), one needs to know the following information to determine the number of deck ovens (32 × 42 in.) required:

- Number of servings—500
- Size of roasting pan—16 × 20 in.
- Size of serving—4 oz
- Number of roasts per pan—2
- Number of pans needed—(500 ÷ 100 = 5)
- Size of roast—18 lb average
- Number of pans per deck—4
- Number of servings per roast—50
- Number of decks needed—2

In another example let us determine the amount of "reach-through" refrigerator space needed for salads, desserts, and other prepared cold food items. For the storage of 200 servings of tossed salad, one would need to know the following:

- Serving size—1 cup
- Dish used—salad bowl
- Height of food and bowl—2½"
- Space between pans—3 in.

- Size of pan—18 × 26 in.
- Number of portions per pan—12
- Number of pans for 100 servings—8⅓
- Number of pans for 200 servings—17
- Capacity per door opening (3 in. spacing)—19
- Total space required—one full-height door opening

For food items that can be prepared in batches, equipment needs may be less than for foods prepared all at one time. For example, the operation may require 12 pans of baked macaroni and cheese, but this is a product that quickly deteriorates in quality if cooked too far in advance. Therefore, a large kettle is required for cooking and mixing, but less space is required for baking since only 2 to 3 pans are needed at a time. Using menu analysis to determine equipment needs is a time-consuming task that is well worth the effort in assuring adequacy in type and amount of equipment required for efficient and effective operation.

With equipment needs established, it is time to look at other factors involved in the selection process, such as performance, materials, construction and design, cost, safety, and sanitation features. The process may begin with a survey of equipment manufacturers to determine what is available.

PERFORMANCE In this context, performance refers to how well the equipment will function over a period of time to produce the volume needed for the operation. Research can be conducted by checking with other foodservice operations with the same equipment. Questions should be asked about the quality of products produced, ease of handling, number and types of repairs needed, availability of parts and promptness of repairs, and other pertinent information that will assist in decision making.

MATERIALS The material used in the construction of the equipment should be suitable for the type of equipment, conforming to applicable standards as determined by the National Sanitation Foundation (NSF). Consider the gauge and finish of metals used for equipment. The gauge or thickness of sheet and plate metal is determined by the weight of metal per square foot. U.S. Standard gauge numbers range from No. 000 with a 0.3750 in. thickness to No. 24 with a 0.0239 in. thickness (Kotschevar & Terrell 1977). The small numbers indicate a thicker metal. Numbers 10 to 14 gauge for galvanized steel and 12 to 16 for noncorrosive metals are generally used for foodservice equipment (West, Wood, Harger, & Shugart 1977). The lighter gauges, above no. 16, are generally used for sides of equipment or in areas where the wear is light.

The finish refers to the degree of polish. For stainless steel, the degree of finish or polish is indicated by nos. 1 to 7. The smaller numbers indicate a dull finish; the larger numbers indicate a high glossy polish. Finish no. 4 has a standard polish and is often used for equipment such as table tops, sinks, and counters. High-luster finishes cost more and should not be used unnecessarily, especially on surfaces not visible to customers. Most kitchen equipment is made of stainless steel because it is durable, easy to clean, resists corrosion, and has a good appearance. The type of stainless steel recommended for foodservice equipment is an alloy, commonly called 18–8 or no. 302. The 18–8 refers to the 18% chromium and 8% nickel it contains (West et al. 1977). Wood has limited use in foodservice operations because it is difficult to maintain proper sanitary conditions. Wood may be used only for single-service articles, such as chopsticks, stirrers, or ice cream spoons. The use of wood as food contact surface under other circumstances is prohibited (U.S. Department of Health and Human Services 1976).

SANITATION AND SAFETY All multiuse equipment should have NSF, and Underwriters Laboratories (UL) approval for maximum sanitation and safety. According to the U.S. Department of Health and Human Services (1976), "Multiuse equipment and utensils shall be constructed and repaired with safe materials, including finishing materials; shall be corrosion resistant and nonabsorbent; and shall be smooth, easily cleanable, and durable under conditions of normal use." To make sure that equipment meets required standards, one should check for NSF and UL seals of approval, which are prominently displayed on all approved equipment.

Prior to equipment selection, a comparison can be made for all major equipment. In making an equipment survey, list all desirable features and compare models, as shown for reach-in freezers in Table 10-8. The features, as listed in the comparison of reach-in freezers, refer to low-temperature cabinets for storage of foods that are already frozen. According to Hall (1982), the following recommendations should be considered during the selection process:

1. Insulation should be maximum thickness for retention of cool air. Polyurethane insulation is recommended.

2. Interior capacity should be visually evaluated for usable space. Placement of shelving and blower coils may take away valuable storage space. Top-mounted blower coils are suggested.

3. Feet must be adjustable to allow for possible uneven flooring where equipment is to be installed.

4. Door liners must be durable so as to withstand possible abuse from daily use.

5. Warranties should be carefully evaluated. Seek maximum warranty.

6. Ask to see test results on temperature differentials throughout the cavity for uniformity of air flow.

7. Consider pros and cons of condensate evaporator system. Refrigerant is dispersed through the refrigerator condensate evaporator system by either capillary tubes providing a standard size orifice or an expansion valve that has an orifice that changes in size to allow more or less refrigerant to evaporate as the temperature varies. Although expansion valves can malfunction, they can be repaired and do provide an efficient flow of refrigerant. Capillary tubes have no moving parts, thus providing a completely closed system; however, if malfunction occurs, the total system must be replaced.

General recommendations for the selection of freezers are as follows:

- Polyurethane insulation, maximum thickness
- Top-mounted blower coils
- Adjustable feet
- Exterior thermometer
- Maximum warranty
- UL, NSF approval

Specifications

The writing of specifications was listed as one of the duties of the foodservice consultant, but this task should not be done in isolation. Input from the foodservice director and possibly from the employees who will have responsibility for the smooth functioning of equipment must be considered.

Specifications are written by the buyer and list in clear statements what is

Table 10-8. Comparison of Reach-In Freezers: Single Section, Full Length[a]

	Delfield	Hobart	Nor-lake	McCall	Traulsen	Victory
Model no.	6125–S	HA–F1	TF27 ASSD	4020F	GL T–1–32 WUT w/stainless steel door	AF–22–SA
Insulation thickness	2 in. Poly-urethane	2 in. Poly-urethane	Door—2½ in. Polyurethane Sides—3½ in. Fiberglass	2¾ in. Poly-urethane	2 in. Poly-urethane	2½ in. Poly-urethane
Compressor size	⅓ hp	½ hp	½ hp	½ hp	½ hp	⅓ hp
Condensate evaporator type:						
Capillary tube	×	×	—	—	×	×
Expansion valve	—	—	×	×	—	—
Net interior capacity	23.6 ft³	21.7 ft³	23.2 ft³	22.4 ft³	24.2 ft³	21.32 ft³
Finish	Stainless steel door, aluminum sides	Stainless steel front, aluminum sides	Stainless steel front, enameled sides and back	Stainless steel front, aluminum exterior	Stainless steel door option with anodized aluminum sides	Stainless steel front, aluminum exterior
Shelves per section	Three	Three	Four	Three	Three	Three
Door handle	Vertical	Horizontal	Vertical	Vertical	Horizontal	Vertical
Magnetic gaskets, hand replaceable	×	×	×	×	×	×
Blower coil location	Top mounted	Top mounted	Top mounted	Top mounted	Top mounted	Ceiling mounted within cabinet
Adjustable feet	×	×	×	×	×	×
Exterior thermometer	Interior thermometer	×	×	×	Optional	Optional
Door liner	ABS molded plastic	High impact plastic	ABS plastic	Aluminum	Anodized aluminum	Stainless steel
Warranty–standard	1 year parts, 30 days labor	1 year parts and labor, includes travel time and expenses, 4 year additional on compressor	90 day labor, 1 year parts	90 days labor, 1 year parts, 5 year compressor	—	1 year parts, 90 days labor
Warranty–optional	5 years, optional	—	5 year compressor	1 year labor	1 or 2 years parts, and labor, 5 years compressor	9 month labor additional, 5 year compressor
Air flow system	Interior molded such that air flows behind shelves	Ducts located on side of door	Side walls ducted to assure temperature uniformity	Ducts located on right side	Top mounted vent, air flows from top to bottom	—
Options:						
Half doors	—	×	×	×	×	×
Casters	Standard	×	×	×	×	×
Rear panels	Standard	×	×	Standard	×	×
Extra shelves	×	×	×	×	×	×
Shelf finishes	Vinyl coated, shelves standard	Zinc galvanized, standard, stainless steel, optional	Chrome plated, standard, stainless steel, optional	Chrome plated standard, stainless steel and epoxy coated, optional	Chrome plated standard, stainless steel, optional	Iron zinc plated, standard stainless steel, optional
UI	×	×	×	×	×	×
NSF	×	×	×	×	×	×
List price[a]	$2380	$3320	$3080	$2820	$3060	$2850

[a]From Hall (1982).
[b]Prices will vary depending on dealer discount.

desired and under what conditions. The written statement, if accepted by a purveyor or manufacturer, represents a contract between the two parties. Unnecessary wording makes for a cumbersome specification and increases the possibility of error on the part of the writer. The responsibility for writing specifications is part of the foodservice consultant's duties, with input from management.

___ Type of Specifications _____

According to Harris (1981), specifications can be classified into four categories:

1. *Closed specification.* One in which the description is so detailed that only one product can qualify. The closed specification may be desirable when new materials or equipment must match existing equipment or decor, such as in renovation projects.

2. *Open specification.* One that allows a competitor to supply a number of products or materials that are considered equal or acceptable. If the "or equal" clause is used, it should be worded "or approved equal," meaning that substitutions are subject to administrative approval.

3. *Manufacturer's specification.* One that is written by manufacturers in such a way as to sell their particular product. The best qualifications are presented, and in most cases the specification fails to mention any deficiencies.

4. *Performance specification.* One written in a manner that stipulates all of the requirements that the installation or product must meet, but does not state how. It allows the methods and sometimes the materials to be selected by the contractor, who then assumes responsibility for desired results.

It may be necessary to combine one or more types of specifications to get the desired results.

___ Guidelines for Specification Writing _____

The most important aspect of specification writing is to explain exactly what is to be done in the most simple, clear, and concise manner. To assist the foodservice director in meeting responsibilities for specification writing, the following list should be beneficial (Avery 1978):

1. Is the specification free of any possible misunderstanding? Is the language used to describe details similar to that used by manufacturers?

2. Are all desired features included in the specification?

3. Is the specification free of all frivolous requirements? Anything that is different from the standard manufacturer's specification sheet should be reviewed for absolute necessity. As a rule it will cost more, and in many cases manufacturers of quality equipment are hesitant to bid on the equipment since they have not tested the modification and will not want their brand name on something they have not tested.

4. Are gauges, finishes, and composition of materials described using standard terminology (such as 302 corrosion-resistant steel, 12-gauge metal thickness, and no. 4 finish)?

5. Is the design well balanced? Is the frame adequate to support the top specified? Is the weight compatible with the floor on which the equipment will rest? Are hinges adequate for the size and weight of door? Will the drawer size carry the drawer weight plus contents? Has a table with an adequate gauge top been properly balanced with lightweight side panels?

6. Are all construction details uniform so that several parts of similar purpose and design are described in identical terms?

7. Are greater quality, more expensive metal, heavier gauge, or finer finish being used than is warranted based on anticipated equipment use?

8. Does the specification indicate who will or will not provide associated equipment (faucets, valves and traps for sinks, electrical connections for work tables and similar equipment)?

9. Who is responsible for installation? If dealer is to install, does the responsibility include preparing the equipment location and bringing in utilities and drains?

10. Is workmanship defined?

11. If the successful bidder is to install equipment, is he or she required to submit proposed installation plans for approval?

12. Is it specified that construction details, particularly those relating to water and drains, conform to local regulations? Does construction conform to Occupational Safety and Health Administration (OSHA) regulations?

13. The terminology "good commercial practice" should be used to cover any details of construction that may have been overlooked.

14. Are provisions made in the equipment design for easy access to parts on which repair or adjustments will have to be made?

15. If the intent is to encourage a number of bidders, the specification should be written loosely enough so that a number of manufacturers can comply with specification details. If specification is written so that only one piece of equipment can comply with all of the details, the price may be high.

In addition to the above guidelines, the following information should be considered by the specification writer;

1. State that all equipment shall be approved by the appropriate agency, such as NSF, UL, AGA (American Gas Association).
2. Stipulate that bid prices should include taxes, shipping, and other related charges. If the facility has a tax-exempt status, it should be stated in the general information specification.
3. Specify delivery and shipment conditions, dates for arrival, and method of shipping.
4. Specify exact destination—for example, delivery is to be made to an off-site warehouse until ready for installation.
5. State who is responsible for equipment assembly, training in use and care.
6. Specify whether warranty is to be for both parts and labor, and length of warranty.
7. Specify the length of time in which parts will be available if model is discontinued; it should be at least 10 years.
8. Specify time span for service and repair of equipment, such as within 48 hours.

Layout Design

Having analyzed the menu to determine equipment needs, it is time to put the individual pieces of equipment into a layout design that will promote smooth, efficient operation. The complete layout is composed of work centers and sections (Kotschevar & Terrell 1977).

___ Work Centers _____

A work center is the smallest area planned in the facility. It is an area where a group of related tasks are performed. Attention should be given to:

1. *Functions to be performed.* The functions may include pre-preparation, preparation, storage, setup, service, and clean-up. For example, in the salad-sandwich work center, the amount of pre-preparation depends on whether all vegetables are cleaned and cut in the salad area or whether this work is accomplished in the ingredient room. If the functions are performed in the ingredient room, then there is no need for equipment such as a slicer or vegetable cutter. Space is required for mixing and dishing of salads and for assembling materials for sandwiches.

2. *Volume to be prepared.* The largest amount of food required at any one time will affect layout design of the work center. It may be necessary to have all salads and sandwiches ready at the beginning of patient tray setup and enough portions ready for cafeteria service to get started with batch making throughout the service period.

3. *Number of employees.* The number of employees is related to the functions and volume. Each employee requires a certain amount of space to perform tasks without bumping into another person and without excessive reaching and traveling.

4. *Kind and amount of equipment.* The menu dictates the kind and amount of equipment needed. Equipment needs for the salad-sandwich area will include tabletop space with sink and garbage disposal. Consider a U shape with the sink at the bottom of the U. Unless cooked foods are prepared in the main cook's area, a trunion-type kettle is required for foods such as cooked dressings, hard-cooked eggs, boiled shrimp, and hot water for jellied salads. Refrigerated space is required for holding salads and sandwiches.

The space allotted to a work center should be adjusted to take into account the above factors. For a medium-size worker, work center space should be approximately 15 ft^2, measuring about 2½ ft deep by 6 ft long (Kotschevar & Terrell 1977). Solicit the aid of workers to assist in designing work centers. Employees are more familiar with the work to be done and can offer useful suggestions on the placement of equipment that will reduce both time and energy in performing tasks. The use of paper, cardboard, or plastic templates, as shown in Figure 10-1, can be used to provide a visual presentation prior to final drawings. Templates are scaled representations of the actual size and shape of equipment. The standard scale is ¼ in. equals 1 ft. If the template represents only the shape and size, allow space for workers and equipment clearances, such as bending, opening drawers and oven doors. With the use of templates, modifications can be made as work centers develop into sections, and sections develop into the complete layout.

___ Work Sections _____

A work section is composed of one or more work centers, such as vegetable and meat cookery in the main cooking section. The sections are formed based on the interrelationship of work activity performed in the work centers. The sequence of work, used to plan work centers, applies to the joining of work centers into sections. Prime considerations are principles relating to travel time and energy expenditure on the part of employees; dual use of equipment, where possible; use of mobile equipment; and safety and sanitation standards.

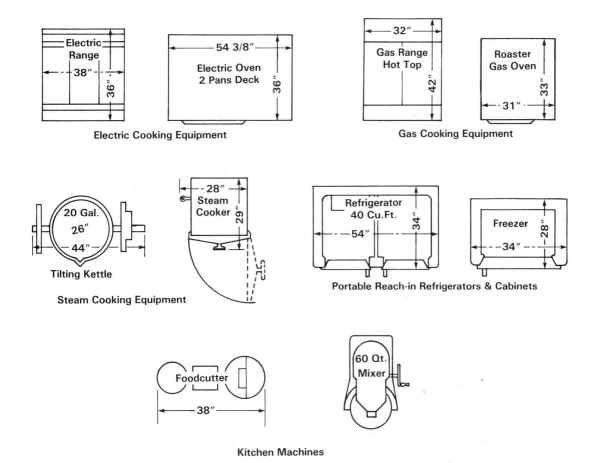

Figure 10-1. Equipment templates for layout design.

The Layout

When planning is implemented into a complete layout, consideration must be given to the flow of materials, workers, and customers, and to the interrelationships of work activities within each section. Layout design is a compromise between a number of factors and is frequently complicated by the diversity and the number of functions, quality and cost control requirements, and the specific needs of the operation. The ideal layout cannot always be achieved, but certain principles and concepts should be considered. Major concerns relate to the flow of food products and the interrelationship of work sections.

Concept of Flow

The layout is guided by the basic concept of flow. Functions in proper sequence should follow the most direct and quickest route without crisscrossing, backtracking, interference, or delay. The arrows in Figure 10-2 indicate the flow of materials in a logical, efficient manner. As a rule, when the flow of materials is minimized, the flow of employees is also minimized. The planner of flow should have a knowledge of production and service functions in order to effectively plan the layout. As suggested by Kotschevar and Terrell (1977) there are eight principles to consider in establishing flow for efficient work accomplishment:

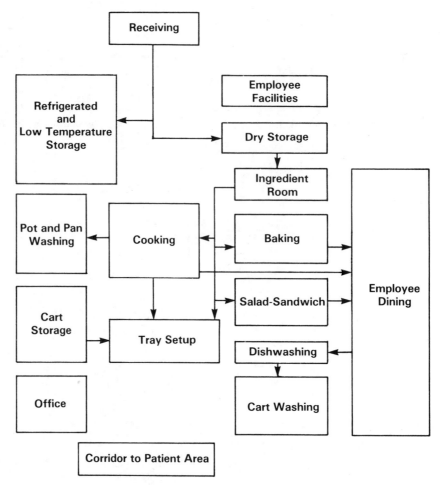

Figure 10-2. Food product flowchart.

1. Functions should proceed in a direct, straightforward sequence with a minimum of crisscrossing and backtracking.
2. Seek smooth, rapid production and service, with minimum of time and energy expended by workers.
3. Delay and storage of food in processing and serving should be eliminated, as much as possible.
4. Travel distance for workers and materials should be minimized.
5. Handling of materials and tools should be minimized, as should worker attention in regard to equipment.
6. Seek maximum utilization of space and equipment.
7. Seek quality control at all critical points.
8. Seek minimum cost of production.

It is important to keep in mind that even though the layout may include labor-saving equipment that is conveniently arranged, there can still be a waste of worker time and energy unless effective employee training is carried out.

___ Work–Activity–Section Relationship ___

It is important to seek a high amount of interrelationship between sections to form the complete layout. Activities related to food materials, as they flow through the facility, are as follows: (1) receiving, (2) storing, (3) preparing, (4) cooking, (5) distributing, and (6) serving. In order to perform these activities in a safe and sanitary manner, other areas must be considered, such as dishwashing, pot and pan washing, and trash removal.

RECEIVING The location of the receiving area should be convenient for the type of deliveries being made, whether by truck or car. The receiving platform should be at truck-bed height to avoid excessive lifting and handling of materials. In large facilities, nonperishable items may be stored in central stores with other hospital supplies or stored in a separate central storage area for foodservice items only. When a central storeroom is used, space for a daily storeroom must be provided near the production area. Doors for the receiving area must be large enough for bins, trucks, and other large equipment to pass through. Space for scales, receiving tables, trucks and carts used for transporting, desk, files, and tools for opening crates and cases must be provided. Adjacent to the receiving area should be space for the storage and disposal of trash and garbage. A separate outside entrance is suggested to avoid possibility of cross contamination. A compactor and a can washer may be required in the garbage–trash area.

STORAGE AREA A dry storage area is required for staple food items, linen, paper supplies, and excess equipment (small utensils, dishes, silverware, silver service, glasses, banquet tables, folding chairs, floral arrangements, and other seasonal decorations). A separate storage area is required for cleaning supplies. Plan for small storage areas in each work section, unless an ingredient room is planned. With the use of an ingredient room, the need for individual storage areas is eliminated. Space utilization is increased with adjustable shelves. The use of mobile bins for dry products and drums with pumps or cradles for oils and other liquids is suggested. Space is needed for other equipment—such as a table, chair, and file cabinet—if an inventory system is maintained in this area. Consider ventilated storage space for items such as underripe fruits and vegetables.

Bulk refrigerated and low-temperature storage (walk-in types) should be located near the receiving area to eliminate distribution problems and to promote forward flow of products. Other refrigerated and low-temperature storage may be located throughout the production and service areas. There may be a need for other types of refrigerated and low-temperature storage such as reach-in, pass-through, counter refrigeration, under-counter refrigeration and freezer, or portable ice cream freezers. Consider the pros and cons of combination coolers where the frozen food section opens into the refrigerated section instead of directly into the production area. If the production system is ready-serve, there will be a need for blast freezing, with temperatures of about $-30°F$ instead of $0°F$ for low temperature. Thawing refrigerators are suggested for the safe thawing of frozen foods. During the thawing process, the food softens but the temperature of the food product never rises above safe refrigerator temperature of $40°F$. The food is thawed under controlled temperatures in approximately 12 hours compared to 2 to 3 days for regular refrigerated thawing.

PRE-PREPARATION Pre-preparation tasks may take place at the individual work centers, or the activity may be accomplished in a separate work center such as a butcher shop or ingredient room. For operations using the carcass or wholesale cuts of meat, pre-preparation is done in a butcher room. For operations using retail cuts and preportioned meat items, the pre-preparation can be done in the ingredient room, along with other food items. One work table with a sink should be used for meats, and another work table with a sink should be used for fruits and vegetables. The two activities should be separated to avoid cross contamination. The ingredient room is the area where all measuring, trimming, grinding, shaping, chopping, and similar activities take place. The location of the ingredient room should be convenient to dry, refrigerated, and low-temperature storage, and in direct flow to the production areas. Equipment required in the area may include scales, slicer, shredder, patty shaper, grinder, cuber, chopper, vegetable cutter, and reach-in and pass-through refrigerated space. The pass-through refrigerator, with roll-in racks, is used for storage of portioned and measured food items. Portion scales (32-oz capacity with ½-oz gradations) are suggested for spices, and bench-type counter scales (30-lb capacity with 1-lb gradations) are required for weighing larger quantities. The number of each needed depends on the volume demand of the operation.

COOKING–BAKING The cooking and baking areas may be combined in small operations, and in those large operations where a minimum amount of baked products are prepared from scratch. The major advantage in combining the two areas is the dual use of equipment such as mixers and ovens. Depending on the menu and volume, a separate bakery area will require much of the same equipment as the main cooking area, such as steam kettle, ovens, deep-fat fryer, mixer, and scales. In addition, specialized equipment such as yeast proofer and dough cutter will also be needed. Workers in the bakery area tend to work independently of other employees and prefer to have a separate washing section for pots and pans to avoid mixing of equipment. Consider the flow of materials from dry and refrigerated storage to the work area and finally to the service area. When the bakery area is combined with the cooking of other foods, a separate table is required for panning and finishing of products. Mobile racks are required for storage and transport of finished products, such as a roll-in refrigerator type.

The most frequently used layout pattern for the cooking area is to have all dry heat and moisture-producing equipment grouped together under one ventilating hood. The parallel back-to-back arrangement is used with or without a wall separating the equipment. The arrangement is economical and may provide for good supervision of the work area if walls are eliminated. In the back-to-back arrangement, dry heat equipment such as ovens, fryers, broilers, and griddles are placed on one side, and steam equipment placed on the other. Work tables are placed in front of equipment on both sides. The amount of pre-preparation equipment required will depend on the use of an ingredient room. The use of partially or fully prepared foods will increase the need for refrigerated space. Efficient layout of this space is the key to the entire production and service areas. Consider the inflow of materials from storage or the ingredient room, and the outflow to serving areas and pot and pan washing.

SALAD–SANDWICH The salad-sandwich section should be located near the serving areas, with direct flow from storage or the ingredient room. The amount of equipment required depends on the menu volume, and whether pre-preparation is performed in the area. The flow of materials may be from storage or the ingredient room to the cooking area (roast meat for sandwiches), or the vegetable cooking section (handling potatoes, hard-cooked eggs, and similar items). A table with sink and garbage disposal is required, along with other table top equipment such as slicer, chopper, hot plate, and steam equipment—if the required food is not prepared in another section. Refrigerated space is required for bulk and portioned food items.

PATIENT TRAY SETUP The tray line setup should have direct flow from the cooking, bakery, and salad–sandwich areas, as well as from storage for direct deliveries. The tray setup location should be near the dietitian's office for supervision, and near the dumbwaiter, vertical conveyor, or exit to the elevator for distribution to the patient area. In addition to a horizontal conveyor for tray setups, mobile equipment is required for holding hot and cold foods. The type and amount of equipment needed depends on the menu variety, volume, and amount of preparation performed during serving, such as toast, eggs, and other foods that lose quality from extended holding. Space is required for storage of food carts, if used. To avoid cross contamination, the return of soiled carts should proceed directly to the dishroom and cart washing areas without travel through the production and service areas.

CAFETERIA SERVICE The cafeteria service area should be placed as close to production areas (main cooking, salad–sandwich, and bakery) as possible. The use of pass-through refrigeration and warming cabinets promotes efficiency for both kitchen and cafeteria personnel. Counter space is determined by menu variety, shape of the serving area, customer load, and anticipated traffic pattern. Counters may be arranged in a straight line, L shape, square, or a combination of the various types. The scatter or scramble arrangement is a popular system because it allows traffic to flow freely in a square area with various counters arranged around the perimeter. Space is provided in back of counters for workers and preparation equipment such as deep-fat fryers, broilers, and griddles. The arrangement chosen should prevent delays and bottlenecks at the cashier station, self-dispensing beverage area, salad bar, condiment station, and cook-to-order counters.

DISHROOM The dishroom should be conveniently located for return of customer trays and the return of food carts from patient areas. Equipment should be arranged to avoid cross contamination at the clean end of the dishwashing machine. The use of self-leveling dispensers for dishes and glasses is encouraged.

POT AND PAN WASHING The area for pot washing should be convenient to all production areas. Space is required for storing clean equipment. A three-compartment sink is required for pot washing done by hand; a pot-washing machine may be considered, if volume justifies the use.

EMPLOYEE FACILITIES Locker rooms and toilets may be in the front or rear of the building. The important factor is that these facilities should be situated near an entrance so that employees will not have to travel through the production and service areas in outside clothing.

OFFICE SPACE A number of sites throughout the facility are appropriate for office space, depending on the nature of activity. Office space for supervisors should be close to the area being supervised. The dietitian's office should be near an entrance, a location that is convenient for consultation with foodservice employees and personnel from other departments. Consider privacy and environmental factors, especially excessive noise.

Emphasis has been placed on flow, but other important factors of layout need to be considered:

1. *Efficient use of utilities.* Group equipment according to type of utility as much as possible. All equipment requiring steam may be placed together, thereby reducing cost because fewer pipes are needed for installation.
2. *Efficient use of equipment.* Promote dual use by placing equipment in a central location, if stationary, or use carts with wheel locks for moving equipment from one location to another.

3. *Efficient use of personnel.* Arrange equipment for minimum movement and travel for skilled personnel. If a choice of travel is between two employees of different skills and pay levels, then the longer distance should be traveled by the less skilled and lower-paid employee.
4. *Safety.* Layout based on flow only may prove to be dangerous to workers in the area. For example, high temperature equipment placed next to a traffic aisle, or doors opening to block traffic aisle.
5. *Sanitation.* An awareness of activities conducive to cross contamination cannot be overlooked.
6. *Environmental factors.* Lack of consideration may affect production, as discussed in the next section

Environmental Factors in Facility Design

Emphasis on environmental factors can have a positive impact on conditions under which employees must work. Even though engineers must comply with established codes and regulations, there is a certain amount of flexibility in facility design. Poor working conditions contribute to decreased productivity, increased labor turnover, absenteeism, and employee fatigue. Employees do their best work in a comfortable work environment. Some factors that have a direct affect on worker efficiency are (1) lighting, (2) temperature, and (3) noise.

Lighting

Consider lighting needs for specific work areas rather than having all ceiling lights with the same light intensity. Light intensity is measured in candlepower (cp), which indicates the strength or force of light going in any direction from the light source. Light meters are used to measure footcandles (fc), which indicate the amount of light concentrated on a surface area. Light quantity is measured in lumens (lm). Kotschevar and Terrell (1977) use the following calculation to derive the footcandle (fc) value: "If a lamp gives off 100 lm, 60% of which strikes a 10-sq-ft surface (60 lm), the footcandles per square foot equals 6 fc." As a member of the planning team, the foodservice director needs to be somewhat familiar with light science technology in order to understand how engineers derive certain figures.

As reported by Myers (1979), the Illuminating Engineering Society suggests 30 fc throughout the kitchen; 70 fc at points where inspection and pricing is done, and 15 fc in storage areas. The foodservice director is familiar with activities to be performed in each work area and is therefore in a position to offer suggestions on light intensity. Guidelines for minimum footcandles of light in various areas are offered in Table 10-9.

One of the problems associated with lighting is that of glare. The source of glare can be the color of walls, ceilings, or floor coverings, or reflections from bright stainless steel equipment. According to Avery's report (n.d.) on human engineering in kitchen design, the upper walls should be pale green, buff, light gray, or light blue, and should reflect 50–60% of the light that strikes them. Ceilings may be white, off-white, yellow, ivory, or cream and should reflect 80–85% of the light. Lower walls should be darker shades of green, brown, gray, or blue. Floors should be light enough to reflect back 30–35%; equipment should reflect 30–50%.

Table 10-9. Minimum Footcandles of Light for Various Areas [a]

Type Area	Footcandles
Baking mixing room	50
Cashier	50
Detail work area	70–100
Fillings and other preparation	30–50
Food checker	70
Food counters and displays	50
Loading platform	20
Office, general	100
Other kitchen areas	30
Oven area	30
Reading or work area	30
Storage area, active	20
Storage area, inactive	1–5
Storeroom	10

[a]From Kotschevar and Terrell (1977).

Temperature

In many of the newer facilities, both the dining and production areas are air-conditioned. Since the cost of air-conditioning may be prohibitive for some operations; thus a sensible compromise is an effective ventilating system. The objective is to provide a comfortable work environment with temperatures ranging from 75° to 80°F, with a relative humidity of 50%. For proper ventilation, there needs to be a balance of air exhaust and air input. The two methods most frequently used to determine exhaust air flow requirements are (1) the air change method, and (2) the fixed air velocity method (Myers 1979). The air change method is based on proper sizing of the exhaust system to provide a given number of air changes per hour. The theory is that if the air volume of a kitchen is exhausted every 2 or 3 minutes and replaced with fresh air, the kitchen temperature will be at a comfortable level and the air velocities will be high enough to remove cooking odors and vapors. The second method is based on maintaining a fixed air velocity across the entire area of the hood opening. Both methods require a balancing of the ventilation system so that fresh air is introduced in such a proportion as to maintain a slight negative pressure in the kitchen.

Noise

Careful attention should be given to possible noise that may be generated in the work areas as the various activities are performed. In planning work sections, consider isolating high-noise-level areas, such as dishwashing, can crushing, and areas where noise is generated from power motors. An office where concentration is required should not be located near a high-noise-level activity such as dishwashing. High noise levels that are generated from improper handling of equipment (banging), improper equipment maintenance (squeaking), loud talking, and loud music can be controlled through proper and continuous employee training. According to West et al. (1977), noise over 40 decibels is considered a nuisance and disturbing.

Equipment Use and Care

Major equipment used for production and service of food may be classified as noncooking, cooking, storage, serving, and cleaning.

Noncooking Equipment

The *food cutter* is a common noncooking piece of equipment. One of the most popular types of cutters is the table model commonly known as the *buffalo chopper* (Fig. 10-3). The equipment consists of a bowl that revolves rapidly around stationary blades. The blades and part of the bowl are covered with a hood for safety. The uncovered section of the bowl is used to add food, and continues to revolve until it is manually shut off. Limited amounts can be cut at one time in bowl sizes ranging from 8 to 14 in. in diameter. The cutter may be purchased with added features for slicing, grinding, cubing, and shredding. For cleaning, the cover lifts up and the bowl can be removed. All electric equipment should be disconnected before cleaning begins.

The *vertical cutter/mixer* (Fig. 10-4) is larger, faster, and more versatile than the buffalo chopper. This cutter is capable of mixing and chopping large quantities of vegetables such as cabbage and lettuce in approximately 30 seconds. For example, to make coleslaw, the cleaned cabbage quarters, carrots or other ingredients, including dressing, can all be put in at the same time. In less than a minute, the coleslaw is ready for portioning. The machine is also used for mixing doughs and batters, blending, emulsifying, and pureeing with similar speed. The equipment should be located near a water supply and drain. In cutting lettuce, water is added to prevent bruising. This equipment is often referred to as a cutter/mixer because of the many functions it can perform. The equipment is available in sizes ranging from 25 to 130 quarts.

Food slicers are available in a variety of models from the conventional to the fully electronically controlled machines. For simple slicing tasks, a conventional type with a rotating blade is sufficient. For large volumes or more complicated tasks, the angular automatic slicer may be more suitable. Where portion control is stressed, a slicer with a scale attached is available. This slicer will automatically stop when the predetermined amount has been sliced. The machine is equipped with a graduated dial or lever that adjusts the thickness desired. For cleaning, the power source must be disconnected and the blade control set at zero. All removable parts should be washed, rinsed, and sanitized, and the clean knife guard should be replaced as quickly as possible to cover the exposed blade. Stationary parts may be cleaned with a long brush and wiped with a clean, thick cloth.

Mixers are available as table or floor models (Fig. 10-5), with capacities ranging from 5 to 140 quarts. Two agitators are considered standard: (1) the beater, used for mashing, creaming, and blending, and (2) the whip for egg form, whipped cream, and frosting. Other agitators are available such as the dough hook, pastry knife, and sweet dough arm. With the use of a universal hub, many attachments are available for chopping, grinding, and slicing. The equipment should be cleaned following each use by removing the bowl and attachments and washing with a mild detergent. If an egg mixture or flour ingredient was used, soak the bowl and attachments in cold water before washing.

Peelers are often referred to as potato peelers because potatoes are the main item prepared with this machine. The equipment is used to peel potatoes and other root vegetables with minimum waste by the action of a revolving abrasive disk. Potatoes and other vegetables should be loaded into the peeler according to size to avoid an uneven removal of peelings. Waste will result if the peeler continues to run until all eyes are removed. The machine should be located near

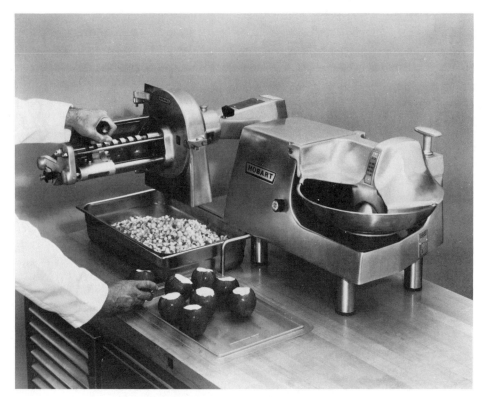

Figure 10-3. Food cutter. *From Hobart Corporation*

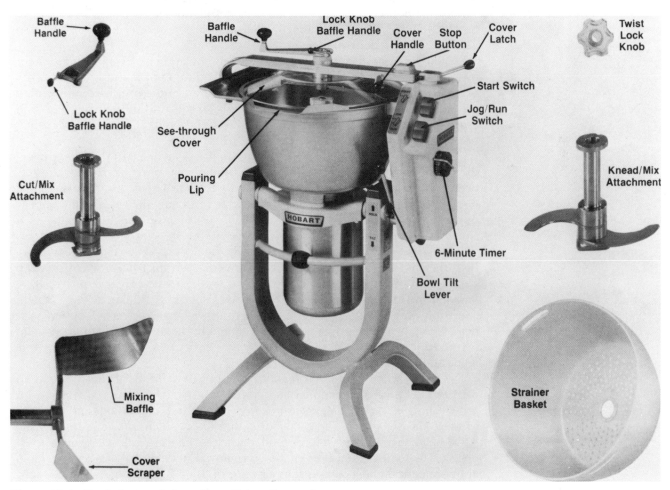

Figure 10-4. Vertical cutter/mixer. *From Hobart Corporation*

a water source and sink so that vegetables can be emptied directly into sink for further preparation. Vegetable peelers are available in tabletop models and floor models, ranging in capacity from 15 to 50 pounds. After each use, the inside of the peeler and disk should be flushed with water to remove all parings and sediment. Rinse and sanitize the peel tray and allow all parts to air-dry.

Cooking Equipment

Most of the equipment found in he kitchen falls into the broad category of cooking equipment.

Ovens are one of the most useful pieces of equipment in a medical foodservice operation. Ovens are used to bake cakes and pastries, to roast meats, to oven-broil or oven-bake portion cuts of meat, and to rethermalize food items at the point of service. The *conventional oven* is available in the single or deck variety. The single units are usually located under a range top, with a solid door and separate heat control. Deck ovens are stacked two to four decks high with separate heat controls for each oven. Compartment heights range from 8 in. for baking to 15 in. for roasting large cuts of meat. The *convection oven* (Fig. 10-6) operates by forced-air heating with a fan. Multiple racks are used in each deck to allow rapid circulation of air and even heat distribution to all food items. Convection ovens are designed to fully utilize all available space, thus more food can be cooked in a shorter period of time. When conventional recipes are used, the temperature should be adjusted by reducing the thermostat by approximately 30%. The convection oven is available in a variety of sizes and styles. In one variety, the bottom rack can be removed as a rollout to allow full racks of food to be rolled in and out at one time. Smaller units are used to rethermalize food in ward kitchen or floor pantry.

The convection combo (Fig. 10-7) is a combination convection and steamer oven. Combo cooking refers to the controlled addition of moisture to the cavity while cooking. This combination of fan-forced air and steam is recommended for baking, roasting, oven braising, steaming, reconstituting, wet roasting, and crusty baking. Optional features include cook and hold, and proofing capabilities. The unit is approved and listed by UL and NSF.

The *rotary* and *reel ovens* operate on similar principles. In the rotary oven, the hearth rotates around a vertical axis similar to a merry-go-round; the reel oven rotates in a fashion similar to a ferris wheel. For both types, there is a single door opening where food is loaded on the revolving shelves as they appear opposite the opening. The ovens are suitable for large-quantity baking in a single facility or in a commissary-type operation.

Microwave ovens are small units, used primarily to rethermalize food from both the chilled and frozen state. Food is cooked in microwave ovens by deep penetration of microwave energy into the food product. Heat is provided by magnetron tubes inserted in the ovens. The energy is similar to that used in television and radar. There are no thermostats. The degree of doneness is determined by the length of time food remains in the oven. When only one item is cooked in the oven, all of the microwave energy is concentrated on the one item, and thus cooking time is reduced.

Ovens should be cleaned regularly to prevent build-up of charred food on interior surfaces. Conventional and convection ovens may be purchased with self-cleaning elements. The *catalytic self-cleaning* oven is continuous and operates as the food is cooked. The catalytic coating of the oven interior prevents the build-up of grease and spilled food particles. The *pyrolytic self-cleaning* oven operates by setting a dial after all food is removed. When the dial is set, the doors are automatically locked and temperature of 1000°F burns off all grease and food spills. The oven must be wiped clean after the self-cleaning process is

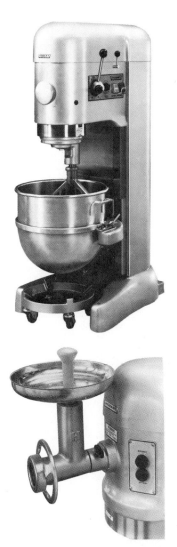

Figure 10-5. Floor model mixer (*above*) with chopping attachment (*below*). *From Hobart Corporation*

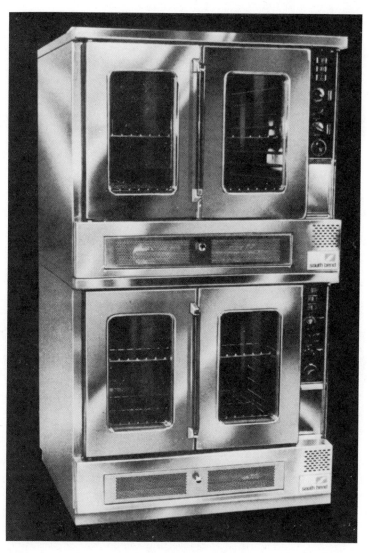

Figure 10-6. Double-deck convection oven. *From Hussman Foodservice Company, Southbend Division.*

completed. Microwave ovens should be wiped clean after each use with a cloth soaked in mild soapy water.

Steam equipment is clean, efficient, and fast. The use of steam equipment has practically eliminated the top-of-range cooking in medical foodservice operations. The *steam-jacketed kettle* is used for foods with a high liquid content or for food mixtures requiring a sauce or gravy. Models are available for mounting on a table, wall, or floor. The kettle may be full or two-thirds jacketed, and powered with direct steam or self-generated steam. The cooker/mixer models are equipped with an automatic stirrer, making it convenient to stir a large mass of food. Kettle sizes range from 10 quarts to 150 gallons. The cavity of the kettle may be shallow or deep. Cooking temperatures range from 215°F at 1-psi pressure to 298°F at 50 psi of pressure. The *trunion kettle* is so called because it is mounted on trunions. The most popular model is the small, tilting type (1 qt to 10 gal) mounted on stainless steel tables with a drain. The hand tilting mechanism may be locked in several positions. The *compartment steamer* is an upright type with one to four compartments. Food is placed in perforated or solid baskets, placed on compartment shelves, and cooked at 5 psi of pressure by direct contact of food with steam. The steamer is equipped with a safety valve for

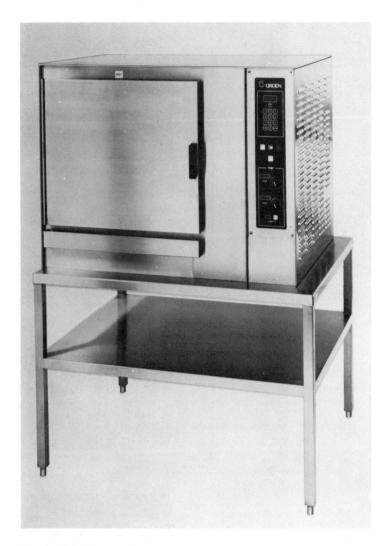

Figure 10-7. Convection combo oven. *From Groen, A Dover Industries Company*

the manual release of pressure, if necessary. The equipment is used primarily for large-batch cookery. Power may be direct steam or self-generated. *High-compression steamers* are smaller units, using at least 15 psi of pressure, and they cook food in a shorter period of time. The equipment is most suitable for small-batch cookery. A 2½ or 3-pound package of vegetables can be cooked in 2 to 3 minutes. Most units operate on self-generated steam. *Pressureless steamers* cook food by steam that is not under pressure. The unique feature of the pressureless steamer is that the door can be opened at any time during the cooking process. The chambers are practically void of air because of the continuous and rapid venting of the steam. The steam transfers heat to the food product by convection. Pressureless steam cooking is faster than other types and produces food of good color and flavor, even when more than one type of food is cooked in the same chamber. Steam equipment should be cleaned on a daily basis. A water source and drains should be provided near all steam equipment for ease of cleaning all compartments, shelves, and gaskets.

Gas or electric broilers are available in a variety of designs. The grid may be above or below the heat source and can be adjustable to various positions. The *char-broiler* is designed with grids above the heat source. As fat drips from the meat, it burns and produces a smoke flavor in the meat. Counter broilers vary in

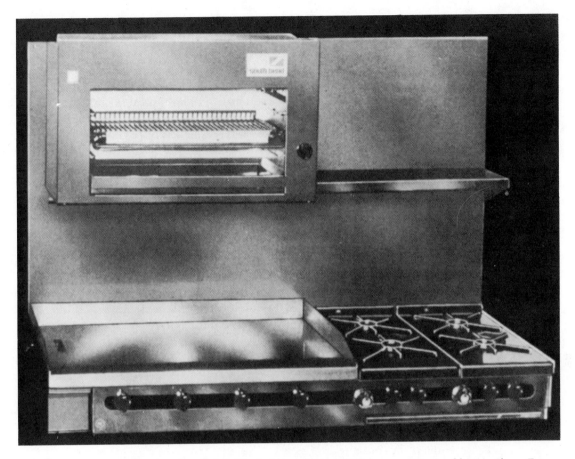

Figure 10-8. Infrared broiler (salamander)–griddle–range top cooking section. *From Hussman Foodservice Company Southbend Division*

grid sizes from 1.4 to 5.2 ft^2. An *infrared broiler* (salamander) is located above a cooking area, such as a range. As shown in Figure 10-8, the combined broiler, griddle, and open range top make a compact cooking section.

Griddles are constructed of one-piece cast iron or polished steel, with raised edges, and a grease trough. The equipment is frequently installed on a counter, back bar, or as part of a range top. Griddles are used for short-order cooking of individual portions of food. Griddles vary in thickness from ½ to 1 in. There is a minimum temperature drop when frozen foods are placed on the thicker griddles. There should be a separate thermostat for temperature control when different foods are cooked at the same time. Uniform heating surface and speed of temperature recovery are important features. It is necessary to season a new griddle prior to use and after each cleaning. To season, preheat griddle to 400°F and spread with a thin film of fat. Wipe off excess fat and repeat the procedure again, allowing the fat to remain on the griddle for 1 to 2 minutes. Wipe off excess fat. To clean the griddle, use pumice or griddle stone and grease, and rub while the equipment is warm. Rub with the grain of the metal, then wipe clean with a damp cloth. Do not use steel wool. Remove grease trough and clean with detergent and water. Dry thoroughly.

Fryers range from the small 11 × 11-in. table model to the automatic, continuous conveyor model. The *conventional fryer* may have single or multiple units and is suitable for single operations such as cooking fried foods on an occasional basis. The ease of cleaning and safety of the equipment are key features to check. Most fryers are equipped with automatic shutoff when the thermostat is not operating properly, or when the fat reaches a certain temperature. Other features include a cold zone for excess crumb accumulation, signal lights to indicate when heat is on, and controls to indicate when desired temperatures have been reached. Single-unit *pressure* fryers are available with safety lock covers. This equipment produces food that has a crisp outer surface, yet the flesh retains a desirable amount of moisture. The tightly sealed lid allows the moisture from the food to build up a steam pressure of 9 to 14 psi. Cooking time is considerably less than in conventional fryers. The entire cooking time for any food is within 10 minutes because the temperature of the fat is held between 310°F and 325°F. An *electronic computerized fryer* is also available. Food is automatically lowered with a push of a button. When the cooking cycle is completed, the basket is automatically raised to a drain position. The *conveyor fryer* is suitable for commissary or other systems where large quantities are produced at a given time. Automatic conveyor types are available in combination with a breading machine. The raw portions are put in at one end of the machine, the food is automatically breaded and fried, and the cooked portions are lowered into the serving pans.

For cleaning, fat should be filtered after each shift, or at the end of the day if the fryer is used continuously. Reusable fat should be refrigerated until ready for use. Commercial deep-fryer cleaning solutions can be used to remove carbon build-up.

The *braising pan* is one of the most versatile pieces of equipment used in medical foodservice operations. The pan is used as follows:

* As a griddle to prepare foods such as eggs, french toast, pancakes, and hash browned potatoes.
* As a fry pan to cook fish, chicken, doughnuts, and other foods requiring deep-fat cooking.
* As a kettle for stews, chili, chop suey, gravies, sauces, and most combination dishes.
* As a steamer for vegetables. As shown in Figure 10-9, the pan can be converted into a pressureless atmospheric steam cooker. The lightweight insert pans are easily removed for stacked storage. The complete unit includes pans, covers, and snap-on handles for removing pans.
* As an oven for roasting meat and poultry, by placing products on wire racks. With the cover closed, the cooking action is same as conventional oven.

The braising pan is equipped with ⅜-in.-thick stainless steel–clad plate to provide an even-temperature cooking surface. Thermostatic control enables the pan to shut off automatically when the desired temperature is reached and to turn on when the product temperature falls below the desired setting. The temperature range of 100°F to 425°F, flat surface, and even cooking capacity provide unlimited cooking performance. The tilting mechanism eliminates lifting, transferring, and the use of extra utensils. The unit is available in both the electric or gas model. Electric model should be UL and NSF approved; gas model should be AGA Design Certified.

Cold-Storage Equipment

Cold-storage equipment may be classified according to temperature: medium or regular temperature at 35°F to 45°F; low temperature at 0°F; and rapid freeze at −20°F to −40°F. Medium-temperature cold storage include refrigerators such as the large walk-in, reach-in, reach-through, under-the-counter, roll-in, refrigerated counters, and thaw refrigerators.

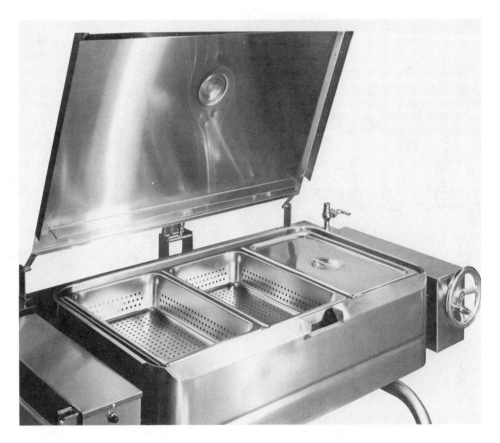

Figure 10-9. Tilting braising pan with steamer insert assembly. *From Groen, a Dover Industries Company*

Walk-in refrigerators are used for bulk storage of food, usually in case lots. Separate walk-ins are used for produce, dairy foods, and prepared foods requiring no further heat treatment. Features should include a door latch with an interior safety release, and easy-to-read thermometer placed outside the door, and adequate insulation. Added features may include a glass-paneled door and an alarm to indicate when the refrigerator is malfunctioning. The equipment should be approved by NSF.

Reach-in refrigerators (Fig. 10-10) provide greater flexibility in terms of location and shelving. Reach-in refrigerators are located in the various production and service areas, and in ward pantries. Adjustable shelving is available to allow for various heights of prepared food stored on trays. The *reach-through refrigerator* is located between production and service areas to allow prepared foods to be put in from one side and removed from the other side. The dual door openings prevent excessive walking by service personnel in replenishing the serving line. *Under-the-counter refrigerators* are convenient when located underneath a high-compression steamer, microwave oven, or service counter. These units are frequently referred to as refrigerated drawers. The major disadvantage of under-the-counter refrigeration is that the height is not convenient for cleaning. *Roll-in refrigerators* (Fig. 10-11) are convenient for loading and transporting multiple trays of food at one time. The roll-in units may be purchased to fit into convection oven or to roll into a refrigerator in another location. *Refrigerated counters* are used in the service areas for salads and desserts requiring refrigeration. It is considered more sanitary to use these units than crushed ice, which may come into contact with food products. *Thaw refrigerators*

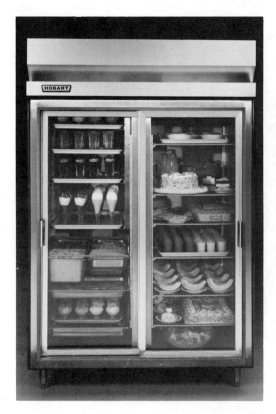

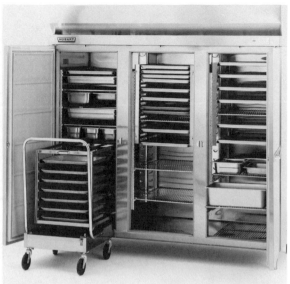

Figure 10-11. Reach-in refrigerator with roll-in unit. *From Hobart Corporation*

Figure 10-10. Reach-in refrigerator with full-length glass door. *From Hobart Corporation*

operate under controlled humidity and temperature to protect food products from bacteria-conducing temperatures while thawing. The thaw refrigerators reduce thawing time from the 2 to 3 days it normally takes to approximately 12 hours. The controlled environment thaws without the use of temperatures over 45°F. When thawing is completed, the refrigeration system automatically changes over to standard refrigerator operation.

Low-temperature storage equipment is frequently referred to as freezers. The more appropriate label should be frozen-food holding cabinets, since freezers are not used to freeze food but to hold food that is already frozen. For institutional use, low-temperature equipment is available in walk-in and reach-in types. The walk-ins may be installed so that the frozen food unit opens into a medium-temperature section, instead of directly into the production area. Low-temperature walk-ins may also be installed outside the building.

Rapid-freeze equipment is used to freeze food quickly and efficiently. Although there are a number of freezing methods used by commercial manufacturers, *blast freezing* is most often associated with the freeze-and-serve production in medical foodservice operations. Food is quickly frozen to temperatures of −40°F, which is an acceptable level for most food products. Quality loss can occur if food is overfrozen and becomes brittle. In blast freezing, food travels on a conveyor belt through a freezing chamber in which air circulates at high velocity by a mechanical unit. A Freon-type refrigerant is used. Other types of rapid-freeze equipment have not been used as extensively or with the efficiency that the blast-freeze type has. Nitrogen freezing was planned for the Walter Reed Army Medical Center in Washington, but had to be canceled because of mechanical problems (Riggs 1981). Initially, a large-capacity cryogenic freezer was intended to handle rapid freezing for the center's ready-food production system. Problems arose when attempts were made to pipe liquid nitrogen, which was stored a considerable distance away, to the freezer. It was found that the temperature at the freezer was not low enough to meet freezing requirements. The operation was converted to blast freezing.

Cleaning and Sanitizing Equipment

Dishwashers are available in single- and multiple-tank varieties. The heat may be supplied by steam, gas, or electricity. The *single-tank dishwasher* is used in small operations serving 100 meals or less. Dishes are prerinsed, loaded into racks, and manually pushed through the machine. Only one tray of dishes is washed at a time, taking approximately 2 minutes for the complete wash-and-rinse cycle. The single-tank unit is also available with a conveyor belt that moves racks through the machine automatically. Doors are used on each end of the manually operated unit; curtains are used on the conveyor type, which makes for faster operation. Multiple-tank dishwashers are available in the rack or flight type. In the *multiple-tank rack machine,* dishes are prewashed by hand or a prewash unit can be specified. Scraped dishes are arranged in racks and placed on a conveyor belt, which moves the trays through the wash, rinse, and final rinse cycle. With the increased length of the machine, there is less spillover of water from one tank to another. There should be a rack-return section so that racks are never placed on the floor. The *flight dishwashing machine* (Fig. 10-12) is designed to be used with or without racks. The distinguishing feature of the flight-type machine is that dishes of various sizes can be placed directly on conveyor drive prongs. Since silverware, cups, and glasses must be racked for washing, it is both practical and economical to select a machine that can accommodate both operations. The *rack-a-round dish machine,* shown in Figure 10-13, provides added versatility for dishwashing. The machine is a combination of the rack and flight types, featuring continuous operation. Desirable specifications of the dish machine include a soak or prewash sink with spray-rinse hose, a sorting table, a

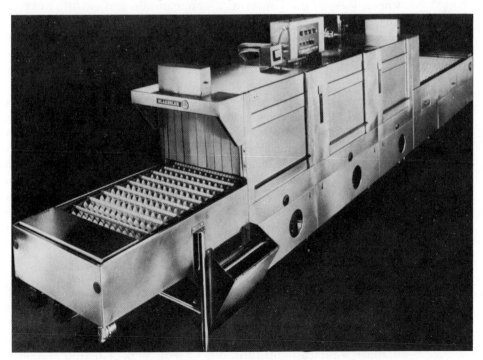

Figure 10-12. Flight-type dishwasher. *From Blakeslee, Division of Blako, Inc.*

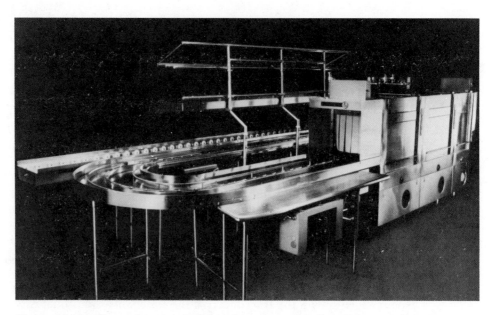

Figure 10-13. The rack-a-round dishwasher. *From Blakeslee, Division of Blako, Inc.*

slanted shelf above the loading section, and a booster heater to ensure 180°F water temperature for final rinse. All machines should be NSF approved. An *automatic tray unloader* is available and is considered practical for operations using disposable serviceware. The unit can be a separate tray-washing machine, or can be designed to wash dishes and other silverware then convert to a tray washing machine. To operate the automatic tray unloader, place the empty tray cart at unloading end of dishwasher. As trays are deposited from dishwasher onto the self-leveling tray cart, a tray carrier will descend and engage an actuating lever or limit switch that stops the conveyor when the cart is full. When the full cart is wheeled away, the conveyor is automatically turned off, to be automatically turned on when the next tray cart is wheeled into position.

Low-temperature dishwashers are available with minimum temperature of 120°F for both wash and rinse. A chemical sanitizer, chlorine or iodine base, is used instead of the high temperature of 180°F for final rinse. Federal sanitation guidelines require a wash temperature of 150°F to 165°F, and a final rinse temperature of 180°F. The low-temperature machines with sanitizers were introduced as energy savers. Foodservice directors should check state and local sanitation codes before purchasing this type of dishwashing machine. One manufacturer has developed dishwashing machines that can operate within a wide range of washing and rinsing temperatures, with or without chemical sanitizers. The ability to vary the wash and rinse temperatures from 120°F to 180°F provides flexibility for the operation. There is some concern that detergents are ineffective in removing animal fat from serviceware at temperatures below 130°F, and there may be problems with the use of chemical agents on silverware and pewter. Machines with dual operation provide flexibility for the foodservice director in deciding when to use a chemical or a 180°F hot-water rinse.

Dishwashing machines should be cleaned after each use. The strainer baskets should be carefully removed to avoid spills into the tank and cleaned of all food particles. Drain all water and rinse the interior with a hose. If the water is hard, a deliming agent may be required periodically. Rinse and air-dry curtains Remove washarms and flush out all sediments. Turn off the heat source and leave the side doors up so that machine can air-dry.

Pot, pan, and utensil washing is accomplished manually in small operations. A three-compartment sink is required for wash, rinse, and final rinse. A chemical sanitizer is used in the final rinse sink with a minimum water temperature of 75°F. Drain boards are required and a garbage disposal is desirable. *Pot and pan washing machines* may be used for large facilities.

Energy Management Related to Equipment Planning

Energy conservation should not compromise effective and efficient operation. Consider the following suggestions in terms of both energy savings and high quality standards.

1. Avoid sliding glass doors in refrigeration equipment, if possible. The slide clearance does not allow a good, tight seal.
2. Use full loads with dishwashers so that the machine can operate at full capacity. An automatic shutoff control that automatically turns the machine off when no dishes are being washed may be a sound investment.
3. Use a rinse-saver device in the final rinse on flight-type machines to prevent the use of unnecessary 180°F water when there are no dishes to be rinsed.
4. Locate refrigerators and freezers away from heat-producing appliances.
5. On dish machines with gas heat, adjust the burners and gas pressure for maximum efficiency and install a gas-pressure-reducing valve.
6. Select correct size for all equipment, insofar as possible. Unused space that must be heated is considered a waste.
7. Specify see-through doors on refrigerators to prevent constant opening for inspection.
8. Compare the use of gas versus electricity for cooking equipment. Gas is considered more efficient and less costly to operate.
9. Consider a low-temperature dishwashing system, using a sanitizing solution. The system reduces the amount of hot water required for the final rinse; however, extra funds are spent for the sanitizing solution. Check local codes on use of low-temperature system.
10. Specify electronic ignition on gas equipment instead of a pilot light.
11. Energy demand is increased when all lights and all equipment are turned on at the same time. Stagger start-up times. Discourage cooks from turning on all equipment at the beginning of shift.
12. Use fluorescent lighting rather than incandescent. Avoid frequent turning on and off of incandescent lights. Leave fluorescent lights on unless they are to be off for 15 minutes or more.
13. Install automatic light controls in walk-in refrigerators and freezers.
14. Each compartment of a warming or serving table should be controlled by a separate thermostat.
15. Thick oven installation conserves energy. Specify 4 in. or more insulation.
16. The deck oven with bottom rack near the floor may constitute a waste of oven space, because employees will use the more convenient waist-high cavity.

17. Convection ovens bake at temperatures 20°F to 50°F lower and are 10% to 15% faster than deck ovens.
18. Establish an ongoing employee training program for proper use and care of equipment.

A gas convection oven introduced in the 1980s has a specially inserted tube that captures hot air that is normally vented immediately. These ovens are converted to direct-fired operations, eliminating the need for heavy, heat-absorbing parts used in direct-fired convection ovens. The new ovens use an input of only 60,000 British thermal units (Btu) and do the same job as gas convection ovens requiring 100,000 Btu.[1]

Manufacturers of deep-fat fryers offer the following developments in equipment design: (1) a built-in filter that enables the operator to strain the frying oil in a matter of seconds, at any time during the day; (2) an intermittent ignition device that eliminates the necessity for a standing gas pilot; (3) built-in computerized time and temperature controls that eliminate the guesswork, guarantee precise and consistent cooking of fried food, and minimize energy consumption; (4) fryers with a deep-cold zone that places food sediment out of the cooking temperature range to prolong fat life; and (5) a modified pressure fryer that increases efficiency by covering the heating well, thus retaining heat that might otherwise be lost.

New, more efficient gas griddles offer grooved surfaces for grid-marked meats, or the flexibility of a smooth surface when needed. Some new gas griddles are zoned to permit partial shutdown in slow periods and to provide for cooking more than one kind of food at a time.

The Gas Research Institute (8600 W. Bryn Mawr, Chicago, IL 60631), formed in 1977, works with gas utilities equipment manufacturers, the Department of Energy, and others to improve new gas equipment and to devise new concepts.

Safety Features of Equipment Planning

Safety is an important aspect of the manager's job. The following list will help ensure safety in the kitchen.

1. Use mobile carts with wheel locks for equipment that must be moved to various locations within the department.
2. Plan for adequate electrical outlets. Avoid use of extension cords that may result in accidents if people trip over them.
3. Consider how stationary equipment can be operated and cleaned in the same location.
4. Make sure all electric equipment is grounded.
5. Install plastic covers over light switches near walk-in refrigerators and freezers.
6. Arrange equipment so that doors do not open into traffic aisles.
7. If swinging doors are used, one should be clearly labeled "in" and one labeled "out."
8. Electric equipment should have signal light o indicate when electricity is on or off.

---

[1] A Btu is a unit for measuring heat. It is the amount of heat necessary to raise the temperature of a pound of water 1 degree Fahrenheit.

Computers in Facility Design

The foodservice industry has been feeling the impact of the computer as an effective device for equipment planning and kitchen design since the 1960s. At present, the initial investment can cost anywhere from $100,000 to more than $2 million for a top-of-the-line custom-designed system. The cost is prohibitive to most kitchen design and consulting firms. Although the price is high, the possibilities are endless for using this tool in the foodservice industry. Since the cost factors in most computer equipment and software are decreasing, we may look forward to major cost breakthroughs in the future.

Using the computer, a draftsman can sit at the video display terminal and enter a command to see floor plans of kitchens designed in the past. In seconds the entire layout is on the screen with all equipment and utility specifications. Using a new fiber optic pen, the plan can be rearranged and adapted for a new project. A steam table, mixer, or work station can be touched with the pen and moved anywhere on the screen. Then, through use of the keyboard, a wall can be moved and a room changed in dimensions. While these changes are being initiated, the computer will automatically alter and adjust the layouts for plumbing and electrical specifications to match the new arrangement. The system just described is called Computer Aided Design and Drafting (CADD). As reported in *Restaurant Hospitality* (DeLuca 1982), it is very popular among kitchen design consultants and architects.

One of the most time-efficient advantages of CADD is its ability to do the tedious job of drawing and changing dimensions and specifications of equipment and layout, thus allowing the draftsman time to think about and manipulate the design. He or she merely types in a number and a piece of equipment appears on the screen. The biggest disadvantage to a program such as CADD is economic. Although the product ensures better quality control and a shorter response time, the expense of the computer is such that a cost savings to the operator is not realized. Even though CADD is more convenient and efficient to use, it is just a tool and does not save money in the process. Until large decreases in equipment and programming take place, CADD will only be cost-efficient on the largest projects.

A computer has many other adaptations for kitchen planning. As reported by Wilkinson (1969), it can be programmed, for example, to produce a layout that minimizes the physical movements of employees between various pieces of equipment in the preparation of menu items. Such a program is based on menu items to be produced, production sequence for each item, frequency of production, and the distance between the pieces of equipment.

A foodservice manager might also consider using a computer to organize the maintenance of equipment, sanitation, repair, and service functions. A computer program with directions for use, repair, and maintenance of all equipment in a foodservice operation could be established. Records of inspections and repairs could be entered and printouts of information made available to the maintenance department when needed. Another program explaining operating instructions and the care and use of equipment could be made available to foodservice employees. Research on establishing methods for use of computers in sanitation are being investigated.

Agencies Related to Equipment Management

Familiarity with regulatory agencies and laws related to equipment management is a responsibility of the foodservice director. Basic knowledge of the following agencies and organizations can greatly enhance communications, both internally and externally, throughout the planning stages.

National Sanitation Foundation (NSF)

The NSF is an independent non-profit organization dedicated to the improvement of public health and the environment. Activities of the foundation include (1) providing liaison between industry, the public health professions, and the general public; (2) conducting research and establishing standards on health related equipment, processes, products, and services; (3) disseminating research results; and (4) issuing official NSF seals for display on equipment and products tested and found to meet NSF standards. Each standard is a detailed statement of what the equipment or product must be, or must do, in order to protect the public health. A booklet is published periodically which lists all manufacturers and their equipment having NSF approval.[2]

Occupational Safety and Health Administration (OSHA)

The purpose of the Occupational Safety and Health Act of 1970 is to ensure safe and healthful working conditions. The law, which created OSHA, provides that each employer has the basic duty to furnish employees a place of employment that is free from recognized hazards that may cause death or serious physical harm (Michigan Department of Labor 1978). A specific standard, relating to facility planning and use, is that aisles and passageways must be kept clear and in good repair, with no obstruction across or in aisles that could create a hazard. (U.S. Department of Labor 1972). The OSHA standards are carried out through the Department of Labor in each state. For compliance and other information, contact the OSHA division at the state level.

Underwriters Laboratories (UL)

Underwriters Laboratories is concerned with safety of electrical equipment and is operated similar to NSF in that participation is on a voluntary basis. Products that have been tested and found to meet the rigid safety standards are authorized to use the UL seal.[3] Each product is tested and approved for use and certified to be safe from electrical shock, hazard, and fire.

Other Professional Organizations and Agencies

In addition, the foodservice director should be familiar with federal, state, and local codes and ordinances for assistance in planning for a safe and sanitary workplace. Other helpful sources include professional organizations and utility companies such as:

1. American Hospital Association
2. American National Standards Institute (Plumbing codes)

---

[2]For additional information on specific equipment or for an NSF publication list, write NSF Testing Laboratory, Inc., P.O. Box 1468, Ann Arbor, MI 48106.
[3]For additional information, write to Underwriters Laboratories, 207 East Ohio Street, Chicago, IL 60611.

3. American Society of Mechanical Engineers
4. American National Safety Institute
5. National and Local Restaurant Associations
6. National Fire Protection Association
7. National Safety Council
8. American Gas Association
9. Electric utility companies

References

American Hospital Association. (1977). *Guidelines for Selecting a Consultant in Food Service Equipment and Layout for Hospitals and Related Health Care Institutions*. Chicago: AHA.

Avery, A. C. (1979). Principles of Kitchen Design. In *Commercial Kitchens*, J. R. Myers, ed. Arlington, VA: American Gas Association.

Avery, A. C. (1978). Writing Specifications. *Food Mgt. 13*(3), 1–42, 66, 68

Avery, A. C. (n.d.). Human *Engineering in Kitchen Design*. Washington, DC: U.S. Department of the Navy, Bureau of Supplies and Accounts.

De Luca, M. (1982). Designing with Computers. *Restaur. Hospitality, 66*(2), 54.

Hall, L. R. (1982). Equipment Comparison. *Stokes Report, 2*(10). Atlanta: Judy Ford Stokes & Associates.

Harris, R. D. (1981). The How's and Why's of Preparing Renovation Specifications. *Hosp. Top. 59*(4).

Kotschevar, L. H, and Terrell, M. E. (1977). *Food Service Planning Layout and Equipment*. New York: Wiley.

Michigan Department of Labor. (1978). *Employer and Employee Responsibilities and Rights, Michigan Occupational Safety and Health Act 154 of P.A.* Lansing: Bureau of Safety and Regulations.

Myers, J. R. (1979). *Commercial Kitchens*. Arlington, VA: American Gas Association.

Riggs, S. (1981). How Well Has Walter Reed's "Revolutionary" Food System Worked? *Restaur. Inst. 88*(1), June 1, 73–75.

U.S. Department of Health and Human Services. (1976). *Sanitation Manual*. Washington, DC: USDHHS.

U.S. Department of Labor. (1972). *Recordkeeping Requirements Under the Williams-Steiger Occupational Safety and Health Act of 1970*. Washington, DC: USDL, Occupational Safety and Health Administration.

West, B. B., Wood, L., Harger, V. F., and Shugart, G. S. (1977). *Food Service in Institutions*. New York: Wiley.

Wilkinson, J. (1969). The Finishing Kitchen. Chicago: *Inst. Mag.*

Chapter 11

Subsystem for Food Purchasing

Food purchasing is based on the planned menu. The process is complex and diverse, requiring a high degree of proficiency on the part of the buyer. The most important factor is that the desired product must be purchased at the right time, in the right amount, and at the level of quality specified.

Organization of the Purchasing Unit

The actual purchasing functions may be performed in-house by the foodservice director or a designee, or the purchasing may be done by the purchasing agent who is responsible not only for food and supplies required by the foodservice department but also for purchasing needs of all other departments within the organization. Regardless of who is responsible for the actual purchasing, the foodservice director is responsible for the end product and therefore must be able to project needs of the department in an organized, efficient, and effective manner. The foodservice director needs a basic knowledge of the following:

- Food quality
- Food processing
- Food grades and yields
- Food availability and marketing conditions
- Purchasing systems
- Product testing and evaluation
- Specification writing
- Ordering, receiving, and storing techniques
- Production and service techniques

In addition to the required basic knowledge, the individual responsible for purchasing must have time available for researching new products, monitoring storeroom procedures, making visits to the market places and food plants, conferring with salespersons and purveyors, and soliciting and analyzing bids. Considering the varied and complex duties, it may be advantageous to have this purchasing function performed by a central agent.

Foodservice directors have complained that central purchasing agents are not familiar with the uniqueness of medical foodservice operations and therefore are not sensitive to their needs. Establishing lines of authority and effective two-way communication can do much to minimize the problem. The amount of authority and how it is used by the purchasing agent affect the relationship with the using departments. Friction may develop when too much or too little authority is given or if the lines of authority are not clear to all concerned. Effective communication implies that the foodservice director will supply the necessary information to the purchasing agent so that intelligent purchasing decisions can be made and that the purchasing agent will provide prompt feedback to the foodservice director on decisions made. For both in-house and central purchasing, all policies and procedures should have administrative approval as part of the internal communication network. The external communication network involves relationships with food purveyors and other food-related professional organizations and agencies. When the purchasing function is done by central purchasing, the entire process should be included—from ordering through inventory. The central storeroom may be in a remote area, with only a small daily storeroom in the foodservice department. Feedback from central stores on daily deliveries and issues should be prompt so that the foodservice director can be aware of food cost at all times.

Qualifications of the Purchasing Agent

The individual responsible for purchasing wields a great deal of power in view of the amount of money involved and the contacts made within and outside of the organization. How the power and contacts are used to fulfill the responsibilities of the position will affect not only the foodservice department but the image of the entire organization. Qualification for purchasing agent should include, but not be limited to the following: (1) educational background, (2) business background, and (3) personal characteristics (Swindler 1978).

Educational Background

The educational background of purchasing agents may be as varied as the number of positions. There are few college or university programs that prepare students for the highly specialized and unique job of purchasing for a medical facility. The responsible individual should have general knowledge of medical terminology and specific knowledge about each of the departments, within the medical facility, with regard to purchasing needs. Because of the accounting and other business activities associated with purchasing, students with a background in business administration are often appointed to the position. A program offered through a school of business administration may or may not offer any courses dealing with food purchasing and other related needs of a foodservice department. Faced with this situation, it is imperative that the foodservice director is able to communicate departmental needs in a clear and concise manner in order to obtain desired results.

The purchasing agent is responsible for:

1. Soliciting and awarding bids and contracts.
2. Placing purchase orders.
3. Supervising personnel in receiving, storing, and issuing food and other products.
4. Establishing and maintaining an inventory system.
5. Training staff in accounting and cost procedures.
6. Conducting research and testing of new products.
7. Keeping up-to-date on changing economic and political conditions.
8. Maintaining open lines of communication, both internal and external.

The educational process is ongoing so as to enable the purchasing agent to acquire and maintain current information—essential for intelligent decision making.

Business Experience

In addition to accounting and budgeting, any business experience relating to medical operations will be helpful to the purchasing agent. The individual must be thoroughly acquainted with the needs of the departments involved and the marketing conditions. In areas where the individual may be deficient, extra effort must be expended to learn as much about specific needs as possible whether through formal courses, on-the-job training, seminars, lectures, or other sources.

Personal Characteristics

The purchasing agent's personal characteristics are equally as important as technical knowledge and skills. The following traits are considered most relevant.

1. *Cooperation.* The individual must be able to work in a cooperative manner with all department heads, higher administration, and subordinates.

2. *Initiative.* He or she must display initiative and creativity in searching for new products and alternate supply sources.

3. *Tact.* The person must be tactful in suggesting substitutes that will perform the same function without antagonizing the department involved or the relationship with the purveyor.

4. *Dependability.* The other departments must be able to rely on products or items being available at the time needed and in the correct quantity and quality.

5. *Industriousness.* The agent must be able to seek out information that will assist him or her in doing a better job, whether the knowledge is acquired from purveyors, from reading marketing newspapers and product brochures, from attending conventions and seminars, or from visiting manufacturing plants and purveyor sites.

6. *Accuracy.* The purchasing agent must give attention to detail of the job such as reading and understanding all contracts and warranties. Neglect of such day-to-day routines can be costly.

7. *Human relations.* He or she must be able to adjust to a wide variety of personalities both inside and outside of the organization. The ability to establish close working relationships without being unduly influenced is an asset.

8. *Ethical standards.* The exposure to opportunities for dishonest or unethical personal gain is prevalent. The individual must have a sense of what is right and wrong. He or she should resist gifts, kickbacks, or bribery, which may eventually affect the quality of products received, the cost of products, or business relationships with purveyors as a result of obligations on the part of the buyer. The purchasing agent must avoid any appearances of unethical dealing, even refusing small gifts at Christmas or other times during the year. A common practice of asking purveyors to sponsor or contribute to various departmental activities may obligate the buyer to favor one purveyor over another. Gifts or discount coupons, offered for doing business with the purveyor, should be for departmental use only.

To summarize, the personal characteristics of the buyer should ensure that none of his or her actions tarnishes the reputation or image of the individual buyer or the organization.

Purchasing Systems

The most common types of purchasing systems may be classified as either *one-stop buying* or *competitive buying.*

___ One-Stop Buying _____

In one-stop buying, the purchaser orders all products or items from one purveyor. The one-stop purveyor may handle products for more than 100 distributors. The combining of products results in a reduced number of orders to place, reduced number of deliveries, and reduced number of bills to pay by the purchasing department. One-stop companies spend an exorbitant amount of time and effort in marketing their services. For example, one such company provides menu planning, marketing data, financial planning, inventory control techniques, merchandising ideas, and technical problem solving.

The one-stop buying system is frequently used by small operations to eliminate cost involved for small deliveries from several purveyors. The one big disadvantage to using this type of system is that the buyer has no control over the prices paid since there is no competition.

___ Competitive Buying _____

In competitive buying, more than one purveyor has an opportunity to bid on the desired products or items. The competition may be on an informal or formal basis. Informal bidding is less complicated than formal bidding and also requires less time. Informal bidding may take place by telephone or be processed through the mail. In *telephone bidding*, the buyer lists all items on a sheet with space for item needed, item description, amount needed, delivery date, and price quotations from selected purveyors. As shown in Figure 11–1, emphasis is put on a full description of the item needed so that purveyors will know exactly what the buyer wants, plus it ensures that all purveyors are bidding on the same item. The amount needed is important because it may affect the unit cost, depending on the size of the order. The delivery date will let the purveyor determine whether the time request can be met. The bid is awarded to the bidder with the lowest price quote. To provide a written record of the transaction, a purchase order is mailed to the purveyor or is picked up by a sales representative. It is considered poor business practice to place the order by telephone except in emergency situations.

For *informal bidding by mail,* specification sheets and a cover sheet of instruction are mailed to selected purveyors. The price quotations are returned by mail, according to a prescribed time schedule. The bids are opened and evaluated, and items are assigned to the lowest bidder. Mail bidding is more time-consuming than telephone bidding and can be used only if prices remain stable for the period of time required to complete the transaction.

Formal bidding is more complex. An invitation to bid is mailed to selected purveyors. If completed and returned by the bidder, it is considered a legal, binding contract. All pertinent information relating to bid opening date, delivery date, payment terms, how bids are awarded, nonconformance, legal requirements, and liability and other general information are mailed to all bidders. Specifications, with detailed information on each item, are also mailed to the bidders. Bids are returned in sealed unmarked envelopes to protect the identity of the bidder until purchasing decisions are made. Formal bidding is usually reserved for stable items that can be stored over a period of time. If larger quantities are purchased and stored by the purveyor, then the additional cost for storage must be considered. Because of prevailing economic conditions and other factors that may affect cost (weather, union strikes, etc.), most long-term bids are set up on a fluctuating price basis.

Contract bidding is a formal, competitive type of purchasing. In this system, the contract is frequently awarded for a period of 3 to 12 months for items such as bread, coffee, milk, ice cream, and similar foods that are used on a daily basis. The contract terms usually stipulate the purchasing of a minimum amount for a

Quantity	Food Item Description	Delivery Date	Quotations		
			1	2	3
100 lb	Roast—Ready Rib no. 103	10-10-89	1.70	1.75	1.72

Figure 11-1. Telephone quotation sheet.

stated period. The daily or weekly orders may vary, but the total amount for a given period should equal or exceed the minimum bid.

__ Group Purchasing _____

More and more independent foodservice operations are participating in cooperative buying ventures as a means of reducing food cost. Many hospital administrators involved in group purchasing today would not have given the idea a serious thought 10 years ago. The fear of losing their autonomy and having to accept foods of a lower quality were the main reasons why some foodservice directors were reluctant to join purchasing groups. To combat such fears, most purchasing groups have formed committees with representatives from each participating facility. Committee members are responsible for research, testing, and evaluating products prior to purchasing arrangements. When a consensus has been reached on a particular product or item, specifications are written and submitted to selected purveyors as part of the bidding process. Each participating facility is responsible for placing its own purchase order. The product or item is delivered directly to the individual facility or to central warehousing for storage. With central storage, there is a reduced delivery charge since the purveyor can make use of "drop shipments." Each participating facility orders and picks up from central storage as needed.

One of the problems associated with group purchasing is that a purveyor may be awarded a contract based on expected volume and later find that the participating hospitals are not ordering in the amounts expected—possibly because of multiple membership by some facilities. Instead of membership in only one group purchasing organization, the hospital may belong to several groups and utilize the service of the group offering the lowest price. As reported by Richards (1982), a recent trend in group purchasing is the change to committed-volume contracting, which provides a quantity guarantee for the purveyor. The price quotation is based on guaranteed volume.

The latest development in group purchasing is the banding together of purchasing groups into what are known as *supergroups*. Although the supergroups were formed primarily to establish a capital equipment purchasing program, food purchasing groups are expected to follow the trend. The rationale behind this trend is that the higher the volume, the more negotiating power is afforded the purchasing group.

The advantages of group purchasing far outweigh any disadvantages that may be associated with the purchasing system. In addition to the savings, there is the sharing of information on food quality, processing techniques, marketing conditions, and availability of new products. The disadvantage may be that of standardization. However, hospitals can and do exert their individuality by purchasing some items outside of the group purchasing program. Items with the highest participation rate are canned fruits and vegetables, milk products, bread, paper supplies, and other disposables.

Specifications

A specification is a written statement in clear, concise terminology that states what is desired by the buyer. For a food product, the specification refers to the quality, size, and other factors needed to obtain the right item. The advantages of well-written specifications are as follows:

1. Indicates that the buyer has given careful consideration to departmental needs.
2. Ensures compliance with facility and departmental standards of quality.
3. Eliminates misunderstandings between the purveyor and purchasing agent on exactly what is required.
4. Eliminates misunderstandings between the purchasing agent and the department making the request.
5. Serves as a cross-check for the receiving clerk.
6. Lowers bid prices because purveyors know exactly what is desired and what they are bidding on.

Specifications are not passed from one institution to another since they reflect the quality standards for a specific operation. The standards set by the federal government and other marketing agencies should be complied with, but they should be tailored to specific needs. Deviations from standard specifications can be costly and should not be practiced without valid justification. An exception is when specifications are written for convenience-modified diet foods to meet caloric, nutrient, or other restrictions.

Types of Specifications

Specifications may be classified as general or specific. *General specifications* refer to arrangements with purveyors on such factors as method of payment, billing procedures, submission of samples for testing, failure to perform, rejection of products, delivery and receiving policies, and other pertinent information. General specifications are given to all purveyors doing business with the organization, including both food and supplies. The issues of billing and method of payment are crucial if the organization is to maintain a good credit rating with purveyors. Most purveyors will allow bills to be paid within 30 days. Even large accounts may be dropped if bills are not paid in a timely manner.

Specific specifications refer to one particular product or a group of related products. Exact descriptions are used to specify the desired product for such factors as grade, size, thickness, and count. Specifications are sent only to the purveyors providing a particular item. The following information should be included in each specification:

- The common, trade, standard of identity, or other name of the item.
- The quality desired, using government, trade, or other grades, brand or other standards.
- The marketing form, such as fresh, chilled, frozen, canned, or dried.
- The weight, thickness, count or size of the item, such as minimum and maximum weight range, number of units per case, crate, or carton.
- The degree of ripeness.
- The unit on which price is quoted (e.g., 50-lb sack, six no. 10 cans).
- Additional statements needed for clarity of exact item desired, such as Blue Lake, Michigan, or Midwest green beans.

Specifications should be written for all food items purchased, but especially for those items that comprise a large percentage of the food dollar. It is estimated that approximately 50% of the food dollar is spent on meat, seafood, and poultry. Fruits, vegetables, and dairy products are the next highest in cost. Therefore, the following discussion will cover specification writing for meats, poultry and eggs, seafoods, processed fruits and vegetables, and fresh fruits and vegetables.

___ Meat Specifications _____

The purchaser needs a knowledge of meat source and classification in order to determine the degree of tenderness, juiciness, flavor, yield, and other advantages or disadvantages of buying various cuts.

A knowledge of basic carcass structure is especially helpful when it is necessary to substitute one cut for another in the preparation of a food item. To know that the bottom round of beef (inside round) is less tender than the top round (outside round) may mean the difference between patient satisfaction and complaints. In reviewing the charts for beef (Fig. 11-2), veal (Fig. 11-3), lamb (Fig. 11-4), and pork (Fig. 11-5), it is well to remember that there is a difference in the color of the meat and the size of the cut, but the muscle and bone structure of the four meats are alike.

Many of the problems associated with meat specification have been eliminated with the development of national standards. Meat standardization began with the establishment of a voluntary "acceptance service" by the U.S. Department of Agriculture (USDA). The acceptance service, which certified meat grades and other characteristics, was paid for by the buyer. Each institution using the government service wrote its own specifications. During the mid-1950s a set of uniform specifications called Institutional Meat Purchasing Specifications (IMPS) was developed for use under the USDA Acceptance Service. The IMPS are published in a series of booklets for the following categories:

Title	Series (no.)
General Requirements	
Fresh Beef	100
Fresh Lamb and Mutton	200
Fresh Veal and Calf	300
Fresh Pork	400
Cured, Cured and Smoked, and Fully Cooked Pork Products	500
Cured, Dried, and Smoked Beef Products	600
Edible By-products	700
Sausage Products	800
Portion-Cut Meat Products	1000

During the 1960s the National Association of Meat Purveyors (NAMP), in cooperation with the USDA, developed the *Meat Buyer's Guide to Standardized Meat Cuts* (National Association of Meat Purveyors 1960) and the *Meat Buyer's Guide to Portion Control Meat Cuts* (National Association of Meat Purveyors 1967). Later NAMP combined the two books into one entitled *Meat Buyer's Guide* (National Association of Meat Purveyors 1976). Both IMPS and NAMP use the same numbering system. For example, the IMPS standard specification number for wholesale cut of beef short loin is no. 173—series 100; the standard NAMP number for a T-bone steak, prepared from a beef short loin, is no. 1173A. Each cut, both wholesale and portion cut, is fully described. In addition to the standardized number, the buyer must indicate specifics such as grade, thickness, and other factors relating to various classifications of meat.

BEEF CUTS For beef portion cuts and roasts, the buyer must specify the (1) grade, (2) thickness and portion weight for steaks or weight range in pounds for roasts, and (3) state of refrigeration. A partial listing of roasts and suggested weight range is given in Table 11-1. For steaks, the buyer may specify the weight range of the trimmed meat cut from which the portions are to be produced. Common portion sizes for many beef steaks are given in Table 11-2. A buyer

RETAIL CUTS OF BEEF

WHERE THEY COME FROM AND HOW TO COOK THEM

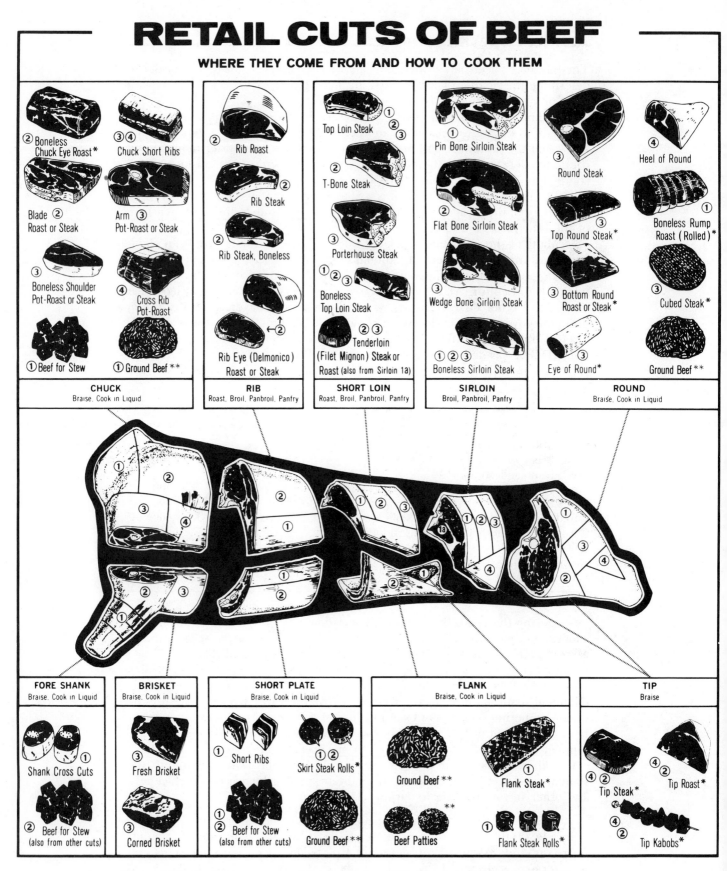

CHUCK
Braise, Cook in Liquid

- ② Boneless Chuck Eye Roast*
- ③④ Chuck Short Ribs
- ② Blade Roast or Steak
- ③ Arm Pot-Roast or Steak
- ③ Boneless Shoulder Pot-Roast or Steak
- ④ Cross Rib Pot-Roast
- ① Beef for Stew
- ① Ground Beef**

RIB
Roast, Broil, Panbroil, Panfry

- ② Rib Roast
- ② Rib Steak
- ② Rib Steak, Boneless
- ② Rib Eye (Delmonico) Roast or Steak

SHORT LOIN
Roast, Broil, Panbroil, Panfry

- ①② Top Loin Steak
- ② T-Bone Steak
- ③ Porterhouse Steak
- ①②③ Boneless Top Loin Steak
- ②③ Tenderloin (Filet Mignon) Steak or Roast (also from Sirloin 1a)

SIRLOIN
Broil, Panbroil, Panfry

- ① Pin Bone Sirloin Steak
- ② Flat Bone Sirloin Steak
- ③ Wedge Bone Sirloin Steak
- ①②③ Boneless Sirloin Steak

ROUND
Braise, Cook in Liquid

- ③ Round Steak
- ④ Heel of Round
- ③ Top Round Steak*
- ① Boneless Rump Roast (Rolled)*
- ③ Bottom Round Roast or Steak*
- ③ Cubed Steak*
- ③ Eye of Round*
- ③ Ground Beef**

FORE SHANK
Braise, Cook in Liquid

- ① Shank Cross Cuts
- ② Beef for Stew (also from other cuts)

BRISKET
Braise, Cook in Liquid

- ③ Fresh Brisket
- ③ Corned Brisket

SHORT PLATE
Braise, Cook in Liquid

- ① Short Ribs
- ①② Skirt Steak Rolls*
- ①② Beef for Stew (also from other cuts)
- ①② Ground Beef**

FLANK
Braise, Cook in Liquid

- ** Ground Beef**
- ① Flank Steak*
- Beef Patties**
- ① Flank Steak Rolls*

TIP
Braise

- ④② Tip Steak*
- ④② Tip Roast*
- ④② Tip Kabobs*

Figure 11-2. Beef chart approved by the National Live Stock and Meat Board. *Cuts from high quality beef may be roasted, broiled, panbroiled, or panfried. **Cuts may be roasted, baked, broiled, panbroiled, or panfried. *From National Live Stock and Meat Board*

182

RETAIL CUTS OF VEAL
WHERE THEY COME FROM AND HOW TO COOK THEM

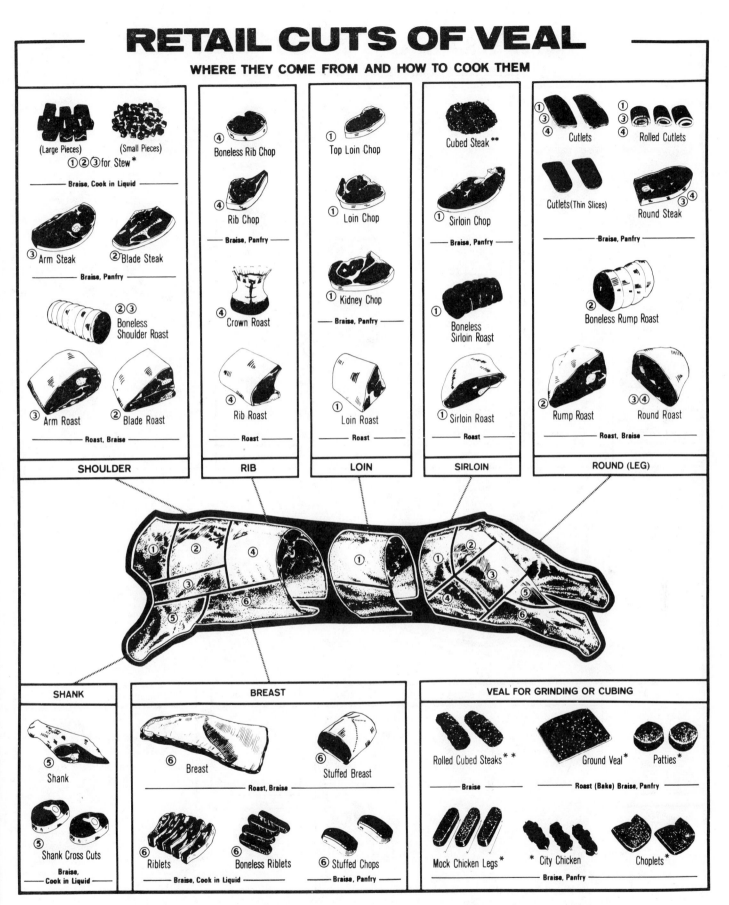

Figure 11-3. Veal chart approved by the National Live Stock and Meat Board. *Veal for stew or grinding may be made from any cut. **Cubed steaks may be made from any thick solid piece of boneless veal. *From National Live Stock and Meat Board*

RETAIL CUTS OF LAMB
WHERE THEY COME FROM AND HOW TO COOK THEM

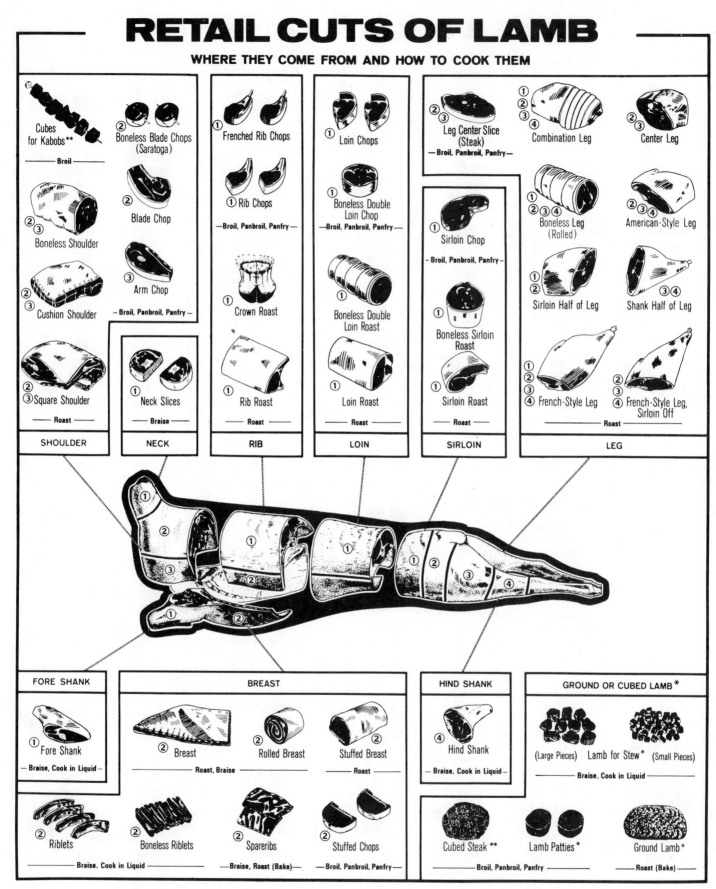

Figure 11-4. Lamb chart approved by the National Live Stock and Meat Board. *Lamb for stew or grinding may be made from any cut. **Kabobs or cubed steaks may be made from any thick solid piece of boneless lamb. *From National Live Stock and Meat Board*

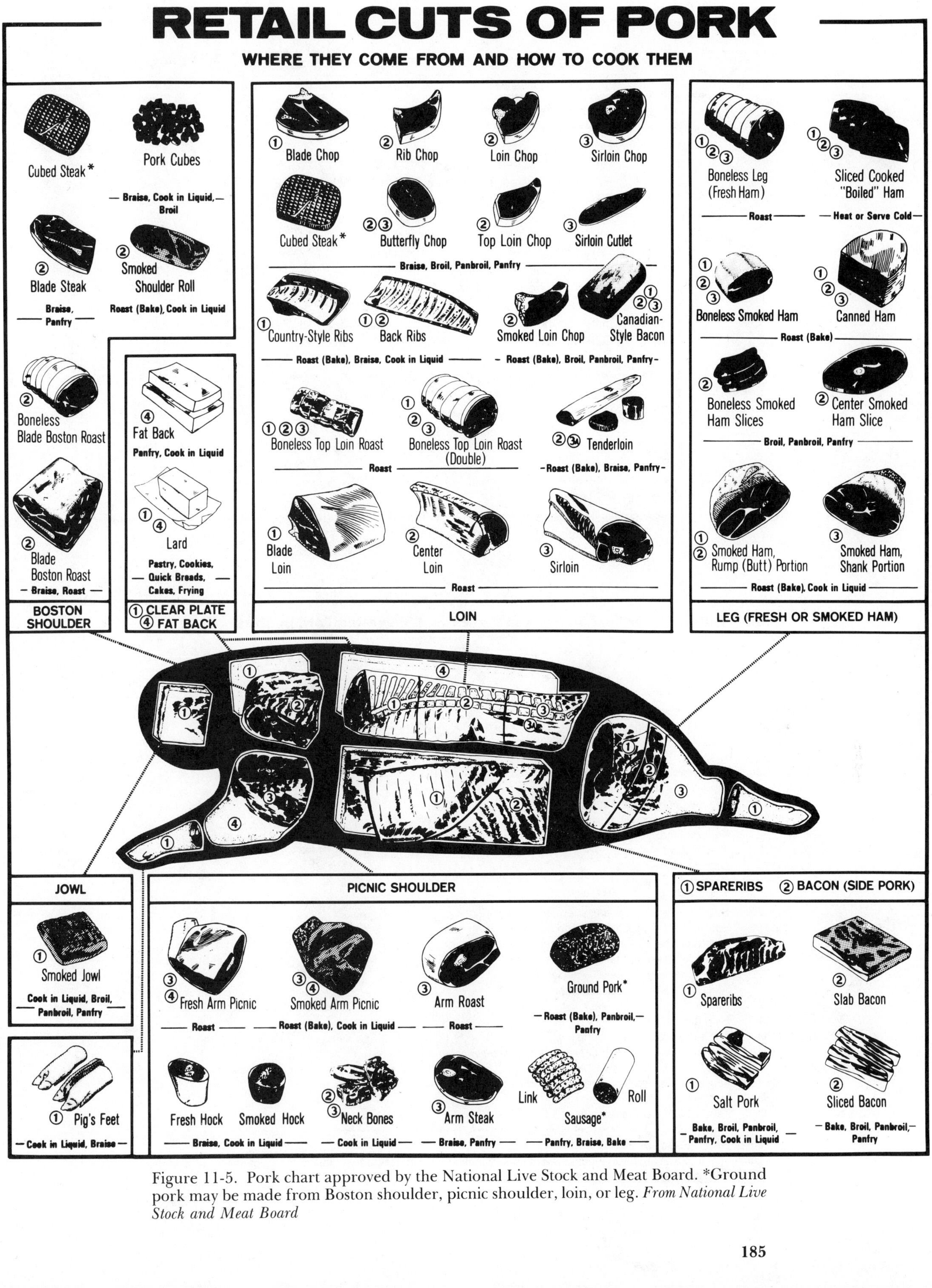

RETAIL CUTS OF PORK

WHERE THEY COME FROM AND HOW TO COOK THEM

BOSTON SHOULDER

Cubed Steak*

Pork Cubes

— Braise, Cook in Liquid, Broil —

② Blade Steak

② Smoked Shoulder Roll

Braise, Panfry

Roast (Bake), Cook in Liquid

② Boneless Blade Boston Roast

② Blade Boston Roast

— Braise, Roast —

① CLEAR PLATE ④ FAT BACK

④ Fat Back

Panfry, Cook in Liquid

① ④ Lard

Pastry, Cookies, Quick Breads, Cakes, Frying

LOIN

① Blade Chop

② Rib Chop

② Loin Chop

③ Sirloin Chop

Cubed Steak*

②③ Butterfly Chop

② Top Loin Chop

③ Sirloin Cutlet

— Braise, Broil, Panbroil, Panfry —

① Country-Style Ribs

①② Back Ribs

② Smoked Loin Chop

①②③ Canadian-Style Bacon

— Roast (Bake), Braise, Cook in Liquid —

— Roast (Bake), Broil, Panbroil, Panfry —

①②③ Boneless Top Loin Roast

①②③ Boneless Top Loin Roast (Double)

②③Ⓐ Tenderloin

— Roast —

— Roast (Bake), Braise, Panfry —

① Blade Loin

② Center Loin

③ Sirloin

— Roast —

LEG (FRESH OR SMOKED HAM)

①②③ Boneless Leg (Fresh Ham)

①②③ Sliced Cooked "Boiled" Ham

— Roast —

— Heat or Serve Cold —

①②③ Boneless Smoked Ham

①②③ Canned Ham

— Roast (Bake) —

Boneless Smoked Ham Slices

② Center Smoked Ham Slice

— Broil, Panbroil, Panfry —

①② Smoked Ham, Rump (Butt) Portion

③ Smoked Ham, Shank Portion

— Roast (Bake), Cook in Liquid —

JOWL

① Smoked Jowl

Cook in Liquid, Broil, Panbroil, Panfry

① Pig's Feet

— Cook in Liquid, Braise —

PICNIC SHOULDER

④ Fresh Arm Picnic

④ Smoked Arm Picnic

③ Arm Roast

Ground Pork*

— Roast —

— Roast (Bake), Cook in Liquid —

— Roast —

— Roast (Bake), Panbroil, Panfry —

Fresh Hock

Smoked Hock

③ Neck Bones

③ Arm Steak

Link Roll Sausage*

— Braise, Cook in Liquid —

— Cook in Liquid —

— Braise, Panfry —

— Panfry, Braise, Bake —

① SPARERIBS ② BACON (SIDE PORK)

① Spareribs

② Slab Bacon

① Salt Pork

② Sliced Bacon

— Bake, Broil, Panbroil, Panfry, Cook in Liquid —

— Bake, Broil, Panbroil, Panfry —

Figure 11-5. Pork chart approved by the National Live Stock and Meat Board. *Ground pork may be made from Boston shoulder, picnic shoulder, loin, or leg. *From National Live Stock and Meat Board*

185

Table 11-1. Index of Beef Roasts and Stew and Suggested Weight Ranges[a]

Item No.	Item Names	Suggested Weight Ranges (lb)[b]				
1107R	Rib, bone–in, short cut	Under 20	20–23	24–26	27–30	31–up
1108R	Rib, boneless, tied, short cut	Under 17	17–19	20–22	23–25	26–up
1109R	Rib, bone–in, tied, roast ready	Under 17	17–19	20–22	23–25	26–up
1109AR	Rib, bone–in, tied, roast ready, special	Under 17	17–19	20–22	23–25	26–up
1110R	Rib, boneless, tied, roast ready	Under 14	14–16	17–19	20–22	23–up
1112R	Rib eye roll	Under 7	7–8	9–10	11–12	13–up
1114R	Shoulder clod, roast ready	Under 16	16–18	19–21	22–24	25–up
1116R	Chuck roll, boneless, tied	Under 15	15–17	18–21	22–25	26–up
1167R	Knuckle, boneless	Under 10	10–up			
1168R	Inside round	Under 18	18–20	21–23	24–26	27–up
1169R	Outside round	Under 11	11–13	14–16	17–19	20–up
1170R	Gooseneck round	Under 18	18–20	21–23	24–26	27–up
1180R	Strip loin, boneless, short cut	Under 8	9–10	11–12	13–14	15–up
1184R	Top sirloin butt, boneless	Under 8	8–10	11–13	14–up	
1186R	Bottom sirloin butt, boneless, trimmed	Under 4	4–6	7–up		
1189R	Full tenderloin, regular	Under 5	5–7	7–9	9–up	
1195	Beef for stewing	Amount	Specified			

[a]From USDA (1967).

[b]Because it is impractical to list all weights for roasts that purchasers may desire, those included in the index table are suggested only. Other weight ranges may be ordered if desired.

Table 11-2. Index of Beef Steaks and Patties and Suggested Portion Sizes[a]

Item No.	Item Names	Suggested Portion Sizes[b] (oz)												
		3	4	6	8	10	12	14	16	18	20	24	28	32
1100	Cubed steaks, regular	×	×	×	×									
1101	Cubed steaks, special	×	×	×	×									
1102	Braising steaks, boneless (Swiss)		×	×	×									
1103	Rib steaks (bone-in)				×	×	×	×	×					
1103A	Rib steaks (boneless)		×	×	×	×	×							
1112	Rib eye roll steaks		×	×	×	×	×							
1136	Ground beef patties, regular	×	×	×	×									
1137	Ground beef patties, special	×	×	×	×									
1167	Knuckle steaks	×	×	×	×	×								
1168	Inside round steaks	×	×	×	×	×								
1169	Outside round steaks	×	×	×	×	×								
1173	Porterhouse steaks						×	×	×	×	×	×	×	×
1173A	T-Bone steaks					×	×	×	×	×	×	×	×	
1177	Strip loin steaks (bone-in), intermediate					×	×	×	×	×	×	×	×	
1178	Strip loin steaks (boneless), intermediate					×	×	×	×	×	×	×	×	
1179	Strip loin steaks (bone-in), short cut					×	×	×	×	×	×	×		
1179A	Strip loin steaks (bone-in), extra short cut					×	×	×	×	×	×	×		
1179B	Strip loin steaks (bone-in), special					×	×	×	×	×	×	×		
1180	Strip loin steaks (boneless), short cut			×	×	×	×	×	×	×				
1180A	Strip loin steaks (boneless), extra short cut			×	×	×	×	×	×	×				
1180B	Strip loin steaks (boneless), special			×	×	×	×	×	×	×				
1184	Top sirloin butt steaks (boneless)			×	×	×	×	×	×	×	×	×	×	
1184A	Top sirloin butt steaks (boneless), semi-center cut			×	×	×	×	×	×	×				
1184B	Top sirloin butt steaks (boneless), center cut			×	×	×	×	×	×					
1189	Tenderloin steaks, close trim		×	×	×	×	×	×						
1190	Tenderloin steaks, special trim	×	×	×	×	×	×	×						

[a]From USDA (1967).

[b]Because it is impractical to list all portion weights for steaks that purchasers may desire, those identified by × in the index table are suggested only. Other portion weights may be ordered if desired.

186

Table 11-3. Federal Classification, Grades, and Yields for Meats

	Class	Grades	Yields
Beef	(steer, heifer, cow[a])	Prime, Choice, Good, Standard, Commercial, Utility, Cutter, Canner	1,2,3,4,5
	(bullock)	Prime, Choice, Good, Standard, Utility	1,2,3,4,5
Veal		Prime, Choice, Good, Standard, Utility	1,2,3,4,5
Lamb[b]	(yearling mutton)	Prime, Choice, Good, Utility, Cull	1,2,3,4,5
	(mutton)	Choice, Good, Utility, Cull	1,2,3,4,5
Pork	(barrows and gilts)	U.S.no. 1, U.S.no. 2, U.S.no. 3, U.S.no. 4, U.S. Utility	
	(sows)	U.S.no. 1, U.S.no. 2, U.S.no. 3, Medium, Cull	

[a]Cows are not graded as prime.
[b]Federally graded lamb and mutton may be graded for either quality or yield or both.

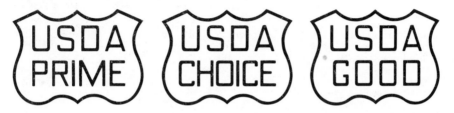

Figure 11-6. Quality and yield grades for meat. *From Agricultural Marketing Service (1975)*

may desire to purchase beef rib steak (bone-in), which may be cut from the chuck end of the rib or the loin end of the rib. If only steak from the loin end is desired, it must be so specified.

The buyer must specify one of the quality grades as shown in Table 11-3. Meat inspection is mandatory, but federal meat grading is voluntary. The quality grade stamp (Fig. 11-6) is routinely rolled on the top three grades; yield grades can be rolled on with the quality grade or stamped on each wholesale cut. All federally graded beef must be graded for both quality and yield; therefore, the buyer may also specify the yield. The yield grades, nos. 1–5, indicate the percentage of usable meat in a specific carcass. The lower grades have a higher percentage of available meat than carcasses graded no. 4 or no. 5. For example, a 600-lb USDA no. 1 beef carcass yields approximately 80% of its weight in trimmed cuts, compared to an approximate yield of 63% of its weight in trimmed cuts from a 600-lb USDA no. 5 carcass.

For portion weight items, the actual portion weight desired must be specified. Unless indicated by the buyer, dependent upon the portion weight specified, tolerances are permitted as follows: less than 6 oz, $\pm \frac{1}{4}$ oz; 6–8 oz, $\pm \frac{1}{2}$ oz; 12–18 oz, $\pm \frac{3}{4}$ oz; over 18 oz, ± 1 oz. The thickness of portion cuts may also be specified with tolerances; 1 in. or less, $\pm \frac{3}{16}$ in.; more than 1 in., $\pm \frac{1}{4}$ in.

The surface fat limitations for steaks, chops, and roasts vary. Unless indicated in specifications, the allowances given in Table 11-4 are permitted.

To indicate the state of refrigeration, the buyer should specify chilled or frozen. Portion cut meats to be delivered frozen may be produced from frozen cuts of meats that were previously accepted by federal meat graders. The meat must be maintained in excellent condition and be packaged, produced, and promptly returned to the frozen state.

The finest veal is milk fed, and the flesh has a pinkish hue. The buyer must specify the (1) grade and class, (2) thickness, and (3) state of refrigeration. Suggested portion and weight ranges are shown in Table 11-5.

Table 11-4. Allowable Surface Fat for Steaks, Chops, and Roasts[a]

Item	Allowable Surface Fat
Steaks	Fat must not exceed an average of ½ in. in thickness and the thickness at any point must not be more than ¾ in.
Chops, cutlets, and filets	Surface fat, where present, must not exceed an average of ¼ in. in thickness and the thickness at any point must be not more than ⅜ in.
Roasts	Average surface fat is ¾ in. with a maximum of 1 in. at any one point or ½ in. with a maximum of ¾ in. at any one point.

[a]From National Association of Meat Purveyors (1967).

Table 11-5. Index of Veal and Calf Steaks, Chops, Cutlets, Roasts, and Stew and Suggested Portion Sizes and Weight Ranges[a]

Item No.	Item Names	Suggested Portion Sizes and Weight Ranges[b]											
		3 oz	4 oz	5 oz	6 oz	8 oz	10 oz	12 oz	16 oz	lb	lb	lb	lb
1300	Cubed steaks, regular	×	×	×	×	×							
1301	Cubed steaks, special	×	×	×	×	×							
1306	Rib chops	×	×	×	×	×	×						
1309	Shoulder chops	×	×	×	×	×	×						
1310	Shoulder clod steaks	×	×	×	×	×							
1332	Loin chops	×	×	×	×	×	×	×	×				
1336	Cutlet, regular	×	×	×	×								
1336A	Cutlet special	×	×	×	×								
1309R	Chuck, square-cut, boneless, tied									Under 10	10–15	16–22	23–up
1310R	Shoulder clod, roast ready									Under 6	6–8	9–10	11–up
1311R	Chuck, square-cut, clod out, boneless, tied									Under 6	6–8	9–10	11–up
1335R	Leg, boneless, tied, roast ready									Under 10	10–15	16–22	23–up
1395	Veal for stewing	Amount specified											

[a]From USDA (1967).
[b]Because it is impractical to list all portion weights for chops and all weight ranges for roasts that purchasers may desire, the portion weights identified by × and the weight ranges for roasts are suggested only. Other portion weights and weight ranges may be ordered if desired.

LAMB CUTS Grading factors for lamb are similar to those for beef. Unlike beef, which must be federally graded for both quality and yield, federally graded lamb and mutton may be graded for either quality or yield, or both. Quality lamb is well fed, is finely grained, and has a pinkish red color. The purchaser must specify grade and class. Unless otherwise specified in the individual item specification, chops must be in full slices in a straight line, reasonably perpendicular to the outer surface and at the approximate right angle of the length of the meat cut from which chops are produced. Suggested portion sizes and weight ranges for lamb chops and roast are given in Table 11-6.

PORK CUTS Grades for pork are based on a combination of quality and yield. Purchaser should specify U.S. no. 1 or U.S. no. 2. Unless otherwise specified in the individual item specifications, filets, chops, and steaks must be cut in full slices in a straight line reasonably perpendicular to the other surface and at an approximate right angle to the length of the meat cut from which the filets, chops, or steaks are produced. Suggested portion sizes and weight ranges for pork cuts are given in Table 11-7.

Table 11-6. Index of Lamb, Yearling Mutton, and Mutton Chops, Roasts, and Stew and Suggested Portion Sizes and Weight Ranges [a]

Item No.	Item Names	|← Suggested Portion Sizes And Weight Ranges [b] →|											
		3 oz	4 oz	5 oz	6 oz	7 oz	8 oz	9 oz	10 oz	lb	lb	lb	lb
1204	Rib chops	×	×	×	×	×	×	×	×				
1204A	Rib chops, frenched	×	×	×	×	×							
1207	Shoulder chops		×	×	×	×	×						
1232	Loin chops		×	×	×	×	×	×	×				
1208R	Shoulder, boneless, tied									Under 4	4–6	7–8	9 and up
1234R	Leg, partially boneless									Under 6	6–8	9–11	12 and up
1234AR	Leg, boneless, tied									Under 6	6–8	9–11	12 and up
1295	Lamb for stewing	Amount specified											

[a] From USDA (1967).

[b] Because it is impractical to list all portion weights for chops and all weight ranges for roasts that purchasers may desire, the portion weights identified by × and the weight ranges for roasts are suggested only. Other portion weights and weight ranges may be ordered if desired.

Table 11-7. Index of Pork Filets, Steaks, Chops, and Roasts and Suggested Portion Sizes and Weight Ranges [a]

Item No.	Item Names	|← Suggested Portion Sizes And Weight Ranges [b] →|									
		3 oz	4 oz	5 oz	6 oz	8 oz	10 oz	4–6 lb	6–8 lb	8–10 lb	10–12 lb
1400	Pork filets	×	×	×	×						
1406	Boston butt steaks, bone-in		×	×	×	×					
1407	Shoulder butt steaks, boneless	×	×	×	×	×					
1410	Pork chops, regular	×	×	×	×						
1410A	Pork chops, with pocket		×	×	×	×					
1410B	Pork rib chops, with pocket		×	×	×	×					
1411	Pork chops, bladeless	×	×	×	×	×					
1412	Pork chops, center cut	×	×	×	×	×					
1412A	Pork chops, center cut, special	×	×	×	×	×					
1412B	Pork chops, center cut, boneless	×	×	×	×	×					
1413	Pork chops, boneless	×	×	×	×	×					
1402R	Fresh ham, boneless, tied								×	×	×
1406R	Boston butt, boneless, tied							×	×		
1413R	Pork loin, boneless, tied								×	×	×

[a] From USDA (1967).

[b] Because it is impractical to list all portion weights for chops and all weight ranges for roasts that purchasers may desire, the portion weights and weight ranges identified by × are suggested only. Other portion weights and weight ranges may be ordered if desired.

Poultry Specifications

Specifications for fresh poultry should include the grade, class, size, and state of refrigeration. It should also include the part if cut-up poultry is specified. Poultry must be federally inspected for wholesomeness before it can be graded for quality. Often the grade shield and the inspection mark appear together (Fig. 11-7). Both inspection and grading are mandatory.

The inspection mark on poultry and poultry products shows that they have been examined for wholesomeness under government supervision in an officially approved processing plant. Not all poultry that has been inspected carries the mark. The exception is that if chilled poultry is packed in large boxes, the box carries the seal.

The highest quality is U.S. Grade A. You may find the shield on any kind of chilled or frozen ready-to-cook poultry or poultry parts. Grade A poultry is

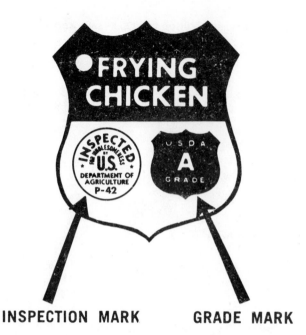

INSPECTION MARK   GRADE MARK

Figure 11-7. Poultry inspection mark and grade shield. *From USDA (1968)*

Table 11-8. Classification for Poultry[a]

Class	Description
Young chickens	May be labeled young chicken, Rock Cornish hen, broiler, fryer, roaster, or capon.
Young turkeys	May be labeled young turkey, fryer, roaster, young hen, or young tom.
Young ducks	May be labeled duckling, young duckling, broiler duckling, fryer duckling, or roaster duckling.
Mature chickens	May be labeled mature chicken, old chicken, stewing chicken, or fowl.
Mature turkeys	May be labeled mature turkey, yearling turkey, or old turkey.
Mature ducks, geese, or guineas	May be labeled as mature or old.

[a]From USDA (1968).

fully freshed and meaty, well finished, and attractive in appearance (Fig. 11-8). The U.S. Grades apply to five kinds of poultry: chicken, turkey, duck, goose, and guinea. The grade does not indicate how tender the bird is; the age (class) is the determining factor. Poultry classifications are given in Table 11-8. Young birds are more tender than older ones. If the poultry is not young, the label will carry the words *mature, old,* or similar terms to indicate the age.

POULTRY PARTS The purchase of chicken parts is equivalent to purchasing portion cut meats such as steaks, chops, and cutlets. The USDA quality grades are the same as those for the whole bird; specific standards on how each part is to be cut are also included. The USDA standards (U.S. Department of Agriculture 1972) exist for the following parts:

- Breast—may be split, or cut into three pieces.
- Breasts with ribs—split or cut into three pieces with part of ribs attached.

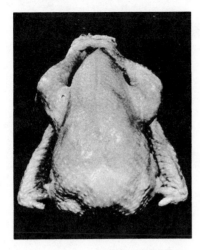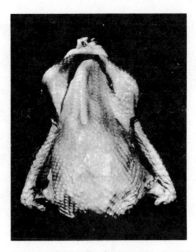

Figure 11-8. Comparison of Grade A (left) and Grade B (right) poultry.
From USDA (1968)

- Leg—includes whole leg (thigh and drumstick).
- Wings—include whole wing with all muscle and skin intact (wing tip may be removed).
- Drumsticks—separated from thigh by cut through knee joint.
- Thigh—disjointed at hip joint, may include pelvic meat but not bone.
- Halves—full-length back and breast split.
- Quarters—split as for halves, then cut crosswise to form quarters.
- Backs—include the pelvic bone and all vertebrae posterior to the shoulder joint.
- Necks—separated from the carcass at the shoulder joint, with or without skin.
- Giblets—approximately equal number of hearts, gizzards, and livers.

Chicken parts are the most popular marketing form used in quantity food service. The breast is especially well liked by patients and employees who prefer all light meat; moreover, it can be prepared in a variety of ways and is easy to serve. The buyer should specify U.S. Grade A. To determine whether chicken parts are a good buy, the purchaser is referred to Table 11-9. For example, the table shows that breast halves with ribs at $1.02 a pound, drumsticks and thighs at $0.88 a pound, drumsticks at $0.86 a pound, thighs at $0.93 a pound, and wings at $0.50 a pound provide as much lean meat for the money as ready-to-cook whole chickens at $0.73. The purchaser pays for the convenience of having whatever parts of a chicken are desired. A similar comparison can be made for turkey parts as shown in Table 11-10.

PROCESSED CHICKEN A variety of processed poultry products are available including canned, frozen, cooked, or partly cooked dishes (Fig. 11-9). Many of these products are combination dishes, with vegetables, pasta, gravy, or other foods added. Federal standards exist for the minimum percentage of meat that manufacturers must include in combination dishes, but the minimum may not be sufficient to meet the protein requirement for menus in a medical foodservice operation. (See Appendix Table E-4 for combination foods containing poultry.) If these products are used, the buyer will have to specify the ratio of poultry to the other ingredients of the combination dish. If the percentage of meat is inadequate, the product must be served with other protein foods such as cheese or eggs.

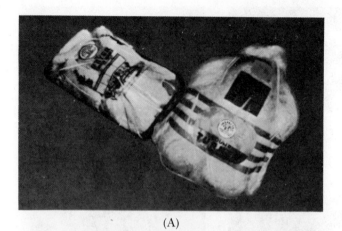

(A)

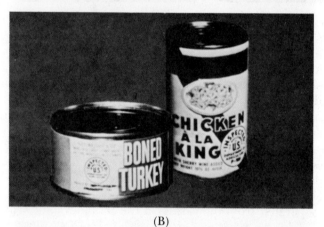

(B)

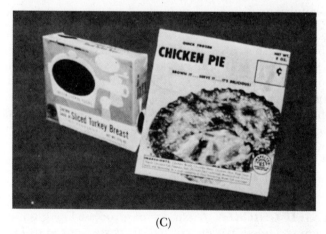

(C)

Figure 11-9. Processed chicken products. (A) Fresh-chilled or frozen ready-to-cook whole birds. (B) Canned poultry products. (C) Frozen cooked or partly cooked dishes. *From USDA (1959)*

___ Egg Specifications ___

There are three consumer grades for eggs: U.S. Grade AA (or Fresh Fancy), U.S. Grade A, and U.S. Grade B. Graded eggs have been examined by an authorized grader to determine factors such as the condition of the white and yolk and the cleanliness and soundness of the shell. Electronic equipment is used for *flash scanning* or *flash candling*, where eggs are placed on a continuous

Table 11-9. Cost of Chicken, Whole and Parts[a]

Price[b] per Pound (in Dollars) of Whole Fryers, Ready to Cook	Chicken Parts Equally Good Buy at This Price per Pound (in Dollars)						
	Breast Half (with Rib)	Drumstick and Thigh	Drumstick	Thigh	Wing	Breast Quarter	Leg Quarter
0.45	0.63	0.54	0.53	0.57	0.31	0.54	0.52
0.47	0.65	0.57	0.55	0.60	0.32	0.56	0.54
0.49	0.68	0.59	0.57	0.62	0.33	0.59	0.57
0.51	0.71	0.61	0.60	0.65	0.35	0.61	0.59
0.53	0.74	0.64	0.62	0.67	0.36	0.64	0.61
0.55	0.77	0.66	0.65	0.70	0.38	0.66	0.64
0.57	0.79	0.69	0.67	0.72	0.39	0.68	0.66
0.59	0.82	0.71	0.69	0.75	0.40	0.71	0.68
0.61	0.85	0.74	0.72	0.77	0.42	0.73	0.71
0.63	0.88	0.76	0.74	0.80	0.43	0.76	0.73
0.65	0.91	0.78	0.76	0.83	0.44	0.78	0.75
0.67	0.93	0.81	0.79	0.85	0.46	0.80	0.78
0.69	0.96	0.83	0.81	0.88	0.47	0.83	0.80
0.71	0.99	0.86	0.83	0.90	0.49	0.85	0.82
0.73	1.02	0.88	0.86	0.93	0.50	0.88	0.85
0.75	1.04	0.90	0.88	0.95	0.51	0.90	0.87
0.77	1.07	0.93	0.90	0.98	0.53	0.92	0.89
0.79	1.10	0.95	0.93	1.00	0.54	0.95	0.92
0.81	1.13	0.98	0.95	1.03	0.55	0.97	0.94
0.83	1.16	1.00	0.97	1.05	0.57	1.00	0.95
0.85	1.18	1.02	1.00	1.08	0.58	1.02	0.98
0.87	1.21	1.05	1.02	1.10	0.59	1.04	1.01
0.89	1.24	1.07	1.04	1.13	0.61	1.07	1.03
0.91	1.27	1.10	1.07	1.16	0.62	1.09	1.05
0.93	1.30	1.12	1.09	1.18	0.64	1.12	1.08
0.95	1.32	1.15	1.11	1.21	0.65	1.14	1.10
0.97	1.35	1.17	1.14	1.23	0.66	1.16	1.12
0.99	1.38	1.19	1.16	1.26	0.68	1.19	1.15

[a]From USDA (1982). Based on yields of cooked chicken meat without skin, from frying chickens that weighed about 3 lb.
[b]Price based on weight of chicken with neck and giblets.

conveyor system and mechanically rotated over strong light. The egg size, which ranges from jumbo to peewee, is not related to egg quality (Table 11-11).

The U.S. Grade AA (or Fresh Fancy) is the top USDA consumer grade for shell eggs. The broken-out egg covers a small area. The white is thick and stands high, the yolk is firm and high. Eggs with this grade are suitable for poaching, frying, or other uses where appearance is important.

The U.S. Grade A is the second-highest USDA grade for shell eggs. The broken-out egg covers a moderate area. The white is reasonably thick and stands fairly high; the yolk is firm and high. Grade AA and A shields are shown in Figure 11-10.

The U.S. Grade B is the lowest consumer grade for eggs. The white is thinner than U.S. Grade AA and U.S. Grade A eggs, and the yolk is somewhat flattened. Grade B eggs are suitable for general cooking and baking, where appearance is not important.

The buyer should specify both grade and size. Grade AA for poaching and frying and Grade A for hard-cooked, scrambled, or other cooking methods. Size depends on use. Compare price and size, as shown in Table 11-12.

PROCESSED EGGS All processed eggs must be pasteurized before processing. USDA inspection is mandatory. Processed eggs may be purchased in a variety of forms. The most popular types are

Table 11-10. Comparative Costs of Turkey Parts[a,b]

Price per Pound (in Dollars) of Whole Turkey, Ready to Cook	Turkey Parts and Products Equally Good Buy at this Price Per Pound (in Dollars)										
							Turkey Roasts		Boned Turkey, Canned	Turkey with Gravy,[e] Canned or Frozen	Gravy with Turkey,[f] Canned or Frozen
	Breast Quarter	Leg Quarter	Breast, Whole or Half	Drumstick	Thigh	Wing	Ready-to-Cook[c]	Cooked[d]			
0.51	0.57	0.55	0.65	0.52	0.62	0.47	0.87	1.17	1.15	0.45	0.19
0.53	0.60	0.57	0.68	0.54	0.65	0.49	0.93	1.22	1.19	0.46	0.20
0.55	0.62	0.59	0.70	0.56	0.67	0.51	0.96	1.26	1.24	0.48	0.21
0.57	0.64	0.61	0.73	0.58	0.70	0.53	1.00	1.31	1.28	0.50	0.21
0.59	0.66	0.63	0.75	0.60	0.72	0.55	1.03	1.36	1.33	0.52	0.22
0.61	0.69	0.66	0.78	0.63	0.75	0.56	1.07	1.40	1.37	0.53	0.23
0.63	0.71	0.68	0.80	0.65	0.77	0.58	1.10	1.45	1.42	0.55	0.24
0.65	0.73	0.70	0.83	0.67	0.80	0.60	1.14	1.50	1.46	0.57	0.24
0.67	0.75	0.72	0.85	0.69	0.82	0.62	1.17	1.54	1.51	0.59	0.25
0.69	0.78	0.74	0.88	0.71	0.85	0.64	1.21	1.59	1.55	0.60	0.26
0.71	0.80	0.76	0.91	0.73	0.87	0.66	1.24	1.63	1.60	0.62	0.27
0.73	0.82	0.78	0.93	0.75	0.89	0.68	1.28	1.68	1.64	0.64	0.27
0.75	0.84	0.81	0.96	0.77	0.92	0.69	1.31	1.72	1.69	0.66	0.28
0.77	0.87	0.83	0.98	0.79	0.94	0.71	1.35	1.77	1.73	0.67	0.29
0.79	0.89	0.85	1.01	0.81	0.97	0.73	1.38	1.82	1.78	0.69	0.30
0.81	0.91	0.87	1.03	0.83	0.99	0.75	1.42	1.86	1.82	0.71	0.30
0.83	0.93	0.89	1.06	0.85	1.02	0.77	1.45	1.91	1.87	0.73	0.31
0.85	0.96	0.91	1.08	0.87	1.04	0.79	1.49	1.96	1.91	0.74	0.32
0.87	0.98	0.94	1.11	0.89	1.07	0.80	1.52	2.00	1.96	0.76	0.33
0.89	1.00	0.96	1.13	0.91	1.09	0.82	1.56	2.05	2.00	0.78	0.33
0.91	1.02	0.98	1.16	0.93	1.11	0.84	1.59	2.09	2.05	0.80	0.34
0.93	1.05	1.00	1.19	0.95	1.14	0.86	1.63	2.14	2.09	0.81	0.35
0.95	1.07	1.02	1.21	0.97	1.15	0.88	1.66	2.18	2.14	0.83	0.36
0.97	1.09	1.04	1.24	0.99	1.19	0.90	1.70	2.23	2.18	0.85	0.36
0.99	1.11	1.06	1.26	1.01	1.21	0.92	1.73	2.28	2.23	0.87	0.37

[a]From USDA (1975).
[b]Based on yields of cooked turkey meat excluding skin, medium to large birds.
[c]Roast, as purchased, includes 15% skin or fat.
[d]Roast, as purchased, has no more than one fourth inch skin and fat on any part of surface.
[e]Assumes 35% cooked boned turkey, minimum required for product labeled "Turkey with Gravy."
[f]Assumes 15% cooked boned turkey, minimum required for product labeled "Gravy with Turkey."

Table 11-11. Egg Size and Weight

Size (Name)	Per Dozen (oz)	Per 30–Dozen Case (lb)[a]
Jumbo	30	56
Extra Large	27	50½
Large	24	45
Medium	21	39½
Small	18	34
Peewee	15	28

[a]Weight includes approximately 4½ lb extra per case for corrugated fiber case and fillers between layers of eggs.

Table 11-12. Calculating the Cost of Eggs[a]

Price per Dozen (in Cents) Large Eggs	Larger of Two Sizes Better Buy if Price Difference per Dozen (in Cents) between One Size and Next Larger Size Less Than
41–48	6
49–56	7
57–64	8
65–72	9
73–80	10
81–88	11
89–96	12
97–104	13
105–112	14
113–120	15

[a]From USDA (1975).

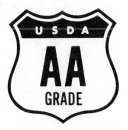
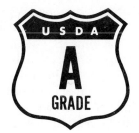

Figure 11-10. USDA grade shields for fresh eggs. *From USDA (1975)*

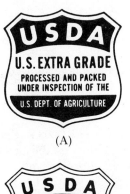

(A)

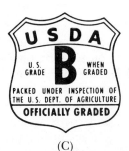

(C)

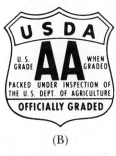

(B)

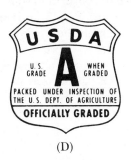

(D)

Figure 11-11. USDA grades for dairy products. (A) Used on instant nonfat dry milk. (B) Highest quality grade for butter and cheddar cheese. (C) Lowest quality grade for butter. (D) Second highest grade for butter and cheddar cheese. *From USDA (1975)*

- Fresh liquid bulk—30-lb can.
- Frozen liquid eggs (whole, yolks, whites)—10-lb and 30-lb cans.
- Frozen hard-cooked eggs (chopped)—packed in plastic bags.
- Frozen egg rolls (yolk is centered, used for slicing or chopping).
- Freeze-dried scrambled eggs—six 3-lb cans per case, 50-lb drums.
- Dried eggs (whole, yolks, or whites).

Processed eggs are used primarily for baking and other cooking needs. Fresh or frozen whole liquid eggs are convenient forms and are used for scrambled eggs.

DAIRY PRODUCTS SPECIFICATIONS Butter and margarine must meet minimum milk fat content of 80%. Butter is made from animal fat; margarine or oleomargarine is made from vegetable or a blend of both vegetable and animal fat. The grading standards range from U.S. Grade AA to U.S. Grade B, as shown in Figure 11–11. The products are sold in ¼-lb or 1-lb prints, 5-lb carton with 72–90 pats per lb, and in 64-lb cubes.

Milk is marketed in a variety of forms. The more common types are fresh, canned, and dried. Standards for Grade A milk are established by state and local governments, as recommended in Public Health Service's *Grade "A" Pasteurized Milk Ordinance* (U.S. Department of Health and Human Services 1965). The milk must come from healthy cows, and be produced, pasteurized, and handled under strict sanitary conditions. The Grade A rating denotes wholesomeness rather than level of quality. *Homogenized milk* has been treated to reduce the size of the milk fat globules, thereby keeping the cream from separating. *Fortified milks* are those with one or more nutrients added. Vitamin D milk is fortified with 400 international units (IU) of vitamin D per quart. Multiple fortified milk can be fortified with substances such as vitamins A, D, multivitamin preparations, minerals, lactose and nonfat dry milk. *Certified milk* denotes that the milk was produced under sanitary conditions. Only certified milk that has been pasteurized should be used in foodservice operations. *Pasteurized milk* means that the product has been subjected to heat treatments at temperatures high enough to ensure pathogen destruction. The following types of milk products are commonly used in foodservice operations.

- *Whole milk* contains a minimum of 3.25% milk fat, with vitamin D added.
- *Low-fat milk* is partially skimmed milk that has between 0.5% and 2% milk fat, depending on state regulations.
- *Skim milk* has less than 0.5% milk fat, the percentage allowed under federal regulations.
- *Chocolate-flavored milk* is made from pasteurized whole milk with sugar and chocolate syrup or cocoa added.
- *Chocolate-flavored drink* is similar to chocolate milk, except that the product does not have to conform to standards of identity established for milk. The product has a lower milk fat content than chocolate milk.
- *Buttermilk* is a cultured milk product made with skim milk fermented mainly by *Streptococcus lactis*.
- *Two percent milk,* as the name implies, contains 2% milk fat.
- *Acidophilus milk* is pasteurized skim milk, cultured with *Lactobacillus acidophilus* and incubated at 100°F. This product is sometimes served to patients with a milk intolerance. It combats excessive intestinal putrefaction by changing the bacterial flora of the intestine.
- *Yogurt* has a consistency resembling custard and is made from fresh partially skimmed milk, enriched and added milk solids. Fermented by a mixed culture of one or more organisms such as *Streptococcus thermophilus, Bacterium bulgaricus,* and *Plocamo-bacterium yoghourtii*.
- *Evaporated milk* is made by heating homogenized whole milk under a vacuum to remove half its water, then sealing it in cans and sterilizing it.
- *Condensed milk* is a concentrated milk with at least 40% sugar added to help preserve it. This canned milk is prepared by removing about half the water from whole milk. It has at least 8.5% milk fat.
- *Dry whole milk* is pasteurized milk with water removed.
- *Nonfat dry milk* is processed to remove the fat and water and pasteurized to destroy microorganisms. It reconstitutes to fluid skim milk.
- *Instant nonfat dry milk* is processed to remove fat and water from pasteurized fluid milk. It is made by a process that produces larger flakes than regular nonfat dry milk, and it dissolves *instantly* in water.

The buyer should purchase ready-to-drink milk in individual cartons as much as possible to prevent cross contamination. Bulk milk for cooking may be purchased in ½-gal or 5-gal containers. Specify grade, type, and container size.

Standards of identity for cream have been established to indicate the minimum fat content. The product must be pasteurized, and if it has less than 18% fat it cannot be called cream. The following types are available and are used in foodservice operation.

- *Light cream* (also coffee or table cream) must have at least 18% milk fat.
- *Light whipping cream* must have at least 30% milk fat under federal standards of identity.

- *Heavy whipping cream* must have at least 36% milk fat.
- *Half-and-half* is a mixture of milk and cream that are homogenized. Under federal requirements, it must have a minimum of 10.5% milk fat.
- *Sour cream* is made by adding lactic acid bacteria culture to light cream. It is smooth and thick and contains at least 18% milk fat.

Ice cream and other frozen dairy dessert-type products must be made from pasteurized milk. Standards of identity are as follows:

- *Ice cream* is made from cream, milk, sugar, flavoring, and stabilizers. It must contain at least 10% milk fat. Overrun (increase from whipping or freezing) is permitted up to 100%. The weight of a gallon of ice cream should be not less than 4½ lb.
- *Ice milk* is made from milk, stabilizers, sugar, and flavorings. It contains between 2% and 7% milk fat.
- *Sherbet* is made from milk, fruit or fruit juices, stabilizers, and sugar.
- *Water ice* is like sherbet except that it contains no milk.

Milk and milk-type products or *imitation milks* are available. They are difficult to define because of differing laws and regulations among the states. Two such products are identified as follows (U.S. Department of Health and Human Services 1969):

1. *Filled milk* is a milk or cream (fluid, frozen, evaporated, condensed, concentrated, or dried) to which a fat other than butterfat has been added. The resulting product resembles milk or cream. A typical formulation consists of skim milk or nonfat dry milk and a vegetable fat. Artificial color or flavoring is frequently added. Under the Federal Filled Milk Act, filled milk may not be shipped in interstate or foreign commerce. *Imitation milks,* which may move in interstate commerce, are products resembling milk but containing no milk ingredients such as skim milk or nonfat dry milk. A typical formulation includes sodium caseinate, vegetable fat, corn syrup or dextrose, artificial color and flavor, and emulsifiers. The product must be labeled as imitation milk.

2. *Coffee lighteners* (or whiteners) are made in much the same manner as the imitation milk products, usually containing sodium caseinate, vegetable oil, and other ingredients.

Cheese is available in a variety of different flavors and textures. Some types bear the "Quality Approved" shield, which assures good quality and sanitary processing. USDA Grade AA cheddar cheese has been graded by a highly trained government grader and has been produced in a USDA-inspected and -approved plant. The USDA Grade A cheese is also of good quality but not quite as good as Grade AA (see Fig. 11-11 for USDA shields).

Natural cheeses is manufactured directly from milk and includes cheddar, cottage, Parmesan, Swiss, blue, cream, Limburger, and hundreds of other varieties. *Pasteurized process cheese* is not a natural cheese; it is a blend of fresh and aged natural cheeses, which are heated and mixed. *Pasteurized process cheese food* contains additional ingredients, such as nonfat dry milk. *Pasteurized processed cheese spread* is like cheese food, except that it has higher moisture and lower milk fat. Club cheese or coldpack cheese is a blend of natural cheeses, like process cheese, except that the cheese is blended without heat.

Natural cheeses are generally classified according to the ripening time. There are six general classifications. *Unripened cheese* includes both soft and firm. Soft unripened cheeses, such as cottage and cream cheese, have high moisture and undergo no ripening. Firm unripened cheeses such as mozzarella are not ripened but have very low moisture, so they may be stored longer. *Soft ripened*

Table 11-13. Characteristics of Commonly Used Varieties of Natural Cheese

Name	Description
American Pasteurized Process	Process (or Pasteurized Process) cheese is made by grinding fine, and mixing together by heating and stirring, one or more cheeses of the same or two or more varieties. American Cheddar Cheese is processed in greatest quantities, but other American-type cheeses, such as Washed-curd, Colby, Granular, Swiss, Gruyere, Brick, Limburger, and others are also processed. Analysis: Moisture, not more than 41 percent; fat in the solids, not less than 49 percent.
Bleu, Blue	Bleu is the French name and Blue is the American name for this blue-veined cheese of the Roquefort type. It is made from cow's or goat milk. The color is white with blue veins throughout. Blue cheese is about 7$\frac{1}{2}$ inches in diameter and weighs from 4$\frac{1}{2}$ to 5 pounds. It is round and flat with a tangy flavor. Analysis: Moisture, not more than 46 percent; fat, 29.5 to 30.5 percent (not less than 50 percent in the solids); protein, 20 to 21 percent; and salt, 4.5 to 5 percent.
Brick	Brick cheese, one of the few cheeses of American origin, is made primarily in Wisconsin. It is a sweet-curd, semi-soft, cow's milk cheese, with a mild but pungent and sweet flavor. The body is elastic and slices well without crumbling. Analysis: Moisture, not more than 44 percent; fat, 31 percent (not less than 50 percent of the solids); protein, 20 to 23 percent; and salt, 1.8 to 2 percent, or slightly more.
Brie	Brie, first made in France, is a soft, surface-ripened cheese made usually from cow's milk but at times from skim or partly skimmed milk. Brie cheese, with its mild to pungent flavor, is made in three pie-shaped sizes: Large (about 16 inches in diameter); medium (about 12 inches in diameter); and small (5$\frac{1}{2}$ to 8 inches in diameter). Analysis: Moisture, 45 to 52.5 percent; fat, 25 to 28 percent when cheese is made with whole milk, and 20 to 22 percent when it is made from partly skimmed milk; protein, 21.6 percent; and salt, 1.5 to 4 percent.
Caciocavallo	Caciocavallo, an Italian plastic-curd cheese, is usually made from cow's milk but sometimes from a mixture of cow's and ewe's. The cured product has a smooth, firm body, and preferably the interior of the cheese is white. Caciocavallo and Provolone are made by almost identical methods with similar sharp flavor. However, Caciocavallo contains less fat and usually is not smoked. Analysis: Moisture, not more than 40 percent; fat in the solids, not less than 42 percent.
Camembert	A soft, surface-ripened, cow's milk cheese, originating in France. Each cheese is 4$\frac{1}{2}$ inches diameter, 1 to 1$\frac{1}{2}$ inches thick, and weighs about 10 ounces. The interior is yellow and waxy, creamy or almost fluid in consistency, depending on the degree of ripening. The rind is a thin, felt-like layer of gray mold and dry cheese interspersed with patches of reddish yellow. Analysis: Moisture, 52.3 percent in domestic Camembert, and 43 to 54.4 percent in imported; fat, 24 to 28 percent (at least 50 percent in the solids); protein, 17 to 21 percent, 17 to 21 percent; and salt, 2.6 percent.
Cheddar	Cheddar cheese originated in England. It is a hard cheese, ranging in color from nearly white to yellow and a flavor ranging from mild to sharp. Cheddar is made from sweet, whole cow's milk, either raw or pasteurized. (If it is made from partly skimmed or skim milk, it must so be labeled). Cheddar cheeses are cured for at least 60 days, usually 3 to 6 months, and in some instances for as long as one year. Analysis: Moisture, 37 to 38 percent (not more than 39 percent); fat, 32 percent (fat in solids, not less than 50 percent); protein, 25 percent; and salt, 1.4 to 1.8 percent.
Colby	Colby cheese, similar to Cheddar, is made from either raw or pasteurized whole cow's milk. It is cured for a shorter period than Cheddar, contains more moisture, and has a softer body and more open texture. For these reasons, it does not keep as well as Cheddar. Analysis: Moisture, not more than 40 percent (usually 38 percent); fat in the solids, not less than 50 percent; and salt, 1.4 to 1.8 percent.

From USDA, 1978. For a complete listing of cheese varieties and descriptions, see USDA (1978) Agriculture Handbook Number 54.

198

Table 11-13. (Continued)

Name	Description
Edam	Edam cheese originated in Holland. It has a mild, clean, sometimes salty flavor and a firm crumbly body, free of holes and openings. Edam is made also in the United States. It usually is shaped like a flattened ball, but in the U.S. it is made also in a loaf shape. The red coating is an identifying characteristic of Edam cheese. Analysis: Moisture, not more than 45 percent (usually 35 to 38 percent); fat, 26.5 to 29.5 percent (not less than 40 percent in the solids); Protein, 27 to 29 percent; and salt, 1.6 to 2 percent.
Feta	Feta, a white cheese, is the primary cheese made in Greece. It is usually made with ewe's milk but is sometimes made from goat's milk. In the United States, it is made from cow's milk. Depending on the ripening process, the cheese is ready to eat in 4 to 30 days.
Gouda	Gouda cheese originated in Holland. The cheese is semi-soft to hard, sweet curd similar to Edam except that it contains more fat. It is made from whole or partly skimmed cow's milk. Gouda is shaped like a flattened sphere and pressed in molds with rounded ends. The flavor is mild, similar to Edam. Cures in 2 to 3 months, but improves in flavor if cured for 5 to 6 months. Analysis: Moisture, not more than 45 percent (usually 36 to 43.5 percent); fat, 29 to 30.5 percent (not less than 45 percent in the solids); protein, 25 to 26 percent; and salt, 1.5 to 2 percent.
Gruyere	Gruyere originated in Switzerland. The cheese is made from whole cow's milk in much the same way as Swiss; but Gruyere is smaller, has smaller eyes, and a sharper flavor. The cheese is cured for at least 90 days. Analysis: Moisture, 33 to not more than 39 percent; fat, 29 to 33 percent (usually 50 but not less than 45 percent in the solids); protein, 26 to 29 percent; and salt, 2 percent.
Monterey (or Jack)	Monterey or Jack cheese originated in California. The cheese is made from pasteurized whole, partly skimmed, or skim milk. Whole milk Monterey is semi-soft; partly skimmed or skim milk Monterey is hard and is used for grating. High-moisture Jack is made from whole milk. Whole milk Monterey is cured for 3 to 6 weeks. Grating-type Monterey is cured for at least 6 months. Analysis: Moisture, not more than 44 percent for whole milk Monterey; not more than 34 percent for grating-type Monterey; and more than 44 but less than 50 percent for high-moisture Jack; fat in the solids, not less than 50 percent for whole milk Monterey and high-moisture Jack; not less than 32 percent for grating-type Monterey; and salt, about 1.5 percent.
Provolone	Provolone, an Italian plastic-curd cheese, was first made in southern Italy, but later made in other parts of Italy and the United States. It is light in color, mellow, smooth, cuts without crumbling, and has an agreeable flavor. The cheese is made with whole cow's milk; raw or pasteurized. If made from raw milk, it must be cured for at least 60 days. Analysis: Moisture, not more than 45 percent (usually 37 to 43.5 percent); fat, 25 to 33 percent (fat in the solids, at least 45 percent and usually 47 percent); and salt, 2 to 4 percent.
Roquefort	Roquefort, a blue-veined, semi-soft to hard cheese, originated in France. The cheese is made from ewe's milk. Roquefort cheese is characterized by its sharp, peppery, piquant flavor and by the mottled, blue-green veins throughout the white curd. The curing period is 2 to 5 months. Analysis: Moisture, 38.5 to 41 percent (not more than 45 percent); fat, 32.2 percent; fat in the solids, not less than 50 percent; protein, 21.1 percent; ash, 6.1 percent; and salt (in the ash), 4.1 percent.
Swiss	Swiss cheese originated in Switzerland. Characterized by a large, hard, pressed-curd with elastic body, the cheese is best known because of the holes or eyes that develop in the curd as the cheese ripens. Swiss cheese is made with low-fat cow's milk. Much of the cheese made in the United States is marketed after curing for 3 to 4 months (2 months minimum). Most of the cheese exported from Switzerland is cured for 6 to 10 months and has a more pronounced flavor. Analysis (Domestic Swiss): Moisture, 39.4 percent (not more than 41 percent); fat, 27.5 percent (not less than 43 percent in the solids); protein, 27.4 percent; and salt, 1 to 1.6 percent.

cheeses are those such as camembert. Curing progresses from the outside to the center. *Semisoft ripened* cheeses, such as brick and Muenster, are less moist than soft ripened cheeses. The cheeses ripen from the interior as well as the surface by using surface growth and bacterial culture. *Firm ripened* cheeses, like cheddar and Swiss, are ripened throughout the entire cheese. The cheese is lower in moisture, thus requiring a long curing time. *Very hard ripened* cheeses are cured very slowly because of their low moisture and high salt content, such as Parmesan and Romano. *Blue-vein mold ripened* cheeses, such as blue and roquefort, are cured by using a mold culture that grows throughout the interior to produce the familiar flavor and appearance. The more commonly used varieties of cheese are shown in Table 11-13.

___ Seafood Specifications ___

Fresh and frozen fish are marketed in various forms or cuts. The edible portion will vary from 45% for whole fish to 100% for fillets. A knowledge of the following cuts is important in buying fish (Fig. 11-12).

* *Whole or round* fish as they come from the water. Edible portion about 45%.
* *Drawn* whole fish that have been eviscerated. Edible portion about 48%.
* *Dressed or pan-dressed.* Whole fish with scales and entrails removed, and usually with the head, tail, and fins removed. Edible portion about 67%.
* *Steaks.* Cross-section slices from large dressed fish, usually about ¾ in. thick. Edible portion about 84%.
* *Fillets.* Sides of fish cut lengthwise from the backbone. Practically boneless and have little or no waste. A fillet cut from one side of a fish is called a single fillet.
* *Butterfly fillet.* The two sides of the fish, corresponding to two single fillets, held together by the uncut flesh and skin of the belly.
* *Sticks.* Elongated pieces of fish cut from blocks of frozen fillets. Each stick weighing not less than ¾ oz and not more than 1¼ oz.
* *Portions.* Uniformly shaped pieces of boneless fish cut from blocks of frozen fillets. A portion cut is larger than a fish stick and has a thickness of ⅜ in.

Fish may be classified as freshwater or saltwater; fat or lean. The amount of fat is important, since it is related to the cooking method. To know the fat content is also important in purchasing fish for modified diets. Table 11-14 provides useful information for the buyer in purchasing the appropriate type of fish.

In determining quality characteristics of fresh whole and drawn fish, the buyer can expect high-quality fish to have (1) firm flesh; (2) fresh, mild odor; (3) bright, clear, and full eyes; (4) red gills; and (5) shiny skin. Fresh fillets and steaks should have a fresh-cut appearance and a firm texture, and should not show traces of browning or a dried-out look. The odor should be fresh and mild.

Frozen fish of good quality has the following characteristics: (1) no discoloration of flesh, (2) little or no odor, and (3) wrapped either individually or in packages of various weights with moisture- or vapor-proof materials and little or no air space between the fish and the wrapping.

The buyer should specify the type, size, and state of refrigeration. Fresh fish should be packed in ice for delivery and still be well iced when received. Frozen fish should be solidly frozen when bought and delivered. The most commonly used containers with net weights of packs are shown in Table 11-15.

A wide variety of canned fish and fish specialty items are available, including canned salmon, tuna, mackerel, cod, herring, shad, sardines, sturgeon, and others. Specialty items include fish balls, chowders, cakes, and roe. The two most

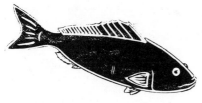

Whole or round fish are those marketed just as they come from the water. Before cooking, they must be scaled and eviscerated (which means removing the entrails). The head, tail, and fins may be removed, if desired, and the fish either split or cut into serving-size portions, except in fish intended for baking. Some small fish, like smelt, are frequently cooked with only the entrails removed.

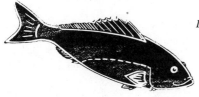

Drawn fish are marketed with only the entrails removed. In preparation for cooking, they generally are scaled. Head, tail, and fins are removed, if desired, and the fish split or cut into serving-size portions. Small drawn fish, or larger sizes intended for baking, may be cooked in the form purchased, after being scaled.

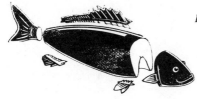

Dressed or pan-dressed fish are scaled and eviscerated, usually with the head, tail and fins removed. The smaller sizes are ready for cooking as purchased (pan-dressed). The larger sizes of dressed fish may be baked as purchased but frequently are cut into steaks or serving-size portions.

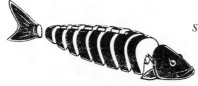

Steaks are cross-section slices of the larger sizes of dressed fish. They are ready to cook as purchased, except for dividing the very largest into serving-size portions. A cross-section of the backbone is usually the only bone in the steak.

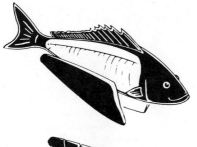

Fillets are the sides of the fish, cut lengthwise away from the backbone. They are practically boneless and require no preparation for cooking. Sometimes the skin, with the scales removed, is left on the fillets; others are skinned. A fillet cut from one side of a fish is called a single fillet. This is the type of fillet most generally seen in the market.

Sticks are pieces of fish cut lengthwise or crosswise from fillets or steaks into portions of uniform width and length.

Butterfly fillets are the two sides of the fish corresponding to two single fillets held together by uncut flesh and the skin.

Figure 11-12. Market forms of fish. *From U.S. Department of the Interior (1964A)*

Table 11-14. Classification of Seafood[a]

Species	Fat or Lean	Usual Range of Weight (lb)	Usual Market Forms
Salt water:			
Bluefish	Lean	1–7	Whole and drawn
Butterfish	Fat	¼–1	Whole and dressed
Cod	Lean	3–20	Drawn, dressed, steaks, and fillets
Croaker	Lean	½–2½	Whole, dressed, and fillets
Flounder	Lean	¼–5	Whole, dressed, and fillets
Grouper	Lean	5–15	Whole, drawn, dressed, steaks, and fillets
Haddock	Lean	1½–7	Drawn and fillets
Hake	Lean	2–5	Whole, drawn, dressed, and fillets
Halibut	Lean	8–75	Dressed and steaks
Herring, sea	Fat	¼–1	Whole
Lingcod	Lean	5–20	Dressed, steaks, and fillets
Mackerel	Fat	¾–3	Whole, drawn, and fillets
Mullet	Lean	½–3	Whole
Pollock	Lean	3–14	Drawn, dressed, steaks, and fillets
Rockfish	Lean	2–5	Dressed and fillets
Rosefish	Lean	½–1¼	Fillets
Salmon	Fat	3–30	Drawn, dressed, steaks, and fillets
Scup (Porgy)	Lean	½–2	Whole and dressed
Sea bass	Lean	¼–4	Whole, dressed, and fillets
Sea trout	Lean	1–6	Whole, drawn, dressed, and fillets
Shad	Fat	1½–7	Whole, drawn, and fillets
Snapper, red	Lean	2–15	Drawn, dressed, steaks, and fillets
Spanish mackerel	Fat	1–4	Whole, drawn, dressed, and fillets
Spot	Lean	¼–1¼	Whole and dressed
Whiting	Lean	½–1½	Whole, drawn, dressed, and fillets
Fresh water:			
Buffalofish	Lean	5–15	Whole, drawn, dressed, and steaks
Carp	Lean	2–8	Whole and fillets
Catfish	Fat	1–10	Whole, dressed, and skinned
Lake herring	Lean	⅓–1	Whole, drawn, and fillets
Lake trout	Fat	1½–10	Drawn, dressed, and fillets
Sheepshead	Lean	½–3	Whole, drawn, dressed, and fillets
Suckers	Lean	½–4	Whole, drawn, dressed, and fillets
Whitefish	Fat	2–6	Whole, drawn, dressed, and fillets
Yellow perch	Lean	½–1	Whole and fillets
Yellow pike	Lean	1½–10	Whole, dressed, and fillets
Shellfish:			
Clams	Lean		In the shell, shucked
Crabs	Lean		Live, cooked meat
Lobsters	Lean		Live, cooked meat
Oysters	Lean		In the shell, shucked
Shrimp	Lean		Headless, cooked meat

[a] From U.S. Department of the Interior (1961).

popular canned fish used in institutional foodservice operations are salmon and tuna.

Salmon canned on the Pacific coast come from five distinct species and are usually sold by their names, which indicate the differences in the type of meat. Salmon differs in color, texture, and flavor. The higher-priced varieties are deeper red in color and have a higher oil content. The grades of salmon are

1. Chinook or king salmon
2. Red or sockeye salmon
3. Medium red salmon

Table 11-15. Commonly Used Containers for Seafood[a]

Seafood	Containers	Net Weights
Fresh fish:		
Whole, drawn, and dressed:		
Most varieties:		
Freshwater	Boxes	25, 40, 50, 60, 100 lb
Saltwater	Boxes	15, 100, 125, 150, 200 lb
	Barrels	125, 150, 250 lb
Some small fish:		
Freshwater	Boxes	10 to 20 lb
Saltwater	Boxes	10 to 30 lb
	Tight barrels	75 lb
Fillets and steaks:		
Freshwater	Tins	20, 25 lb
Saltwater	Tins	10, 15, 20, 25, 30 lb
Frozen fish:		
Whole, drawn, and dressed:		
Most varieties:		
Freshwater	Boxes	60, 70, 100 lb
Saltwater	Boxes	50, 100, 150, 200 lb
Some small fish:		
Freshwater	Boxes	10, 20 lb
Saltwater	Boxes and packages	1, 5, 10, 15, 20, 25 lb
Fillets and steaks:		
Freshwater	Packages	1, 5, 10 lb
Saltwater	Packages	12 oz; 1, 5, 10, 15, 20, 25 lb
Fish portions:		
Unbreaded, breaded and pre-cooked	Packages	8, 10, 12, 14 oz; 1, 3, 4, 5, 6 lb
Fish sticks:		
Breaded and precooked	Packages	8, 10, 12, 14 oz; 1, 3, 4, 5, 6 lb
Shellfish:		
Clams and oysters:		
In shell	Bags	100, 225, 250 lb
Shucked:		
Fresh	Tins	½ pt, 1 pt, 1 qt; ½, 1, 5 gal
Frozen	Tins and packages	12 oz, 5 lb
Crabs:		
Hard: Live	Bushel baskets; barrels	100 lb
Crabs:		
Soft:		
Live	Trunks	60, 80 lb
Frozen	Packages	Up to 1 lb
Dungeness eviscerated		
Frozen	Poly bags	1½–2½ lb
Crab meat, cooked:		
Blue	Tins	1 lb
Dungeness	Tins	1, 5 lb
King	Packages	6 oz, 3 lb
Lobsters, live	Barrels	50, 100 lb
	Boxes	25, 50 lb
Lobster meat, cooked, fresh and frozen	Tins	6 oz, 14 oz; 1, 5 lb
Scallops, sea:		
Fresh meats	Tins	1 gal
	Bags	30, 40 lb
Frozen meats	Tins	1 gal
	Packages	10 oz; 1, 5, 10 lb
Frozen breaded and precooked	Packages	7 oz; 1, 2, 5 lb
Scallops, bay: Fresh meat	Tins	1 gal
Shrimp, headless:		
Fresh	Boxes	100 lb
Frozen	Tins and packages	6, 12 oz;
	Packages	1, 2½, 5, 10 lb
Breaded, frozen	Packages	8, 10, 12 oz; 1, 5 lb
Shrimp meat, cooked peeled and de-veined	Tins and packages	4, 8, 12 oz; 1, 5 lb

[a]From U.S. Department of the Interior (1959).

203

4. Pink salmon
5. Chum salmon

Salmon may be purchased in 3¾-, 7½-, 15½-, and 64-oz cans.

Tuna canned in this country is produced from four species of the mackerel family. They are yellowfin, bluefin, skipjack, and albacore. Tuna is divided into grades according to the type of meat used, as indicated below:

1. *Fancy* or *fancy whitemeat* tuna consists of choice cuts of cooked albacore tuna packed as large pieces of solid meat.
2. *Standard* tuna consists of cooked tuna meat packed in the approximate proportion of 75% large pieces and 25% flakes.
3. *Grated or shredded* tuna is cooked tuna packed in small uniform pieces.
4. *Flaked* tuna is cooked tuna packed in small pieces.

Tuna may be purchased in the following size cans: 3½, 7, and 13 oz. Tuna flakes and grated tuna are packed in 3-, 5-, 12-, and 64-oz cans (U.S. Department of the Interior 1964A)

Some of the more popular species of shellfish are shrimp, clams, oysters, crabs, lobsters, and scallops. Some shellfish are marketed alive. Other market forms (Fig. 11-13), depending on the variety, include cooked whole in the shell, headless, fresh meat (shucked), and cooked meat.

- *Live.* Shellfish, such as crabs, lobsters, clams, and oysters should be alive if purchased in the shell. The exception is for boiled crabs and lobsters, which may be cooked in the shell before marketing.
- *Shucked.* Shucked shellfish are those that have been removed from their shells. Oysters, clams, and scallops are marketed in this manner.
- *Headless.* The term applies to shrimp, which are marketed in most areas with the head and thorax removed.
- *Cooked meat.* The edible portion of shellfish is often sold cooked, ready to eat. Shrimp, crab, and lobster meat are marketed in this way.

The various kinds of shrimp range in color from greenish gray to brownish red, when raw; they differ little in appearance and flavor, when cooked. The

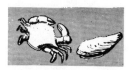

Live

Shellfish, such as crabs, lobsters, clams, and oysters should be alive if purchased in the shell, except for boiled crabs and lobsters.

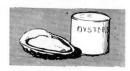

Shucked

Shucked shellfish are those which have been removed from their shells. Oysters, clams, and scallops are marketed in this manner.

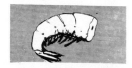

Headless

This term applies to shrimp, which are marketed in most areas with the head and thorax removed.

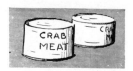

Cooked meat

The edible portion of shellfish is often sold cooked, ready to eat. Shrimp, crab, and lobster meat are marketed in this way.

Figure 11-13. Market forms of shellfish. *From U.S. Department of the Interior (1964A)*

term *green shrimp* does not refer to color, but is a name used in the trade to describe shrimp that have not been cooked. Shrimp are sold on a size basis or by such terms as jumbo, large, medium, and small. The largest size or grade runs 15 or fewer shrimp to the pound. The smallest size runs 60 or more to the pound. The larger sizes are higher priced. Shrimp are sold as

- Fresh or frozen, headless, but with shells on.
- Fresh or frozen, cooked, generally peeled (shells removed and meat deveined).
- Frozen, breaded (raw and cooked) after being peeled and deveined.

The trade term for peeled, deveined, and quick-frozen is PDQ. Most shrimp marketed in the United States are sold as fresh or frozen; canned shrimp are available packed either in brine or dry. The buyer should specify Grade A, count, class (headless, peeled, and deveined), and state of refrigeration (U.S. Department of the Interior 1964B).

Several species of clams are widely used for food. On the Atlantic coast, the marketed species are the hard clams, the soft clams, and the surf clams. The hard-shell clam is commonly called quahog in New England, where *clam* generally means the soft-shell variety. In the Middle Atlantic states and southward, *clam* is the usual name for the hard clam.

Littlenecks and cherrystones are dealer's names for the smaller-sized hard clams, generally served raw on the half shell. The larger sizes of hard clams are called chowders and are used mainly for chowders and soups. The larger sizes of soft clams are known as in-shells, and the smaller sizes as steamers.

On the Pacific coast, the most common market species are the butter, littleneck, razor, and pismo clams. Clams in the shell should be alive and the shells should close tight when tapped lightly. Fresh clams are pale orange to deep orange in color and free of stale odor or taste. Clams are purchased by the dozen in the shell. If shucked, clams should be packed in little or no free liquid. Clams may be purchased in the frozen or canned state. Frozen clams are breaded and may be raw or cooked. Canned clams may be whole, minced, or in combination foods such as chowders and soups (U.S. Department of Interior 1964C).

There are three major species of oysters available. The Eastern oyster is found and cultivated from Massachusetts to Texas; the small Olympia oyster is found on the Pacific coast from Washington to Mexico; and the larger Pacific or Japanese oyster is cultivated on the Pacific coast. Oysters may be purchased in these forms (U.S. Department of Interior 1964D):

1. *Shell oysters.* Oysters in the shell are sold by the dozen and must be alive when purchased. Gaping shells that do not close when tapped lightly indicate that the oysters are dead and therefore should not be used.

2. *Shucked oysters.* These are oysters that have been removed from the shell and are usually sold by the pint or quart. Shucked oysters should be plump, and have a natural creamy color, with clear liquor, and be free from shell particles. Fresh shucked oysters are packed in metal containers or waxed cartons. The Eastern oysters, comprising about 89% of the domestic oyster production, are packed in commercial grades as shown in Table 11-16.

3. *Frozen oysters.* These are shucked oysters that have been quick-frozen. Frozen oysters should not be thawed until ready to use. Once thawed, they should never be refrozen. Frozen, raw, or cooked breaded oysters are also available.

4. *Canned oysters.* Canned oysters packed on the Atlantic and Gulf coast are usually sold in No. 1 picnic cans containing 7½ oz drained weight of oysters.

Table 11-16. Grade and Count for Eastern Oysters[a]

Grade	Oysters per Gallon
Counts or extra large	Not more than 160
Extra selects or large	161–210
Selects or medium	211–300
Standards or small	301–500
Standards or very small	Over 500

[a]From U.S. Department of the Interior (1964D).

Oysters packed on the Pacific coast are usually sold in cans containing 5 or 8 oz drained weight (U.S. Department of the Interior 1964D).

Crabs are one of the popular shellfish because of their tender meat and distinctive flavor. Blue crabs come from the Atlantic and Gulf coastal areas; Dungeness crabs are found on the Pacific coast; king crabs come from the North Pacific off Alaska; and Rock crabs are taken on the New England and California coasts. Blue crabs weigh ¼ to 1 lb. Depending on the season, they can be in the form of Eastern hard-shell crabs or soft-shell crabs. Soft-shell crabs are molting blue crabs taken just after they have shed their hard shells and before new shells are formed. Dungeness crabs weigh 1¾–3½ lb, king crabs weigh 6–20 lb, and rock crabs weigh ⅓–½ lb (U.S. Department of the Interior 1964E).

Crabs are marketed as live, cooked in the shell, cooked and frozen, fresh cooked meat, and canned meat. Fresh hard-shell and soft-shell crabs should be alive at the time of cooking. Cooked hard-shell crabs must be kept refrigerated, iced, or frozen from the time they are cooked until they are used. Frozen crab legs are cooked legs of the king crab. The large legs are either split or cut into sections. Canned crab meat may be from the blue, Dungeness, king, or rock crab. Fresh cooked meat is picked from the hard-shell crabs, packed, chilled, and sold by the pound. Fresh cooked meat is packed in several grades for blue crabs: (1) lump meat is the white meat from the body of the crab, (2) flake meat consists of small pieces of white meat from the rest of the body, (3) lump and flake meat is a combination of body and leg meat, and (4) claw meat is meat with a brownish tint from the claw. Fresh cooked meat from the Dungeness crab is picked from both body and claws, has a pinkish tinge, and is packed as one grade. Fresh cooked meat from the king crab is taken mostly from the legs. Fresh cooked meat from rock crabs is picked from both body and claws and is marketed as one grade.

Lobsters and spiny lobsters should show movement of legs when they are alive. The tail of the live lobster curls under the body and does not hang down when the lobster is picked up. The Northern lobster, caught off the coast of Maine and Massachusetts, is considered the true lobster. Another type, off the coast of California and Florida, is known as the *spiny* or *rock lobster*. The difference is that the Northern lobster has large heavy claws, whereas the spiny lobster has no claws. Frozen spiny or rock lobster tails should have clear white meat, be hard-frozen when bought, and have no odor. Whole lobsters are sold in the shell as fresh, frozen, or cooked and vary in size from ¾ to 4 lb. The buyer should specify lobster size as:

- Chicken, ¾–1 lb
- Quarters, 1¼–1½ lb
- Large, 1½–2½ lb
- Jumbo, over 3 lb

Cooked lobster meat is marketed as fresh pack, frozen, or canned. The meat should be white with deep pink covering and free of any disagreeable odors (U.S. Department of the Interior 1964F).

Scallops are a shellfish, a mollusk possessing two shells, similar to oysters and clams. Unlike other shellfish, scallops are marketed only as dressed meat. Because scallops are active swimmers, snapping their shells together to provide locomotion, an oversized muscle is developed, called the abductor muscle. This muscle is the only part of the scallop eaten by Americans (U.S. Department of the Interior 1964G).

There are two varieties of scallops: the large sea scallop and the smaller bay scallop. The sea scallop is taken from the waters of northern and Middle Atlantic states and measuring about ½ inch across. The bay scallop is taken from in-shore bays from New England to the Gulf of Mexico. Fresh scallops are a light cream color, sometimes varying to a delicate pink. Scallops are available fresh or frozen, but only in the form of dressed meat. Sea scallops are generally opened, packed, and iced at sea. Fresh and frozen scallops when thawed should have a sweetish odor and should be practically free of liquid.

___ Fresh Fruit and Vegetable Specifications ___

The produce market is one of the most difficult markets for the buyer because of variations in grading standards, methods of packaging, and the seasonability of products.

In formulating standards for fruits and vegetables, the Department of Agriculture originally adopted the numerical system of nomenclature for grades, with some exceptions (U.S. Department of Agriculture 1956). The highest grade for a product is U.S. No. 1. Under normal conditions, better than half of the crop usually will be U.S. No. 1 grade. The designation of U.S. No. 2 ordinarily represents the quality of the lowest grade deemed practical to pack under normal conditions. It was found that U.S. No. 1 and U.S. No. 2 designations were not sufficient to represent all of the graduations of quality for a number of specialized products. Many shippers preferred to pack a top-grade product of high color and practically free from defects, for which they would receive premium prices. Thus it was necessary, in some sets of standards, to provide a grade designation for a product superior to that ordinarily termed U.S. No. 1. To meet this need the designation U.S. Fancy was chosen. In a few standards it was necessary to provide a grade designation for quality between U.S. Fancy and U.S. No. 1, as in standards for peaches and potatoes. The designation of U.S. Extra No. 1 is applied to this quality. It was also necessary to provide a grade designation between U.S. No. 1 and U.S. No. 2 for quality not up to U.S. No. 1, but superior to U.S. No. 2 grade. The terms U.S. Commercial and U.S. Combination were adopted. The grade designations prompted criticism that the system was misleading and confusing. In 1976, efforts to standardize grade designations resulted in the use of the following terms: U.S. Fancy, U.S. No. 1, U.S. No. 2, and U.S. No. 3. The U.S. No. 1 grade is generally recommended for institutional foodservice use.

The packaging or unit of purchasing ranges from loose pack by the pound to sacks, crates, cartons, boxes, baskets, lungs, gallons, and bunches (Table 11-17). Price quotations should be based on the pound, rather than the container. The buyer will need to study the specifications for each food item, and visually inspect fresh fruit and vegetables to recognize quality products.

Table 11-17. Container Types and Approximate Weights for Fresh Fruits and Vegetables[a]

Food Item	Type Container	Approximate Weight (lb)	Count
Asparagus	Cartons	15–16 lb	
	Pyramid crates	30–32 lb	
Avocados	Cartons and flats	12–15 lb	
Beans, green or waxed	Basket	28–30 lb	
	Crates	28–30 lb	
	Cartons	28–30 lb	
Broccoli	Crates, wirebound	20 lb	
	Baskets	6 lb	
	Cartons, 14 bu	20–23 lb	
Brussels sprouts	Wooden drums	25 lb	
	Flats, 12 10–oz cups	7½–8 oz/cup	
Cabbage	Crates, 1⅗ bu	50–55 lb	
	Cartons	45–50 lb	
	Mesh sacks	50–60 lb	
Carrots (without tops)	Sacks	50 lb	
	Crates	50 lb	
	Baskets, bu	50 lb	
Cauliflower	Cartons	18–24 lb	(12–16 heads)
	Crates, wirebound	45–50 lb	
Celery	Crates, Florida, 16 in. length	55–60 lb	
	Crates, California, 16 in. length	60–65 lb	
Corn	Crates, wirebound	40–60 lb	4 doz ears
	Mesh bags	45–50 lb	
Cucumbers	Crates, 1⅑ bu	55 lb	
	Baskets, bu	47–55 lb	
	Cartons	26–30 lb	
	Lugs	26–30 lb	
Green, salad (chicory, endive, escarole)	Crates, 1⅑ bu	25–28 lb	
	1⅖ bu	33–40 lb	
	16-in. crate	33–40 lb	
	Cartons	18–22 lb	
	Baskets, 24 qt	16 lb	
	bu	25 lb	
Greens (collards, kale)	Baskets, bu	18–25 lb	
	Crates	18–25 lb	
Greens (spinach, turnip, mustard)	Baskets, bu	18–22 lb	
	Crates,	18–22 lb	
	1½ bu	30–32 lb	
	Cartons, 1⅛ bu	20–22 lb	
Lettuce (head)	Cartons	40–45 lb	2 doz heads
Lettuce (romaine)	Crates, wirebound, 1⅑ bu	28–32 lb	
	Cartons	34–36 lb	2 dozen heads
Lettuce (leaf)	Baskets, 12 qt	7 lb	
	Other containers	5–10 lb	
		20–25 lb	
Okra	Baskets, bu	28–32 lb	
	½ bu	14–16 lb	
	Crates, bu	28–32 lb	
	Los Angeles (L.A.) lugs	17–19 lb	
Onions, mature	Mesh sacks	25 or 50 lb	
	Cartons	48–50 lb	
Parsley	Crates, wirebound	20–22 lb	
	Cartons	20–22 lb	5 doz bunches
Peas, green (pods)	Baskets, bu	28–30 lb	
	Crates, western	28–30 lb	
Peppers	Crates, 1⅑ bu	28–33 lb	
	Baskets, bu	28–33 lb	
	Cartons, 1⅛ bu	28–34 lb	
	Lugs	18 lb	

Table 11-17. (Continued)

Food Item	Type Container	Approximate Weight (lb)	Count
Potatoes, white	Burlap sacks	50 or 100 lb	
	Paper cartons or paper bags	10, 15, 20, 25 or 50 lb	
Radishes (without tops)	Baskets	11¼ lb	
	Cartons	11¼ lb	
	Bags	25 or 40 lb	
Squash (summer)	Baskets, bu	40–45 lb	
	½ bu	20–22 lb	
	Crates, 1⅑ bu	42–45 lb	
	5/9 bu	22–25 lb	
	Cartons	20–25 lb	
	Lugs	24 lb	
Squash (winter)	Baskets, bu	50 lb	
	Crates	40–50 lb	
	Cartons	20–25 lb	
Sweet potatoes	Baskets, bu	50 lb	
	Crates, bu	50 lb	
	Cartons	38–42 lb	
Tomatoes	Cartons	10, 20, 30, or 40 lb	
	Crates	40 lb	
	Lugs	30–34 lb	
	Flats	10–20 lb	
	Baskets (various)	9–20 lb	
Turnips (without tops)	Baskets, bu	50 lb	
	Sacks	50 lb	
	Cartons	40–50 lb	
Apples	Cartons, tray-pack 1 or 1⅛ bu	36–45 lb	113–138 (medium)
	Cartons, cell-pack 1 or 1⅛ bu	36–45 lb	100–140 (medium)
	Cartons, bulk (various)	20–46 lb	50–140 (medium)
	Cartons, boxes bu	36–44 lb	113–138 (medium)
	Cartons, baskets bu	36–44 lb	110–140 (medium)
Apricots	Lugs	25–30 lb	
	Cartons	12–25 lb	
	Cartons or crates, 4 baskets	20–26 lb	
Bananas	Cartons	40 lb	110–125 175–200 (petite)
Berries (blackberries, blueberries)	Trays, 12 pt	9–15 lb	
Cantaloupe	Crates	80–85 lb	27, 36, 45
	Cartons	38–41 lb	12, 18, 23
Cherries, Sweet	Lugs or cartons	12, 14, 15, 18, or 20 lb	
	Crates, 8 qt	12 lb	
Cranberries	Cartons, 24 packs	24 lb (1-lb packs)	
Grapefruit	Cartons, Texas 7/10 bu	40 lb	
	Cartons, Florida ⅘ bu	42 lb	
	Cartons, Western half-box	34–36 lb	

(continued)

Table 11-17. Container Types and Approximate Weights for Fresh Fruits and Vegetables[a]

Food Item	Type Container	Approximate Weight (lb)	Count
Grapes	Lugs or cartons	17–28 lb	
Lemons	Cartons	37–39 lb	140–165 (medium)
Limes	Flats or cartons	10–11 lb	25–35 (medium)
	Boxes or cartons	40–41 lb	
Melons, honeydew	Crates	45–50 lb	6–8
	Cartons	29–32 lb	4–5
Nectarines	Sanger lugs or cartons	19–22 lb	64–82 (medium)
	L.A. lugs	22–29 lb	72–90
Oranges	Cartons, Florida and Texas	43–47 lb	100–125 (small)
	Cartons, California and Arizona—⅘ lb	36–39 lb	88, 113, 138 (medium)
Peaches	Cartons, ¾ bu	35–42 lb	100–125 (medium)
	Crates, ¾ bu	35–42 lb	100–125
	½ bu	22–28 lb	70–90
	Baskets, ¾ bu	35–42 lb	100–125
	½ bu	22–28 lb	70–90
	Lugs	19–29 lb	60–70
Pears	Boxes	45–48 lb	110–150 (medium)
	Cartons	36–48 lb	60–150
	Lugs	21–26 lb	50–65
Pineapple	Cartons or crates	35 lb	9–12
Plums	Cartons, 4 baskets	26–30 lb	
	Crates	24–32 lb	
	Lugs	18–30 lb	
Raspberries	Trays, 12 pt	9–15 lb	
Strawberries	Trays, 12 pt	11–12 lb	
Tangerines	Crates, Florida	45 lb	210–294 (small)
	Cartons, Florida	30 lb	
	Cartons, California	23–30 lb	120–176 (medium)
Watermelon	Whole melon	15–18 lb	(small)
		19–28 lb	(medium)

[a]From Food Purchasing Pointers for School Food Service, USDA (1977).

Processed Fruits and Vegetables

With the use of processed foods, it is not necessary to have seasonal menus, except for economic reasons, because most foods are available year-round. Canned and frozen foods are types most often used in institutional foodservice. Other types of processed foods include vacuum-dried potatoes and onions, and freeze-dried fruits and vegetables.

The specification for canned fruits and vegetables should include the following:

• Name of food item
• Grade
• Size of container
• Style, type, or size
• Other information to obtain desired product, such as variety, drained weight, syrup density, harvest area.

Table 11-18. USDA Grades for Canned Fruits, Vegetables, and Juice

Product	Grade	Score
Fruits	U.S. Grade A or U.S. Grade Fancy	90 and above
	U.S. Grade B or U.S. Choice	80–89
	U.S. Grade C or U.S. Standard	70–79
Vegetables	U.S. Grade A or U.S. Fancy	90 and above
	U.S. Grade B or U.S. Extra Standard	80–89
	U.S. Grade C or U.S. Standard	70–79
Fruit or vegetable juice	U.S. Grade A or U.S. Fancy	85–100
	U.S. Grade B, U.S. Choice, or U.S. Extra Standard	70–84

The USDA Grades for fruits, vegetables, and juices are shown in Table 11.18. The factors used for scoring of products are color, absence of defects, and character. Absence of defects includes uniformity of product, whereas character refers to tenderness, texture, maturity, flavor, and odor. Some fruits and vegetables score at the bottom of the grade, as is frequently the case in meat products. The buyer can request a grade certificate from the purveyor to determine the product score. The buyer can also conduct *can-cutting* experiments to compare quality. The general procedure is to remove all labels from the various brands and code each can prior to opening. Allow all products the same period of time for draining off liquid, usually 2 minutes. Compare products for color, texture, uniformity of products, count, size, and drained weight.

Processed fruits and vegetables must conform to labeling as established by the Food and Drug Administration (FDA); see Friedelson (1967). The following basic information must be on all food labels:

- The name of the product (common or usual)
- Form or style (whole, slices, or halves)
- The net contents or net weight. The net weight on canned food includes the liquid in which the product is packed, such as water in canned vegetables and syrup in canned fruit.
- The name and place of business of the manufacturer, packer, or distributor.

Other information, as required under certain conditions, must also be listed:

1. *List of ingredients.* On most foods, the ingredients must be listed in descending order by weight, with the ingredient present in the largest amount listed first. Any additives used in the product must be listed, but colors and flavors do not have to be listed by name. If the flavors are artificial, this fact must be stated. The labels on butter, cheese, and ice cream do not need to include the listing of artificial color because these foods have a Standard of Identity. The only foods not required to list all ingredients are those that meet FDA *Standards of Identity.* These standards require that all foods called by a particular name (such as catsup and mayonnaise) contain certain mandatory ingredients. These Standards of Identity are published in the Code of Federal Regulations (1984).

2. *Nutrition information.* Under FDA regulations, any food to which a nutrient has been added, or any food for which a nutritional claim is made, must have the nutritional content listed on the label.

3. *Common or usual name.* For example, a non-carbonated beverage that appears to contain a fruit or vegetable juice but does not contain any juice, must

state on the label that it contains no fruit or vegetable juice. Another special label requirement concerns packaged foods in which the main ingredient or component of a recipe is not included. The regulation states that the picture must represent the product, such as cake with icing, chicken casserole, and so on. A statement must be added such as "icing not included," or "you must add chicken to complete the recipe."

As a competitive edge, some manufacturers include voluntary statements such as:

- U.S. Grade
- Size (extra large, small, midget, etc.)
- Descriptive terms (very young, young, mature)
- Serving suggestions (recipes, garnishes, and number of servings). If number of servings are given, the size of serving must also be given.

Container sizes for canned fruits and vegetables are standardized throughout the industry. Except for small servings required for modified diets, the no. 10 can size is used for most fruits and vegetables in institutional foodservice. Other container sizes and their usual weight capacities are given in Table 11-19.

The style, type, or size should be specified in order to obtain the most appropriate food for a particular menu item. Some examples are as follows:

- Peaches—halves, slices
- Beets—whole, slices, julienne
- Corn—whole kernel, cream style, yellow, white
- Carrots—whole, slices, quarters, julienne, dices
- Apples—slices, Northern Spy

The packing medium must be stated on the label and should be part of the specification to ensure appropriateness to the planned menu. The packing medium may be water, natural juice, slightly sweetened juice, light syrup, medium syrup, heavy syrup, or extra heavy syrup. Syrup density refers to the sweetness of the packing medium and is tested by using a Brix hydrometer. As measured, 1 Brix equals 1% sugar. The syrup density, at the time the can is opened, called *cut-out*, is lower than the syrup density at packing which is called *put-in*. The reason is that some of the sugar is absorbed by the fruit, and thus the syrup is less concentrated.

Frozen Fruits, Vegetables, and Juices

Specification factors to consider are the same as those stated for canned products. The USDA Grading system also applies to these foods. For frozen juice concentrates, the buyer should specify the water-juice ratio required for reconstitution. Frozen juice concentrate may be purchased in cans from 6 to 32 oz. Frozen fruits are packed in 1-, 2½-, or 5-lb packages and 6½- to 30-lb cans. Frozen vegetables may be purchased in 2-, 2½-, or 3-lb boxes; and up to 20- or 30-lb bags. See Appendix Table E-11 for purchase units and portion information for various frozen vegetables.

Dealing with Purveyors

The selection of purveyors is not a simple task and should not be taken lightly. The buyer should conduct some investigation prior to contacting a particular

Table 11-19. Common Can and Jar Sizes[a]

| Can Size (Industry Term)[b] | Average Net Weight of fluid Measure per Can[c] | | Average Volume per Can | | Cans per Case (no.) | Principal Products |
	Customary	Metric	Cups	Liters		
No. 10	6 lb (96 oz) to 7 lb 5 oz (117 oz)	2.72 kg to 3.31 kg	12 to 13⅔	2.84 to 3.24	6	*Institutional size:* Fruits, vegetables, some other foods.
No. 3 Cyl	51 oz (3 lb 3 oz) or 46 fl oz (1 qt 14 fl oz)	1.44 kg or 1.36 liter	5¾	1.36	12	Condensed soups, some vegetables, meat and poultry products, fruit and vegetable juices.
No. 2½	26 oz (1 lb 10 oz) to 30 oz (1 lb 14 oz)	737 g to 850 g	3½	0.83	24	*Family size:* Fruits, some vegetables.
No. 2 Cyl	24 fl oz	709 ml	3	0.71	24	Juices, soups.
No. 2	20 oz (1 lb 4 oz) or 18 fl oz (1 pt 2 fl oz)	567 g or 532 ml	2½	0.59	24	Juices, ready-to-serve soups, some fruits.
No. 303	16 oz (1 lb) to 17 oz (1 lb 1 oz)	453 g to 481 g	2	0.47	24 or 36	*Small cans:* Fruits and vegetables, some meat and poultry products, ready-to-serve soups.
No. 300	14 oz to 16 oz (1 lb)	396 g to 453 g	1¾	0.41	24	Some fruits and meat products.
No. 2 (vacuum)	12 oz	340 g	1½	0.36	24	Principally vacuum pack corn.
No. 1 (picnic)	10½ oz to 12 oz	297 g to 340 g	1¼	0.30	48	Condensed soups, some fruits, vegetables, meat, fish.
8 oz	8 oz	226 g	1	0.24	48 or 72	Ready-to-serve soups, fruits, vegetables.

[a]From USDA (1980).

[b]Can sizes are industry terms and do not necessarily appear on the label.

[c]The net weight on can or jar labels differs according to the density of the contents. For example: A no. 10 can of sauerkraut weighs 6 lb 3 oz (2.81 kg); a no. 10 can of cranberry sauce weighs 7 lb 5 oz (3.32 kg). Meats, fish, and shellfish are known and sold by weight of contents.

purveyor. For example, a buyer can check on the reputation of a purveyor by talking with buyers at other foodservice facilities. Questions to ask should deal with (1) company stability, (2) reliability, (3) honesty, (4) ability to meet delivery schedule, (5) product quality, (6) ability to provide large quantities if necessary, and (7) competitive prices. After the list of prospective purveyors has been narrowed down, the buyer should contact the purveyor for an interview. It is preferred that the interview take place at the company facilities so that observations can be made of processing sanitation, storage facilities, and other conditions.

___ Ordering ___

Before an order can be placed, it is necessary to determine the item desired, its quality, and its quantity. The desired item is based on the planned menu; the quality is based on specifications; and the quantity is based on the number of portions needed, through analytical forecasting.

FORECASTING Forecasting is a prediction of how much to buy based on previous records. In a medical foodservice operation, some of the managerial tools used in forecasting are as follows:

1. *Production worksheet.* At the end of each meal, the total amount of food used and the total number of persons served are entered on the production worksheet (See Chapter 12, Fig. 12–3). The totals include food served to patients, personnel, and guests. The information, plus recording data on special events, weather conditions, and other significant factors, can be used as part of the forecasting process.
2. *Patient census.* The average daily patient census for those requiring regular and modified diet food must be calculated.
3. *Menu rotation.* Check the day of the week that the menu item is to be served on the basis of menu rotation. In some medical facilities the patient census is lower on weekends and fewer employees are assigned for duty.
4. *Selective menu.* Consider food preferences. How many patients selected a particular food item during the last menu cycle?
5. *Special activities.* Check calendar for conferences, seminars, meetings, parties, and other activities.

PLACING THE ORDER The actual ordering is a simple process, provided that the necessary groundwork has been done to make an intelligent purchasing decision. A written order form should be used as a matter of recordkeeping. Even when orders are placed by telephone, a written order should follow as a cross-check for receiving personnel. The order form should not be a duplication of the specification, assuming that copies of specifications have been distributed to all purveyors and purchasing personnel. A brief description of items needed may be written on a form similar to that shown in Figure 11–14. The use of common language, such as USDA Grades for fruits and vegetables, and IMPS-NAMP numbers for meats, eliminates the need for full descriptions of each item, yet ensures that the order will be filled correctly.

A purchase order is written only after prices and other factors have been agreed upon between the buyer and the purveyor. The prices may be obtained by use of a telephone quotation sheet like the one shown in Figure 11-1 or from long-term negotiated bids. Instructions for completing a purchase order such as the one in Figure 11-14 are as follows:

1. List all items needed in column 1. If the facility is using the *one-stop* buying system, there may be a mixture of staple foods, fresh foods, and frozen foods.
2. Briefly describe each item, based on specifications, in a clear and concise manner.
3. Specify amounts needed based on the forecast.
4. The amount on hand is recorded by storeroom personnel from the perpetual inventory records.
5. The amount to order is obtained by subtracting the amount on hand from the amount needed. The amount to order may need adjusting if a minimum stock level has been established.

| XYZ General Hospital | | | | | | |
| Purchase Order Form | | | | | | |

Purveyor: _____   Date: _____

(1) Item	(2) Description	(3) Amount Needed	(4) Amount on Hand	(5) Amount to Order	(6) Purveyor Quote	(7) Delivery Date

Figure 11-14. Purchase order form.

6. The purveyor quote is based on prior agreement from telephone quotations, long-term, or contract bids.
7. The delivery date is based on the amount of *lead time* required for thawing, preparation, and other factors related to serving the menu item at the correct time.

Although the process is simple, it requires considerable thought and time. The buyer should never wait until the sales representative is in the office to complete the purchase order form. It should be filled out and ready to place, thus using the time with the salesperson to discuss new products. For daily deliveries of bread, ice cream, milk, and similar items, a standard preprinted order form with carbon copies may be used.

___ Receiving, Inspecting, and Storing ___

The receiving, inspecting, and storing of food are functions of the purchasing department. It is the responsibility of the purchasing director to establish controls to make sure that items received are in accord with items ordered. Receiving personnel should have copies of all specifications and be thoroughly familiar with quality standards. Receiving personnel should also have a copy of all orders placed. When food is delivered, the order form can be used to inspect for quantity. Procedures should be established to handle discrepancies such as shortages, poor quality, and general condition of food as delivered. It is important that only authorized personnel be allowed to receive food. The practice of allowing any foodservice or other employee sign for food is poor practice. These individuals cannot possibly check for quantity or quality with any degree of accuracy. Records of food received must be maintained by the purchasing department on forms such as those shown in Figures 11-15 and 11-16.

Adequate storage of food is essential in order to avoid a waste of the time, energy, and funds expended during the purchasing process. Depending on the purchasing system, all food may be delivered to the foodservice department, all food may be delivered to central storage, or staples may be delivered to central

	Invoice		Description	Cost
Vendor	Date	Number	(Food, Paper, Cleaning, Office)	Cost

Daily Receiving Record

Date Received _____   Received by _____

Figure 11-15. Daily receiving record form.

Date Received _____ Daily Receiving Record Received by _____

| Vendor | Invoice | | Fresh Meat, Fish, Poultry | Frozen Prepared Entrees | Canned Entrees | Frozen Fruits and Vegetables | Canned Fruits and Vegetables | Fresh Produce | Dairy | Bakery | Groceries | Other | Cost |
	Date	Number											
Total													

Figure 11-16. Daily receiving record form.

217

storage while meats and fresh produce are delivered directly to the department involved.

There may be a loss of control when food is delivered to different areas unless trained personnel are available in the different areas to receive the food. The most efficient procedure is to have all deliveries made directly to one area, whether it is the using department or central storage. The food can be promptly and properly stored or distributed immediately to the department involved.

Proper storage of food, from the time it is delivered until it is consumed by the customer, is a managerial function that must be shared by the purchasing department and the foodservice director. When food is received, there should be adequate safe, clean, and sanitary space available for storage at the proper temperature. When personnel are aware of delivery schedules, food stores can be arranged to utilize the *first-in-first-out* (FIFO) system. Table 11-20 provides a detailed description of safe and sanitary handling of stored food. All food cartons can be dated with a marking pen upon arrival. A cleaning schedule should be provided for storeroom personnel so that the areas are clean and orderly at all times.

Food Requisition and Inventory System

All food issued from stores should be accounted for by signed requisitions. It is management's responsibility to establish policies designating who is allowed to requisition food. The procedure varies, depending mainly on the size of the facility. In small operations, the foodservice supervisor or head cook may be responsible for requisitioning all food for all work areas. In large operations, requisitions may be submitted by the various units, such as main production, salad, bakery, patient service, and cafeteria service. At no times should the storeroom be left unattended and unlocked. The practice of leaving the storeroom open and unattended or hanging the storeroom key in the production area, allowing employees to walk in and out all during the day, should be avoided. For security purposes, storeroom keys should be handled by storeroom personnel only and left at the facility when the shift is over. Many of the problems associated with requisitions and distribution of food are eliminated with the use of an ingredient room, as discussed in Chapter 12.

The requisition form, as shown in Figure 11-17, should indicate the item, unit, item description, and amount issued. At the end of the serving period, all items requisitioned and not used should be returned to storage and recorded by storeroom personnel. To determine how much was used, the amount returned is subtracted from the amount issued.

An effective system for recording the amount of food on hand is the use of both the perpetual and physical inventory. In the perpetual inventory method there is continuous or daily posting of all food received and issued. There is a separate card (Fig. 11-18) for each item with space for name of product, minimum stock levels, date, order numbers, amounts received, amounts issued, amounts returned, and amounts on hand. The daily invoices and requisition sheets are used for daily posting. The main advantage of the perpetual inventory is that it provides a running balance of food items, as needed by management.

The physical inventory system involves the actual counting of each item in storage at designated intervals, at least once a month. A sample form for taking physical inventory is given in Figure 11-19. Sometimes a pretyped form may be used listing food items in alphabetical order or according to storeroom arrangement. The inventory is commonly taken by a storeroom employee and a disinterested party. The clerical task of costing may be accomplished by storeroom personnel or the accounting department. The perpetual inventory indicates the

Table 11-20. Safe Storage of Food Products[a]

Food	Suggested Type and Length of Storage
Fresh meats (roasts, steaks, and chops)	Refrigerate at 30°–36°F. Loosely wrapped meats store longer than tightly wrapped. Loosely wrapped: 3–5 days or less. Tightly wrapped: 2 days or less. Never keep meat at room temperature except during actual preparation.
Ground and stew meat	Refrigerate at 30°–36°F. Freeze, unless designated for immediate use. 1–2 days, preferably only 1 day. Longer storage possible if original quality high and refrigerator temperature is low (near 32°F).
Variety meats	Refrigerate at 30°–36°F. Loosely wrapped: 1–2 days.
Hams (tenderized, not fully cooked)	Keep refrigerated at 30°–36°F at all times including storage at vendor's premises. 1 week only for best quality: 1–3 weeks is safe, unless mishandled (left out of refrigerator).
Hams (tenderized, *fully cooked*; mildly cured, sometimes smoked; internal temperature of 150°F reached)	Refrigerate at all times (including at vendor's premises). Storage times same as above.
Bacon (cured)	Refrigerate at 30°–36°F, no more than 1–2 weeks.
Cold cuts (including frankfurters)	Refrigerate at 30°–36°F, wrapped with some access to air. Original quality and moisture content affect keeping quality. High-moisture cuts: 3–5 days; franks, approximately a week. Hard sausage: 2 or more weeks; inspect weekly for molds.
Frozen meats	Freezer-store at 0°F or below. It is good to practice rapid turnover of frozen foods. The limits for storage are these: Beef, lamb; 9–12 months. Pork: 6–9 months. Veal: 4–6 months. Sausage, ham, slab bacon: 1–3 months. Beef liver: 3–4 months. Pork liver: 1–2 months.
Poultry (fresh)	Refrigerate at 30°–36°F loosely wrapped; remove giblets from original wrap, rewrap loosely. 1–2 days (freeze, if storage must be extended beyond a few days).
Poultry (frozen)	Freezer at 0°F or below. Chicken, 6–8 months. Turkey, 4–5 months. Giblets, 2–3 months.
Fish and shellfish (fresh, frozen or smoked)	Fresh fish: refrigerate, loosely wrapped, at 30°–32°F; or pack in ice and refrigerate; or freeze if fish cannot be used within 2–3 days. Fresh shellfish: refrigerate in original, covered container; 1–5 days. Frozen fish and shellfish: hold at 0°F 4–6 months; shellfish, 3–4 months. Smoked fish: if to be held longer than 3 days, freeze.
Canned foods	Cool (50°–60°F), dry storage. Freezing may break seal of can or jar or crack jar; leaks will allow bacteria to enter. Unless cans or jars are damaged, freezing will not make food unsafe. Maximum storage time, 1 year, but 6 months is preferable.
Frozen precooked foods	Freezer at 0°F or below. Length of storage depends on product. Do not store anything over 3 months.

[a]From Longree and Blaker (1971).

Storeroom Requisition and Issue Form

Unit: _____ Date _____

Requisitioned		Description	Amount Issued	Amount Returned	Amount Used	Unit Cost (%)	Total Cost (%)
Amount	Unit						

Requisitioned by: _____ Issued by: _____

Figure 11-17. Storeroom requisition and issue form.

Perpetual Inventory

Date	Order No.	Received			Issued		Amount Returned	Amount on Hand
		Amount	Unit	Unit Cost	Amount	Unit		
1/14/89					4	No. 10	0	36
1/15/89	7214	6	Case	10.40				72
1/15/89					4	No. 10	1	69
1/18/89					4	No. 10	0	65

Stock Level: Minimum 5 cases (30 No. 10 cans)   Maximum 12 cases (72 No. 10 cans)

Item: Peaches, halves, cling	Unit: No. 10	Style: Canned

Figure 11-18. Perpetual inventory form.

		Amount on Hand		Unit	Total	
Unit	Food Item	Physical	Perpetual	Cost	Cost	Remarks

Physical Inventory

Location: _____   Date _____

Value of Sheet: _____   Page _____ of _____

Inventory Taken By:

_____ and _____

Name   Name

_____   _____

Title   Title

Figure 11-19. Physical inventory form.

amount that should be on hand; the physical inventory gives an accurate record of what is actually on hand. If there is a discrepancy in the totals of the two inventories, management should investigate. The discrepancies may be due to pilferage or errors in recording data.

Quality Control

Quality control should be checked at key points throughout the purchasing process: (1) specification, (2) system of purchasing, (3) purveyor selection, (4) food ordering, (5) receiving, and (6) storing. When the stages of purchasing are considered as integral parts of the total purchasing system, then quality can be controlled. Quality control points to remember include the following:

- Specify foods that have been federally inspected and graded.
- Agree on a purchasing system that will support specification standards.
- Do not compromise quality for price in awarding bids and contracts.
- Purchase only from reputable purveyors.
- Visit the purveyor's company to check food handling and general sanitation.

- Buy from sources that comply with all laws relating to food and food labeling.
- Check trucks and other modes of transportation for cleanliness and adequate refrigeration.
- Order all food from approved sources.
- Buy only federally inspected meat and poultry.
- Buy only Grade A pasteurized milk and milk products.
- Buy seafood from approved sources.
- Upon delivery, check all food for signs of spoilage, filth, and damage.
- Accept only clean whole eggs with shell intact and without cracks.
- Reject bulging, leaking, and rusty canned foods.
- Check frozen foods for evidence of thawing.
- Accept fresh and shucked shellfish only in nonreturnable containers.
- Store food separately from poisonous materials.
- Store food at least 6 inches off the floor.
- Keep storage area free from insects, rodents, dust, and leaky overhead pipes.
- Provide adequate storage space (dry and refrigerated) to allow for air circulation.
- Use FIFO system for rotating stored foods.
- Maintain storage areas in clean and sanitary condition.

Computer Assistance in Food Purchasing

In order to purchase food, a forecasting system must be established, recipe ingredients from the menu need to be extended and complied, and a grocery list must be created. All of these processes can be done by using a computer. This procedure will save a foodservice department labor time and money as well as afford closer control over the purchasing procedure.

As indicated in Chapter 9, purchasing by computer can be a continuation of a computer-assisted menu planning program. For example, if the complete menu is entered into the computer, a program should be able to extract all the needed recipes from the menu for a particular day, forecast and extend those recipes, and produce a grocery list for procurement either from the storeroom or an outside vendor.

If the foodservice computer system does not include a computerized menu planning program (most do not), a system for purchasing can be initiated using various data bases such as an inventory file, a census file, and a recipe file. Although the following subsections describe aspects of systems reported in the literature, any actual system should be especially designed for a medical foodservice according to its needs.

Inventory File

The data base or file for a computerized inventory system is a list of every possible item ordered by the foodservice. This includes all food items on the menu, as well as cleaning supplies and other miscellaneous items used by the operation. Each item is coded, and part of the code number indicates a particular category, such as meats or produce.

The foodservice director could include anything in the inventory file that would help with inventory accuracy and control. Some of these items might be vendor name, storage location, and purchase unit or issue unit.

When using a computer to control and record inventory, it is important that employees have access to stock and that they record accurately all foods received and issued. The system is invalid unless the data base always contains the correct number of items in its file. If anyone is lax about record keeping, the system will fail.

Inventory is often the first function to be computerized because of the great potential savings of time and money for a foodservice department. However, the department must be well organized before computers are installed or there will be no savings. Instead, more confusion may be added to what already exists. On the other hand, a well-organized computer operation can save hours of work and substantial amounts of money when used properly.

Although some foodservice operations are still conducting inventories manually, computer assistance has been in practice at other facilities for more than 20 years. A computer-assisted perpetual inventory system, at the University of Missouri Medical Center, Columbia (Anon. 1966), begins with an information-orienting terminal in the dietary office of the main kitchen. A dietary clerk punches information about each transaction into the computer.

Five types of information are recorded: (1) type of transaction (foods requisitioned or removed from the inventory, foods ordered or received); (2) food code (a five-digit number categorizing a food into a group); (3) quantity in number stock units; (4) requisitioning area (main kitchen, cafeteria, diet area), and (5) code number of person recording transaction. Reports generated from this inventory system are in the form of

1. Printouts recommending amounts to buy, showing amounts on hand and on order, the established minimum and maximum amounts to have in stock, and the amounts recommended to buy.
2. Daily or monthly reports on amounts of foods issued, plus costs for each type of food, each food category, and total cost.

Census File

Procurement of food begins with a forecast of demand. Computer-printed purchase requisitions can be created by calculating an order quantity based on a menu item forecast, and comparing this quantity with current inventory stock levels of that item.

A census or forecast file can be created to store information regarding the amounts of each item used the last time it was served on the cycle. For example, if chocolate cake and sliced peaches were selections for dessert on the menu for lunch, the file may have stored the information that the selection percentage for chocolate cake was 90% and 10% for sliced peaches the last time they were served. Therefore, if the projected census estimated for this time is 500, then 450 servings (90% of 500) of chocolate cake and 50 servings of sliced peaches would be needed. In order to ensure accuracy for the next step of making production decisions, updates must be entered in the file daily.

Recipe File

The recipe file consists of all the standardized recipes needed for each item in the cycle menu. After a mathematical forecast has been established, the recipe ingredients will automatically be extended to that number, and a grocery list will be made for purchasing.

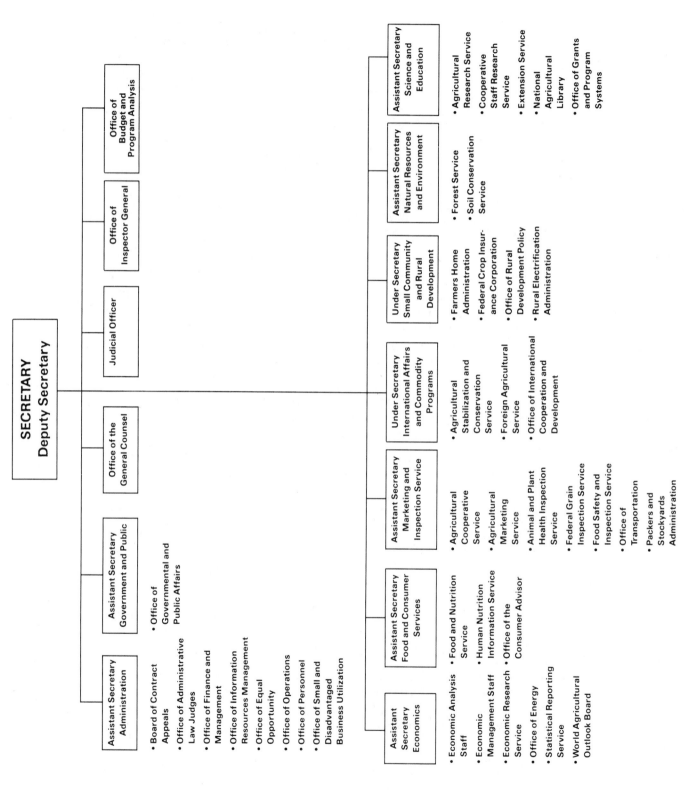

Figure 11-20. Organization of U.S. Department of Agriculture. *From Office of the Federal Register (1964)*

Table 11-21. Federal Agencies Responsible for Food Inspection, Grading, and Other Food-Related Services

Services Provided	Federal Agencies
Inspection	
Meat and poultry	USDA—Animal and Plant Health Service
Dairy products	USDA—Agriculture Marketing Service
Seafood	U.S. Department of Commerce—National Marine Fisheries Service
Fruits and vegetables (fresh and processed)	USDA—Agriculture Marketing Service
Grains	USDA—Agriculture Marketing Service
Grading	
Meat and poultry	USDA
Dairy products	USDA
Seafood	U.S. Department of Commerce—National Marine Fisheries Service
Fruits and vegetables	USDA
Other services	
False advertising	USDHHS–FDA and Federal Trade Commission
Weights, measures and containers	U.S. Department of Commerce—Bureau of Standards
Food additives	USDHHS–FDA
Fair packing and labeling	USDHHS–FDA
Standards of identity	USDA (meats); USDHHS–FDA (all other foods)
Standards of quality	USDHHS–FDA
Standards of fill	USDHHS–FDA
Standards of enrichment	USDHHS–FDA
Sanitation in processing plants	USDHHS–FDA
Food safety pesticides	USDA–FDA
Employee safety in processing plants	U.S. Department of Labor–OSHA
Food specifications	USDA–Food Safety and Quality Service, National Marine Fisheries Service (NMFS)
Inspection acceptance service	USDA–Food Safety and Quality Service

Laws Related to Food Purchasing

There are federal, state, and local laws relating to various aspects of food wholesomeness and quality. State and local laws must be as strict as federal laws, and in most instances the laws are much more stringent. Agencies, as established by law, are responsible for ensuring that all food for human consumption is harvested, manufactured, processed, packaged, stored, and transported in a safe and sanitary manner. Reorganization of the various federal agencies are constantly under way in efforts to strengthen services for consumer protection. Major federal agencies responsible for food and quality are the U.S. Department of Agriculture (USDA) (see Figure 11-20), the U.S. Department of Health and Human Services (USDHHS), and the U.S. Department of Commerce. Other services are provided by the U.S. Department of Labor through the Occupational Safety and Health Administration (OSHA), and the U.S. Department of Public Health. Because of the constant reorganization of the various agencies, it is difficult to classify the present duties assigned each with complete accuracy. The U.S. government agencies responsible for food inspection, grading, and other food-related services are listed in Table 11.21 (current for 1984).

References

Agricultural Marketing Service. (1975). *How to Buy Food* (Agriculture Handbook No. 443). Washington, DC: USDA.

Anon, (1966). Computer Provides Instant Updating of Perpetual Inventory at Missouri Medical Center. *Hospitals 40*(7), 158–160.

Code of Federal Regulations, Food and Drugs. (1984). *Standards of Identity* (Title 21, Parts 130–169). Washington, DC: U.S. Government Printing Office.

Friedelson, I. (1967). *Fair Packaging: Synopsis of Food Packaging and Labeling Regulations* (Reprint from FDA Papers). Washington, DC: U.S. Department of Health and Human Services, Food and Drug Administration.

Longree, K., and Blaker, G. G. (1971). *Sanitary Techniques in Food Service.* New York: Wiley.

National Association of Meat Purveyors. (1960). *Meat Buyer's Guide to Standardized Meat Cuts.* Chicago: NAMP.

National Association of Meat Purveyors. (1967). *Meat Buyer's Guide to Portion Control Meat Cuts.* Chicago: NAMP.

National Association of Meat Purveyors. (1976). *Meat Buyer's Guide.* Chicago: NAMP.

National Live Stock and Meat Board. (1977). *Meat in the Foodservice Industry.* Chicago: NLSMB.

Office of the Federal Register. (1984). *The U.S. Government Manual: 1984–1985. National Archives and Records Service. General Service Administration.* Washington, DC: U.S. Government Printing Office.

Richards, G. (1982). From Light Bulbs to CT Scanners, Group Purchasing is Filling the Bill at a Lower Price. *Hospitals 56*(2), 81–89.

Swindler, J. P. (1978). The Future of the Purchasing Agent: Materials Management as a Profession. *Hosp. Top. 56*(4), 22–26.

U.S. Department of Agriculture. (1956). *Standardization and Inspection of Fresh Fruits and Vegetables* (USDA Agriculture Marketing Service Pub. No. 604). Washington, DC: U.S. Government Printing Office.

U.S. Department of Agriculture. (1959). *Inspection Mark for Poultry.* Washington, DC: U.S. Government Printing Office.

U.S. Department of Agriculture. (1967). *Institutional Meat Purchase Specifications for Portion-Cut Meat Products* (Series 1000). Washington, DC: USDA Consumer & Marketing Service, Livestock Division.

U.S. Department of Agriculture. (1968). *How to Buy Poultry* (Home and Garden Bull. No. 157). Superintendent of Documents, Washington, DC: U.S. Government Printing Office.

U.S. Department of Agriculture. (1972). *Regulations Governing the Grading and Inspection of Poultry and Edible Products Thereof and U.S. Classes, Standards and Grades with Respect Thereto* (7CFR, Pt. 70). Washington, DC: USDA.

U.S. Department of Agriculture. (1975). *How to Buy Food: Lesson Aids for Teachers* (Agriculture Marketing Service. Agriculture Handbook No. 443). Washington, DC: U.S. Government Printing Office.

U.S. Department of Agriculture. (1977). *Food Purchasing Pointers for School Food Service* (Program Aid No. 1160). Washington, DC: USDA Food and Nutrition Service.

U.S. Department of Agriculture. (1980). *Food Buying for School Food Service* (Program Aid No. 1257). Washington, DC: USDA Food and Nutrition Service.

U.S. Department of Agriculture. (1982). *Your Money's Worth in Foods* (Home Garden Bull. No. 183). Washington, DC: USDA Human Nutrition Information Service.

U.S. Department of Health and Human Services. (1965). *Grade "A" Pasteurized Milk Ordinance: 1965 Recommendations of the U.S. Public Health Service* (Public Health Service Publication No. 229). Washington, DC: USDHHS.

U.S. Department of Health and Human Services. (1969). *FDA Fact Sheet: Milk and Milk Type Products.* Washington, DC: Public Health Service, Consumer Protection and Environmental Health Service, Food and Drug Administration.

U.S. Department of the Interior. (1959). *Guide for Buying Fresh and Frozen Fish and Shellfish* (Fish and Wildlife Service Circular 214). Washington, DC: USDI, Bureau of Commercial Fisheries.

U.S. Department of the Interior (1961). *Basic Fish Cookery* (Fish and Wildlife Service Test Kitchen Series No. 2). Washington, DC: USDI.

U.S. Department of the Interior. (1964A). *Fish Cookery for One Hundred* (Test Kitchen Series No. 1). Washington, DC: USDI.

U.S. Department of the Interior. (1964B). *How to Cook Shrimp* (Test Kitchen Series No. 7). Washington, DC: USDI.

U.S. Department of the Interior. (1964C). *How to Cook Clams* (Test Kitchen Series No. 8). Washington, DC: USDI.

U.S. Department of the Interior. (1964D). *How to Cook Oysters* (Test Kitchen Series No. 3). Washington, DC: USDI.

U.S. Department of the Interior. (1964E). *How to Cook Crabs* (Test Kitchen Series No. 10). Washington, DC: USDI.

U.S. Department of the Interior. (1964F). *How to Cook Lobsters* (Test Kitchen Series No. 11). Washington, DC: USDI.

U.S. Department of the Interior. (1964G). *How to Cook Scallops* (Test Kitchen Series No. 13). Washington, DC: USDI.

Chapter 12

Subsystem for Food Production

The planned menu precedes any decision relating to the type of production system to use in a foodservice operation. The decision should be based on an objective evaluation of menu requirements, with full consideration to other subsystems (food purchasing, equipment, distribution and service, personnel, and finances) required for a quality foodservice. Menu factors that may affect the type of production system are as follows:

1. *Menu style or format.* A nonselective menu or a selective menu with two or three choices could be used effectively by all production systems. A restaurant-type menu is more suitable for the cook-freeze-serve system if food items are individually packaged. The bulk packaging used for assembly-serve and for some freeze-serve systems may present problems in patient tray assembly due to the wide variety of menu items offered by a restaurant-type menu. The current trend in using restaurant-type menus is to preplate menu items prior to freezing. One of the problems associated with preplating menu items is that menu combinations may not be acceptable to patients. For example, if entree no. 1 (roast beef) is served with mashed potatoes and Brussels sprouts, the patient may not like the vegetable combination and ask for a substitute. If no substitutions are allowed, the patient is unhappy, resulting in a lower rating for food acceptance.

2. *Menu variety.* Some questions need to be asked concerning system capability. Can the process method accommodate all planned menu items such as hard- and soft-cooked eggs, meats without sauce or gravy, flour- or cereal-based puddings, egg custards, and other similar foods? Can the system accommodate all food served to personnel and guests, for special activities, vending, and coffee shops, as well as patient foodservice? When a system is used for only part of the foodservice required, the use of the system may result in added labor, equipment, and food costs as well as increased pressure on employees.

For a better understanding of how the menu is related to the production system, it is appropriate to discuss the various systems at this time.

Production Systems

Food production systems, currently used in medical foodservice operations, can be classified into four categories: (1) cook-serve, (2) assembly-serve, (3) cook-freeze-serve, and (4) cook-chill-serve. The commissary or food factory, a method of producing food in large quantities, can be applied to all categories of food production systems.

__ Cook-Serve Production System __

This system is sometimes referred to as conventional or *conventional-convenience*. The cook-serve system is characterized by on-premise preparation of food from the raw state (scratch cookery) on a daily basis for each meal. Food is assembled and served with a minimum holding period. Cook-serve is the system most often used in medical foodservice operations. Due to the lack of skilled employees and financial constraints, few cook-serve systems prepare all foods from scratch. Most operations use some form of commercially prepared convenience food. The use of a butcher shop for portioning, grinding, and cubing meat from carcass or wholesale cuts is practically extinct in medical foodservice. Meat is frequently purchased in portion-controlled units, either fresh or frozen. The large bake shops, where all types of bread, rolls, buns, cakes, and pastries were prepared, have practically disappeared. Today there is a dessert preparation area where mixes are used for cakes and cookies; frozen pies or frozen pie shells and canned or frozen fruit fillings are used; and bread, rolls, and buns are purchased from commercial bakeries.

Employees are assigned various duties to prepare all food for a particular meal just prior to serving time. Food is portioned, assembled, and transported to wards for patient service without additional heating. In most operations, employees prepare food for patients and personnel at the same time. After one meal is served and the preparation and service area is cleaned, preparation begins for the next meal. Employees work overlapping shifts of 8 hours each. For a three-meal feeding plan, employees may be scheduled to work from 6:00 A.M. to 2:00 P.M. for the first shift, with responsibility for breakfast and lunch preparation. The second shift may be scheduled to work from 11:00 A.M. to 7:00 P.M., with responsibility to assist with lunch preparation and service and to prepare and serve the dinner meal. The overlap time between 11:00 A.M. and 2:00 P.M. must be carefully planned and monitored for full utilization of employees.

Advantages of the cook-serve system are as follows:

1. The system provides flexibility in menu planning for both regular and modified diets without dependence on outside preparation sources.
2. Although some canned and frozen foods are used, patients and employees tend to equate the cook-serve system with serving of fresh foods.
3. With on-premise preparation, it is easier to cater to individual needs and preferences.
4. Menu variety is not limited by any processing technique associated with the system.

The disadvantages of a cook-serve system are as follows:

1. The rush periods associated with each meal hour may cause undue employee stress.
2. Skilled employees must be scheduled for each shift, 7 days a week.
3. The overlap of work shifts may result in low productivity and high labor cost.

__ Assembly-Serve Production System __

The system is also referred to as *total convenience* and *semiconvenience*. In assembly-serve, all food is purchased in a prepared state from an outside source. The prepared frozen food is in bulk form, packaged in disposable pans. When ready for use, the food is thawed, plated, assembled, and distributed to wards for service to patients. For the employee cafeteria, food may be heated in disposable pans and served from a counter. Fresh produce such as cabbage is purchased in precut form for coleslaw, precut mixed greens for tossed salad, and other forms requiring a minimum of preparation prior to service. Pies, cakes, and pastries are purchased in frozen state and only require thawing and portioning. For a limited number of assembly-serve operations, preplated entree-vegetable combination plates are purchased. In other operations, only the entree item is purchased from commercial sources and all other foods, such as vegetables, salads, and desserts are prepared on the premises. This arrangement is considered a semiconvenience system.

Managerial decisions to convert the operation to assembly-serve should be carefully analyzed not only in terms of cost but also in terms of menu variety, quality, and acceptability. With a full assembly-serve operation, equipment and labor costs are drastically reduced. When disposable serviceware is used, the cost is further reduced. Initial costs may involve additional freezer space, equipment on each ward for thermalizing plated food, purchasing of disposables, and equipment for disposing of disposables.

Menu variety may present a problem. A variety of convenience products are available, but they are not consistent in terms of quality, size, and ingredients from one manufacturer to the other. It will be necessary to write specifications to accommodate the needs of the operation, such as the amount of protein per serving, and the ratio of other ingredients in a particular product. Unless the amount ordered is large enough to justify a change in standard processing techniques, the cost may be prohibitive or the manufacturer may refuse to honor the specification. Most modified diets are multirestrictive, either in caloric or nutritive value. Careful planning is required in order to serve food as prescribed.

Consider food acceptance by patients and employees. Some individuals have a negative attitude towards convenience foods from early "TV dinner" experiences. Better appearance and greater acceptability is possible with the use of china or attractive plastic serviceware and garnishes.

Advantages of the assembly-serve production system are as follows:

1. Reduced labor costs. Skilled cooks are not required for production.
2. Uniformity of product. Food products are the same each time they are served.
3. Reduced waste resulting from excess trimming, overcooking, shrinkage, and spoilage.
4. Portion control is assured. Pans are consistently filled with the same amount.
5. Less equipment is required. Pre-preparation and most cooking equipment can be eliminated. Dishwashers can be eliminated if disposables are used exclusively.
6. Purchasing, inventory, and accounting procedures are easier.

Disadvantages of the assembly-serve production system are as follows:

1. Increased food costs. The price of the product includes the cost of food and the built-in labor costs.
2. Food for modified diets may be limited. Acute care facilities may have problems meeting patient needs because of the complexity of diet prescriptions.

3. Availability of product is not assured. The manufacturer may decide to discontinue certain products or may go out of business.
4. It is difficult to satisfy individual food preferences.
5. Patients may object to convenience foods, especially if food is served on disposables.
6. Loss of control over production. Employees at the manufacturing company may go on strike.
7. Initial equipment cost may be high. There will be a need for thermalizing equipment on each ward and possibly extra freezer space.

── Cook-Freeze-Serve Production System ──

The cook-freeze-serve system is also referred to as *ready-serve* and *ready-food*. In medical foodservice operations, food is prepared on-premise, packaged in individual portions, blast-frozen, freezer-stored, thawed, assembled, distributed cold to wards, rethermalized on wards, and served to patients. As conceptualized by researchers at Cornell's School of Hotel Administration (MacLennan 1968), the system is a *ready-food production system* and is distinguished from other ready-serve foods as follows:

1. *Preparation of food in large quantities.* Master chef and cooks work 5 days per week, preparing 3–4 different foods each day.
2. *Return to classical cooking methods.* Since a single food item is only prepared about 5–10 times a year, extra time can be used to prepare classical foods.
3. *Single-portion packaging.* Portions are rethermalized as needed, thus avoiding long periods on steam tables.
4. *Freezing as a means of preservation and storage.* Food is blast-frozen and freezer stored.
5. *Simplified reheating process.* Both "boil-in-a-bag" and microwave heating methods are used.
6. *On-premise operation.* Since all foods are prepared on the premises, quality standards are controlled.
7. *Ready-foods meet local tastes and portion sizes.* Consumer preferences and portion sizes can be accommodated.
8. *Absence of synthetics and food additives.* Using this system, there is no need for preservatives, antioxidants, sequestrants, surfactants, stabilizers, thickeners, buffers, firming agents, tenderizers, or taste enhancers.

The system was developed for luxury hotel dining places and included foods from appetizers and soups to desserts. Food is cooked, using conventional methods, to varying degrees of doneness. A modified starch is used for dishes that normally require tapioca starch. Single portions are packaged in plastic pouches or plastic airtight boxes, blast-frozen, and then held in frozen storage until ready for use. Special equipment was designed to complement the *cook-in-a-bag* process. Food is rethermalized from the frozen state.

For use in medical foodservice operations, the ready-food system was modified to accommodate the complexities of patient and cafeteria foodservice. In hospitals, the process is the same as originally designed through the blast-freezing stage. Instead of removing individual portions from the freezer as needed, all food required for a meal is removed at least 1 day in advance and placed in a thaw refrigerator. The *thaw refrigerator* is a special type that is capable of thawing food at a much faster rate than a regular refrigerator which takes approximately 3 days. In this refrigerator, food is automatically thawed and maintained at a safe temperature, not exceeding 45°F. The thawed portions are cold-plated according to individual diet requirements or as indicated on the selective menu. Trays are transported to wards in refrigerated carts and remain under refrigeration until serving time. Prior to service, foods requiring heat are removed from the patient tray, rethermalized, returned to the tray along with other foods, and served immediately. Some operations use a tray cart with an electronic component beneath each tray for heating foods requiring heat and for supplying refrigerated air to keep cold food at the proper temperature.

Another variation of hospital cook-freeze-serve production system is the Leeds Cook-Freeze system, developed by United Leeds Hospitals, Leeds, England (Rinke 1976). All food, including entrees, soups, vegetables, starches, egg dishes, casseroles, and desserts, are prepared in the following manner:

1. Foods are slightly undercooked, to allow for further cooking during rethermalizing process.
2. Foods are packed hot in polyethylene molds that hold 6–8 portions.
3. Molds are blast-frozen.
4. Food is removed from molds in the form of frozen slabs.
5. The slabs are heat-sealed in polyethylene bags, and packed in boxes for freeze storage.
6. Food is reconstituted by placing slabs in reusable metal pans that are heated on the wards in specially designed convection ovens.
7. Food is assembled and served from the ward pantry.

As noted, the multiportion frozen molds and the rethermalizing techniques are completely different from methods used in other cook-freeze-serve production systems. The procedure of decentralized heating and plating of food may result in loss of managerial control over the finished product.

It is observed that the use of cook-freeze-serve for medical foodservice operations is designed only for patient service. Although patient foodservice should receive top priority, a dual production system of cook-freeze-serve for patients and a cook-serve for personnel is questionable. The dual production system negates most of the advantages normally expected from a cook-freeze-serve system, such as reduced labor and food costs. For example, with a dual production system, only the cooks assigned cook-freeze-serve can be scheduled for a 5-day Monday-through-Friday workweek. Other cooks responsible for the cook-serve system must be scheduled to work the three meals per day, 7 days per week. MacLennan (1968) advised hotel foodservice operations to either go all the way with ready food or not to use it at all. The advice can also apply to medical foodservice operations in the use of cook-freeze-serve.

As reported by McIver (1970), bulk blast freezing has been used at the Brooklyn (New York) Hospital since 1965. The procedure is as follows:

1. One cook is assigned to produce 1600 portions of a given entree each day Monday through Friday, plus a variety of combination dishes for patient selective menu and personnel cafeteria.
2. Items are prepared in 200-portion units using both the tilting skillet and steam kettles.
3. Completed items are portioned into $9\frac{1}{2} \times 12 \times 1\frac{1}{2}$ inch foil pans with fold-over lids. Each pan is scaled to 5 pounds and is considered a packed unit. Packages are labeled with date of preparation, contents, and reconstituting instructions.
4. Packages are quick-cooled by a cold water cooling jacket that causes the temperature to drop from 212°F to 150°F in 30 minutes, prior to blast freezing.

5. Packages are blast-frozen for 2 to 3 hours, depending on the product.
6. Convection ovens are used to reconstitute food, following time and temperature instructions given on lid of each box.

The system used at Brooklyn Hospital appears to be a practical approach for serving both patients and personnel. When food is reconstituted in the main production area, it is hot-plated and served as described for the cook-serve system.

One of the most revolutionary cook-freeze-serve systems is the one designed and implemented for the 1280-bed Walter Reed Army Medical Center in Washington, DC. Food is prepared for individual or bulk blast freezing. As designed, a monorail system is used to transport food deliveries to dry, refrigerated, or frozen storage, where movable shelving permits the FIFO system of storage and issue. Food, as needed, is programmed to the ingredient room, pre-prepared, and delivered to the production area. In the production area, food preparation is monitored from the production manager's office where computerized audiovisual panels are designed to control equipment, cooking cycle, speed of cooking conveyors, and temperature settings (Anon. 1977). Equipment features include the following:

1. A vegetable and fruit washer built to raise the washed items out of the water.
2. Automatic breading machines for foods such as chops, fish, chicken, and some vegetables.
3. Electrically heated braise-and-simmer kettles to cook up to 26 gallons of stews, sauces, and gravies. The equipment has an ingredient dispensing unit with an instruction card reader that automatically adds ingredients at the proper time.
4. Double-jacketed steam kettles are equipped with self-contained stirrers, mashers, and pureers.
5. Two conveyorized fryer-griddles can produce over 2200 portions of chops, sausage, or hamburger patties in 1 hour.
6. More than 200 pounds of roast can be cooked in each of two rotating self-basting ovens. When a button on the oven is pressed, natural juice is pumped from the bottom of the pan to baste the meat.

Most of the equipment was imported from European manufacturing companies (Simler 1978). The Tricalt revolving hot-food tables were purchased in France; the Kuppersbusch models of continuous conveyor fryer-griddle, self-basting ovens, and semiautomated gravy and sauce makers were purchased from Germany. Blast freezers and the Chill-Therm food carts were manufactured by U.S. companies.

Food is cooked, packaged in either individual portions or bulk containers, and rapidly frozen. Limited quantities of food are requisitioned from freezer storage and thawed as needed. Patient trays are manually preplated (temporary procedure) and transported to patient wards in Chill-Therm carts, which are used to refrigerate and cook foods in dishes on the fully assembled serving tray (see Chapter 13 for a description of the service system).

Advantages cited for use of cook-freeze-serve in medical foodservice operations are as follows:

1. Employee scheduling is easier. Cooks and main production employees are scheduled for one 8-hour shift, Monday through Friday.
2. Large-batch cooking reduces the number of times that a menu item must be prepared during a given period.

3. Employees work in a more relaxed atmosphere without the pressure of meeting culinary schedules three times a day.
4. Peak production workloads are eliminated; thus employees are fully utilized throughout the work shift.
5. Labor costs may be reduced since large quantities are purchased at one time for bulk preparation.

Major disadvantages cited for use of the cook-freeze-serve system are as follows:

1. Equipment cost. There is a large initial outlay of capital for added freezer space, packaging, and rethermalizing. There also may be a renovation cost if operation is converted from one type of system to another.
2. Dual-system operation. When freeze-serve is used for only part of the operation, there is added food and labor cost. There may be friction between employees who are off on weekends and those who are not.

─── Cook-Chill-Serve Production System ───

The cook-chill-serve production system is characterized by the cooking of food in conventional manner, quick chilling, packaging, and chill storing until ready for use. One of the first cook-chill-serve systems to be designed was originated and implemented in early 1960s at Nacka Hospital, Stockholm, Sweden.

As reported by Bjorkman and Delphin (1966), production of food at the Nacka Hospital takes place under bacteriologically controlled conditions, with food samples taken on the day of cooking and the end of the storage period. Personnel, equipment, and materials are carefully checked. Food is prepared for the Nacka Hospital plus other facilities in the Stockholm area, and one facility more than 220 miles away. Prepared food is transported in refrigerated vans to satellite units. The procedure at Nacka Hospital is as follows:

1. Food is conventionally cooked—by frying, boiling, roasting, stewing, or other methods—to a temperature of 176°F.
2. Hot food is transferred to plastic bags, five portions per bag.
3. Air is extracted from bags, and food is sealed airtight by a Cryovac machine.
4. Bags are placed in boiling water (rectangular kettle for rapid heating) for 3 minutes.
5. Sealed bags pass through a tunnel with running water for 1 hour at a temperature of 50°F, then lowered to 37°F.
6. After quick drying, packages are stored in a refrigerated room at 37°F or less.
7. At time of service, bags are placed in boiling water for 30 minutes.
8. Bags are cut open and contents served. Food may be emptied into a steam table pan and served from a counter.

The cook-chill-serve system is currently used by a number of facilities with slightly varied production procedures. Depending on the chilling procedures used, food is stored from 1 day to 3 weeks or more. In the United States, notable cook-chill-serve systems were designed at the University of Wisconsin Hospitals and for a group of hospitals in South Carolina, known as the Anderson, Greenville, Spartanburg (AGS) food production system (McGuckian 1969).

At the University of Wisconsin, food is prepared a day in advance, chilled in bulk, portioned for tray assembly, and transported to patient areas in refrigerated carts (Kaud 1972). The unique feature of this system is the specially designed food carts, which contain refrigerated space for 30 trays, a microwave oven, coffee and hot water dispensers, and storage space for beverage servers and cups. There is a fold-up table attached to the side of the cart where a patient tray can be placed while food requiring heat is thermalized.

The AGS system (McGuckian 1969) is similar to the Nacka system with the following exceptions:

1. Raw or partially cooked foods are placed in pouches, and the cooking process is completed in temperature-controlled water baths.
2. After processing, products are chilled in ice water tanks, then chill-stored at 28°F–32°F.
3. Pouches are delivered to satellite units in covered plastic containers that are surrounded by ice.
4. Before serving, sealed pouches are placed in a hot water bath for 30–40 minutes and heated to 160°F.
5. When plated, entrees and other hot foods are microwaved for 10–20 seconds immediately before distribution to patients.

Both the Nacka and the AGS systems use the pasteurization process of heating pouches prior to chilling, which adds an extra step in the food flow for cook-chill-serve products. Each time food is handled represents a critical point for control of microbial, nutritional, and sensory qualities of the food—a major concern to researchers, managers, and consumers.

Another concern associated with the cook-chill-serve system is how to extend the shelf life of prepared food while maintaining high standards of quality. One system responding to this problem is the Groen Copkold System for kettle-cooked foods. Using the specially designed equipment, food is produced for a cook-chill-serve system as follows:

1. Products to be prepared are cooked in a steam-jacketed kettle equipped with an agitator.
2. Ingredients are added sequentially to ensure proper degree of doneness.
3. When the cooking process is completed, the product, at 180°F, is pumped into the Cryovac casing.
4. Packages of 1 gallon, 5 quarts, 1½ gallons or 2 gallons are sealed with a positive clip closure and labeled.
5. The product is placed in a tumble chiller filled with cold water, 34°F–36°F, and gently agitated in constantly circulated cold water. In less than 1 hour, the product temperature is reduced to 40°F.
6. Cooled casings are immediately placed in the cooler for storage at 28°F–32°F until needed for distribution.
7. The finished product is stored in the casting on open racks or cartons for distribution to satellite units.
8. For serving, products can be heated in the casings in a hot water bath or removed from the casings and heated in any conventional manner.

The filling station (shown on the left in Fig. 12-1) is equipped with a very simple single-lobe pump that gently moves the food from the cooking vessel to the casing. Sanitation is assured since the product is transferred while hot, near pasteurization temperatures, from cooking vessel into the casing, thereby eliminating any chance for human or utensil contamination. The kettle-cooked Copkold system can be used for foods such as stews, casseroles, soups, gravies, sauces, and for uncooked products such as salad dressing.

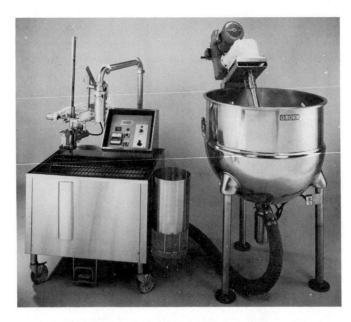

Figure 12-1. Capkold system for kettle-cooked foods. A positive displacement pump-fill station (left) and special inclined agitator kettle with air-operated bottom draw-off are key elements of the Groen Capkold cook-chill Central Commissary System. Kettle cooking then pumps food directly into plastic casings and this ensures fresh flavor and minimizes human and utensil contamination. *From Groen, a Dover Industries Company*

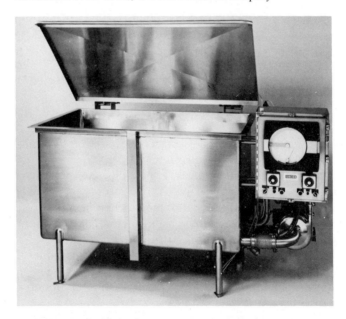

Figure 12-2. Stainless steel cook tank. *From Groen, a Dover Industries Company*

For the processing of meat in quantity, including poultry, pork, corned beef, and spareribs, a stainless steel cook tank (Fig. 12-2) can be used. The cook tank is a self-contained, automatic cooking system that incorporates controlled temperature water to slow-cook meats and other foods automatically in vacuumized bags. The bagged meat, or other food, is placed in one of five wire racks that stack into the tank, five bags to a tray. Large-batch cooking of up to fifty 20-pound roasts can be completed in one cook tank. High quality and higher

Table 12-1.   Recipe for Liver and Onions, Using Cook-Chill Tank[a]

Name of Item: Liver and Onions	Date Prepared:		Batch Number: Size of Batch:
Type of Preparation: Cook in Casing	Serving Size:		Number of Servings: 36 portions (3 1/2 oz slices)

Ingredients	Measures		Method of Preparation
	Weight	Volume	
Liver—3 1/2 oz slices	8 lb		1. Dredge liver slices in seasoned
Browned flour		2 cups	flour, place 12 in each casing.
Salt ⎫ Mix	1 oz		
Pepper ⎭		1 Tbsp	
Bacon, sliced, diced	1 lb		2. Fry bacon until crisp. Add 8-oz
Onions, diced	1 lb		mixture of onions and bacon to
			each casing.
			3. Vacuumize and cook in 180°F
			water for 50–55 minutes
			4. Chill in ice.

[a] From Groen, a Dover Industries Company.

meat yields are produced. The procedure for cooking beef in a cook tank is as follows:

1. *Preparation.* Meat to be cooked is trimmed of excess or discolored fat. Seasonings are applied to the outer surface of the meat as a dry rub, or the meat may be injected up to 10% of its raw weight with a seasoning solution. Only spices or spice blends that carry a manufacturer's certification that they are free of pathogenic microorganisms should be used. Rubs give the meat the desired flavor and oven-roasted appearance.

2. *Packaging.* The trimmed product is placed in a polyolefin casing, with one end preclipped. An air-powered heavy-duty vacuum system extracts the air from the bagged meat cut, gathers the neck of the bag, and applies a rugged clip. If natural meat juices are to be drained from the package after cooking, an additional 6-inch *tail* is left in order to permit revacuumizing and reclipping the original casing.

3. *Cooking.* Meat in vacuum-sealed bags is cooked at controlled temperatures not exceeding 195°F. The cooking process meets USDA guidelines for Cooking Requirements for Cooked and Roast Beef (see Federal Register 1978), which specifies that all products must be cooked to an internal temperature of 145°F (63°C).

4. *Chilling and storage.* After cooking, the product is cooled to arrest any additional interior cooking of the meat. The hot water is drained from the tank, and city water or water from an ice builder is pumped through the tank to arrest the cooking process. Injected beef must be chilled below 40°F within a 6-hour period. Cooked beef that has been injected with spices must be frozen at 0°F for storage and distribution. Beef that is not injected should be stored at 28°F–30°F for refrigerated storage of 6–12 weeks, or 0°F for longer-term frozen storage.

The cook-chill tank is used for a number of other products other than solid cuts of meats, such as liver and onions, meat loaf, salisbury steak, steamed rice, and other entree food items. The procedure for making liver and onions in the cook-chill tank is given in Table 12-1. The extended time for chill-holding of foods makes the cook-chill-serve system a more practical alternative in medical foodservice operations.

Commissary or Food Factory

A commissary is a central location where food is produced using any of the production systems previously discussed. Food may be produced, using the cook-serve, cook-freeze-serve, or the cook-chill-serve system. Food is transported to satellite units, as needed. The food flow for commissary food production is the same as when food is produced in a single facility. There are logical reasons for using a commissary to produce food for several facilities, but certain managerial decisions need careful consideration:

1. *Menu or type of food to be prepared.* Will all satellite units use the same food items during a menu cycle? Will all units conform to standardized portion sizes? Will the commissary prepare food for patients, personnel, and special activities? Will the commissary prepare only hot foods, or both hot and cold?

2. *Type of production system.* Which production system can best meet the needs of all satellite units? Consideration should be given to holding time and temperature in providing safe food.

3. *Delivery schedule.* Depending on the type of production system used and the amount of storage space at the satellite units, food deliveries may be required three times a day, once a day, or once a week. If the cook-serve system is used, the delivery schedule is not at the discretion of management; food must be delivered prior to each meal served with a minimum of holding.

4. *Packaging.* The packaging depends on the state of readiness as food is delivered to the various units. For patient foodservice, food may be packaged as follows:

- Bulk packaging with portioning and tray assembly at satellite unit.
- Individual portions with tray assembly at the satellite unit.
- Individual portions with complete tray assembly at the commissary site.
- Bulk packaging for cafeteria service.

5. *Processing equipment.* Equipment should be appropriate for the type of system selected. Consider equipment that will reduce handling, thus minimizing contamination sources.

6. *Transporting equipment.* For keeping processed food safe, the temperature must be below 45°F or above 140°F. The type of equipment used to transport will depend on the preparation state, such as hot, cold, frozen, or chilled; holding time required; delays; and travel distance and time.

Food Flow

Alternatives to the conventional cook-serve method of preparing food in quantity have reached major proportions since the early 1960s. Not only is the flow of food different, but there is an increase in the number of stages that must be completed before the food is served. Depending on the system, there may be 11 or more stages involved in food production and service. The various stages given for the four systems in Table 12-2 are considered critical control points that may affect microbial, sensory, and nutritional quality of food.

Bobeng and David (1978) applied the Hazard Analysis Critical Control Point (HACCP) to the conventional, cook-chill, and cook-freeze hospital foodservice systems. A system for preventing the deterioration of food quality, HACCP was successfully implemented by commercial food processors. Emphasis is on managerial awareness of microbiological hazards and on identifying the

Table 12-2. Food Flow for Various Production Systems

Cook-Serve	Assembly-Serve	Cook-Chill-Serve	Cook-Freeze-Serve
Purchasing	Purchasing	Purchasing	Purchasing
Receiving	Receiving	Receiving	Receiving
Storage (dry, refrigeration, and low temperature)	Storage (dry, refrigeration, and low temperature)	Storage (dry and refrigeration)	Storage (dry, refrigeration, and low temperature)
Pre-preparation		Pre-preparation	Preparation
Preparation		Preparation	Preparation
		Packaging	Packaging
Prepared holding (chill-hot)		Prepared holding (chill)	Prepared holding (Low temperature)
	Thawing		Thawing
Portioning	Portioning (bulk)	Portioning	Portioning (bulk)
Assembly	Assembly	Assembly	Assembly
Transport/holding (Chill-Hot)	Transport/holding (chill)	Transport/holding (chill)	Transport/holding (chill)
	Rethermalize	Rethermalize	Rethermalize
Serve	Serve	Serve	Serve

process stages at which loss of control could present food safety risks. Each process stage of production is considered a control point.

The study was limited to three on-premise foodservice systems. Control points were studied in relation to (1) ingredient control and storage, (2) equipment sanitation, (3) personnel sanitation, and (4) time-temperature relationships. It was determined that microbiological testing can be done but not in time to take corrective action for the current batch. Because of variations in types, sizes, equipment models, kind and number of employees for each foodservice operation, it was impossible to establish universal critical control point parameters for monitoring equipment and personnel sanitation. The most practical procedure, one that can be applied to all production systems, is the establishment of time-temperature standards. Time-temperature standards developed are similar to those specified by federal regulations for the holding of processed foods.

Food Production

The daily production of food must be organized, regardless of the type of production system used. The most valuable tool for managerial control is the production worksheet (Fig. 12-3). Depending on the size of the operation, a separate production worksheet may be used for each unit, such as cooking, baking, salad–sandwich, and others. In some operations, a separate area with diet cooks assigned is used for preparation of modified diet foods. The production worksheet is completed as follows:

1. *Food item.* The food items listed on the production worksheet are taken directly from the planned menu. Any deviations must have managerial approval.

2. *Amount needed.* The amount needed is based on the projected number of portions required. The amount may be adjusted on the day of service if an increase or decrease in patient census or some other special activity justifies the change. Space is provided for both regular and modified diets. Amounts in the regular column include amounts needed by patients on regular diets and in the cafeteria and for special activities.

3. *Prepared by.* The chef or head cook, responsible for completing the worksheet, refers to the employee duty schedule and assigns work accordingly. When the production worksheet is posted one day in advance of preparation, employees know exactly what their duties will be and can plan work time efficiently.

4. *Time of preparation.* When food is prepared too early, there may be a loss of quality in both taste and appearance. If food is not prepared on time, there may be undue pressure on employees and possibly chaotic situations in a rush to meet culinary schedules. Both situations can be eliminated by indicating the time to begin preparation.

5. *Instructions.* Information in this column may simply state, "Use recipe no. 42" or instructions may be given to serve larger portions of an entree item for a special activity.

6. *Amount used.* To be completed at the end of serving period. Information is obtained from the tray line, cafeteria, and special activities supervisors.

7. *Amount left.* The amount used is subtracted from the amount prepared to equal the amount left. The information is important for use in forecasting the amount to prepare during the next menu cycle.

8. *Disposition.* All leftover foods should be accounted for in some manner. The shift supervisor or person responsible for completing the form must indicate what disposition was made of leftover items, such as chill-stored, freezer-stored, or discarded.

At the end of service, additional information is recorded at the bottom of the worksheet by the shift supervisor, such as unexpected guests, weather conditions, or other significant events affecting the number of persons served. As a control tool, management can readily observe whether there were any irregularities during the preparation and service of the meal, and note the accuracy of forecasting. For example, if enough food were requisitioned and prepared for 500 portions, 450 portions were served, and no portions were left, then management must find out what happened to 50 portions of food. The effectiveness of the production worksheet depends on managerial practices from menu planning and standardized recipes through food purchasing.

── Food Production for Modified Diets ──────

The preparation of modified diet food is often combined with the production of food for regular diet, personnel, and guests. The general practice is to omit seasoning and added fat for a given number of servings to be served to patients on modified diets. All patients are served plain, unseasoned food, regardless of

Production Worksheet

UNIT _____ MEAL _____ DAY _____ DATE _____

(1)	(2) Amount Needed						(3) Prepared by	(4) Time of Preparation	(5) Instructions	(6) Amount Used	(7) Amount Left	(8) Disposition
Food Item	Reg	Ca	Na	Fa	Fi	Li						

Projected Number of Meals: _____ Patients _____ Cafeteria _____ Other _____

Actual Meals Served: _____ Patients _____ Cafeteria _____ Other _____

Comments: _____

Prepared by: _____ Shift Supervisor: _____

Figure 12-3. Production worksheet. Under amount needed, Reg stands for regular; Ca, restricted calories; Na, restricted sodium; Fa, restricted fat; Fi, restricted fiber; Li, full liquid.

what type of diet modification. Cooks in the main production area often do not take the time to prepare tasty, attractive meals for modified diets. The primary purpose of a medical foodservice operation is to provide nutritious, appetizing, and attractive meals to patients; yet emphasis is often put on merchandising food served to physicians, administrators, employees, and others.

In some foodservice operations, there is a separate unit for the preparation of modified diet foods, with specialty cooks assigned. Cooks assigned to this unit have a basic knowledge and understanding of diet modification, and are trained in preparation techniques applicable to the various diets. The advantages of this type of production design are as follows:

1. Assigned personnel will have the time to individualize the preparation of food for the various diets.
2. Cooks can respond to special requests related to complicated or multi-restricted diets.
3. With a knowledge of diet modification, cooks can add allowed seasonings to make diets more appetizing.
4. Cooks will have time to prepare combination dishes, as prescribed, such as beef cubes with vegetables, macaroni and cheese, tuna-noodle casserole, and other foods that are normally served only to patients on a regular diet.
5. Cooks will be able to prepare specialty-type items for patients on restricted diets—for example, the preparation of bread using nonwheat flour for patients with wheat intolerance, pancakes with egg whites for restricted-cholesterol diets, and other special considerations.
6. Cooks will be able to prepare tasty cream soups, restricted-calorie soups, and dressings for salads.

Patients will appreciate the attention given to preparation of food for modified diets, and employees will take pride in preparing food that patients will eat and enjoy.

Nourishments

Nourishments are foods served to patients, either as a supplement or as a part of the regular dietary regimen. Serving time is designated approximately 2 to 3 hours after the regular meal, such as 10:00 A.M., 2:00 P.M., and 8:00 P.M. All patients normally receive the night nourishment; patients on modified diets, such as a diabetic, may receive nourishment three times a day. The nourishment menu should be planned on a rotation basis to ensure that a variety of food is served (Table 12-3). For example, a patient on a clear liquid diet should not receive the same flavor and color of Jell-O for three consecutive times until the prepared batch is used up. The employee assigned to nourishment preparation should have a basic knowledge of foods allowed on various diets and be able to measure and weigh prescribed amounts with accuracy. In a large facility, the preparation of nourishments is a full-time position. Since nourishments are an important part of the patient's total daily food intake, the task should not be assigned to any employee at random.

Special Activities

Medical foodservice operations should agree to provide food for special activities only after due consideration is given to the impact that the increased work load will have on patient foodservice. The handling of special activities for in-house and outside professional groups can enhance the image of the hospital and serve

Table 12-3. Sample Nourishment Menu

Day	Regular	Restricted Calories	Restricted Sodium	Restricted Fat	Restricted Fiber	Full Liquid	Clear Liquid
Sunday	Turkey Sandwich Pear Nectar	FF Turkey Sandwich[a] Pear Nectar	SF Turkey Sandwich[b] Pear Nectar	FF Turkey Sandwich Pear Nectar	Turkey Sandwich Pear Nectar	Ice Cream	Apple Juice
Monday	Lime Sherbet Vanilla Wafers	Diet Gelatin Vanilla Wafers	Lime Sherbet Vanilla Wafers	Lime Sherbet Vanilla Wafers	Lime Sherbet Vanilla Wafers	Lime Sherbet	Lime Gelatin
Tuesday	Cheese and Crackers Grape Juice	Cheese and Crackers Grape Juice	SF Cheese and SF Crackers Grape Juice	Low-fat Cheese and Crackers Grape Juice	Cheese and Crackers Grape Juice	Chocolate Milkshake	Cherry Popsicle
Wednesday	Sugar Cookies Whole Milk	Vanilla Wafers Skim Milk	Sugar Cookies Whole Milk	Sugar Cookies Skim Milk	Sugar Cookies Whole Milk	Vanilla Yogurt	Orange Gelatin
Thursday	Peanut Butter and Crackers Pineapple Juice	Peanut Butter and Crackers Pineapple Juice	SF Peanut Butter and SF Crackers Pineapple Juice	Canned Pears Graham Crackers Pineapple Juice	Canned Pears Pineapple Juice	Orange Sherbet	Grape Popsicle
Friday	Strawberry Gelatin Graham Crackers Orange Juice	Diet Gelatin Graham Crackers Orange Juice	SF Strawberry Gelatin Graham Crackers Orange Juice	Strawberry Gelatin Graham Crackers Orange Juice	Strawberry Gelatin Vanilla Wafers Orange Juice	Strawberry Gelatin Whole Milk	Strawberry Gelatin
Saturday	Canned Peaches Whole Milk	Diet Peaches Skim Milk	Canned Peaches Whole Milk	Canned Peaches Skim Milk	Canned Peaches Whole Milk	Vanilla Milkshake	Ginger Ale

[a] FF indicates fat-free.
[b] SF indicates salt-free.

243

as good public relations, but special activities should not be promoted at the expense of patient care. To operate smoothly, these activities must be well planned.

Staffing, menus, and other arrangements require special attention. A special activities supervisor is needed for facilities catering to special activities on a daily basis. Other employees need to be assigned for table setup, arranging tables and chairs, and transporting food and other supplies to the service areas. Professional waiters and waitresses may work on an on-call basis. If elaborate or large catered functions are planned, it may be necessary to include a catering chef position as part of staffing.

A selection of precosted menus should be available to assist groups in making special requests. Groups can select preferred foods and know exactly how much it will cost. The cost per serving, whether it is for a coffee break or an elaborate dinner, should include all labor, food, and overhead costs. Additional charges may be assessed for alcoholic beverages, special floral arrangements, and other special requests. To allow the requisiting party an opportunity to select preferred combinations, suggested menu items can be grouped as shown in Figure 12.4, using the à la carte pricing method. Standardized recipes, indicating portion sizes, should be used for all catered food items. For example, a sandwich plate recipe may include both the ingredient amounts and a diagram showing how the ingredients should be arranged on the plate.

Record keeping is an important task associated with special activities. There should not be any mix-up concerning dates and times of planned activities. A reservation form, such as the one shown in Figure 12-5, can be used to document requests. Complete arrangements, including table and seating patterns should be agreed upon so that correct charges can be made. All food requested, whether it is a pot of coffee or a gourmet dinner for a large party, should be charged to some account. As shown in Figures 15-8 and 15-9, each request for special activity is charged to an account, approved by administration, and processed for credit to the foodservice department. Copies of the approved reservation should be routed to the following: (1) special activities supervisor, (2) requesting group, (3) accounting office, and (4) foodservice director's office.

Vending Service

Vending services are frequently offered in medical foodservice operations to accommodate employees and guests during hours when the cafeteria is closed. Services may be provided in-house or by outside vendors. Employees scheduled for night shifts often complain about the lack of variety and quality of food available. To resolve the problem, some foodservice operations remain open for 24 hours; other operations prefer vending services. When the vending is in-house, the same high standards of quality should apply as for other services provided by the department. Advantages of in-house vending are the following:

1. A variety of food items can be served, such as fresh fruits and salads. Complete meals can be cold-plated as in the procedure for patient service, using a microwave oven for reheating.
2. Food quality can be controlled by removing unused items and replenishing with fresh food daily.
3. Safety and sanitation is assured. Machines can be cleaned and checked for proper temperature on a daily basis. Preparation dates can be stamped on all perishables to ensure freshness.

	Suggested Menu Items	Cost ($)
Appetizers:	Broiled Grapefruit Half with Cherry	_____
	New England Clam Chowder	_____
	French Onion Soup with Parmesan Cheese Croutons	_____
	V-8 Juice, Lemon Wedge	_____
	Fruit Cup, Mint Garnish	_____
	Jumbo Shrimp Cocktail, Lemon Wedge	_____
Entrees:	Broiled Rib Eye Steak with Mushroom Cap	_____
	Breaded Center-Cut Pork Chop	_____
	Boneless Breast of Chicken Cordon Bleu	_____
	Broiled Filet Mignon, Mushroom Cap, Bordelaise Sauce	_____
	Stuffed Flounder	_____
	Veal Cutlet Cordon Bleu	_____
	Glazed Duck with Plum Sauce	_____
	Stuffed Pork Chop	_____
	Marinated Lamb Chops	_____
	Baked Chicken with Wild Rice	_____
	Veal Parmigiana	_____
Potatoes or Substitutes:	Baked Potato with Sour Cream	_____
	Au Gratin Potato with Colby Sharp Cheese	_____
	Rice Pilaf	_____
	Almond Potato Puff	_____
	Saffron Rice	_____
	Stuffed Baked Potato	_____
	Duchess Potatoes	_____
Vegetables:	French-Style Green Beans Amandine	_____
	Green Peas and Pearl Onions	_____
	Broccoli Spears with Hollandaise Sauce	_____
	Baby Asparagus Spears	_____
	Candied Carrot Logs	_____
	Mixed Vegetables, Oriental	_____
	Harvard Beets	_____
	Whole Green Beans with Walnuts	_____
	Italian Green Beans with Bacon Bits	_____
Salads:	Lemon Jello with Celery, Pimento, and Carrots	_____
	Tossed Salad with Bleu Cheese Dressing	_____
	Cranberry Nut Salad	_____
	Green Salad Bowl with Roquefort Cheese Dressing	_____
	Caesar Salad with Caesar Dressing	_____
	Sliced Tomato and Cottage Cheese	_____
	Lettuce Hearts, Cucumber, Tomato with French Dressing	_____
Desserts:	Parfait, Creme de Menthe or Cherry	_____
	Apple Pie with Colby Cheese or Ice Cream	_____
	Hot Fudge Sundae or Peppermint Ice Cream	_____
	Strawberry Shortcake with Old-Fashioned Brown Sugar Biscuit and Whipped Cream	_____
	Strawberry-Filled Eclair	_____
	Lemon, Strawberry, or Cherry Cheese Cake	_____
	Ice Cream Cake Roll	_____
	Peach Melba	_____
	Apple Crunch à la mode	_____
	Pecan Pie	_____
Breads:	Baking Powder Biscuit with Marmalade or Honey	_____
	Small Onion Rolls	_____
	Cheese Sticks	_____
	Small Dinner Rolls	_____
	Homemade Loaf, Garlic or Parmesan	_____
	Crescent Dinner Rolls	_____
Beverages:	Coffee—Regular, Decaffeinated	_____
	Tea—Iced, Hot	_____
	Milk—Whole, Low-Fat, Skim, Chocolate	_____
	Punch	_____

Figure 12-4. Suggested menu for special activities. *From Detroit-Macomb Hospital Corporation.*

Name of Group _____ Date of Activity _____
Time of Activity _____ Room Assigned _____
Type of Activity (Luncheon, Tea, Coffee Break, etc.) _____
Number Expected _____
Type of Service (Table, Buffet) _____
Type of Serviceware (Disposables, China, Silver Service) _____

Menu:

Seating Arrangement:

Additional Information: (1) Fresh floral arrangement for Buffet. (2) Small vase with fresh flowers at each table.

Requested by: _____   Account No. _____

Approved by: _____   Date _____
               Foodservice Director

_____   Date _____
       Assistant Administrator

Figure 12-5. Special activities reservation form.

   4. Foods provided by an outside vending company are limited to foods with an extended shelf life.
   5. With in-house repair persons, there is less waiting when machines malfunction.

Although there may be improved quality of food served when using in-house vending, there are also certain disadvantages:

   1. Additional staffing is required to prepare food items in an attractive and appetizing manner.
   2. Time must be spent in training and supervising employees to load the machines properly and to rotate food items regularly to ensure freshness.
   3. Additional menu-planning responsibilities are required. Vending menus must be an integral part of menu planning to avoid depending on the use of leftover foods.
   4. Increased supervision is necessary to ensure safety and sanitation. Food items must be dated, machines maintained in a clean and sanitary condition, and temperatures controlled.
   5. There is an increased cost for equipment and supplies. This cost includes the initial cost to purchase or rent machines, the maintenance and repairs, and the paper supplies designed especially for vending machines.

Quality Control

The control of quality is a continuous process and should be closely monitored from menu planning until the food item is served to the consumer. Factors that affect the quality of food during the production stage are (1) cooking time and temperature and (2) the cooking method.

—— Time and Temperature ——————

Control of these two variables is related to the type of product, size, thickness, degree of tenderness, composition of the food, temperature of the food, batch size, type of equipment, and degree of doneness desired. Depending on the qualities to be developed in the end product, some foods are cooked for a short period of time at high temperatures, whereas other foods are cooked at low temperatures for a long period of time.

Most roast meats are cooked at low temperatures to retain moisture and to improve flavor and texture. Thin cuts of meat, such as steaks, may be cooked at high temperatures for short periods of time to produce a brown attractive appearance but not long enough to burn or dry out the meat. Time and temperature charts have been developed as a guideline for meat cookery. As shown in Table 12-4, the cooking time is based on minutes per pound for each roast at refrigerated temperature. As noted, a longer time period is required for boneless, rolled, and tied meat compared to a rib roast with bones included. The chart is based on meat that is cut according to **IMP-NAMP standards.** For other cuts of roast beef, such as a flat cut, which requires less cooking time, the chart may not be an accurate guide.

One of the best methods for determining the degree of doneness is with the use of the meat thermometer (Fig. 12-6). According to standards published in the *Food Service Sanitation Manual* (U.S. Department of Health and Human Services 1976), "a metal-type numerically scaled indicating thermometer, accurate to ±2°F, is the type approved for assuring proper internal cooking, holding, or refrigeration temperature of all potentially hazardous foods." An important aspect of meat cookery is that heat must be applied to all parts of the food to a temperature of at least 140°F. The exception is for rare roast beef, which may be cooked to a rare stage at 130°F. Pork and poultry require a much higher minimum temperature (Table 12-5).

Time and temperature are critical for seafood, since those products are too frequently overcooked. Except for broiled shellfish and oven-fried breaded fish where a brown surface is desired, fish is cooked for a short period of time at moderate to high temperatures (Table 12-6).

Most vegetables can be cooked to a desirable state in a short period of time. Time and temperatures vary depending on the kind of vegetable and the type of

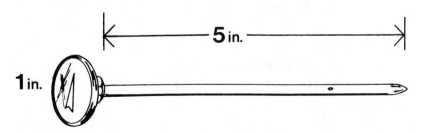

Figure 12-6. Dial face metal probe-type thermometer has an accuracy of ±2°F (±1°C) and a temperature range of 0°F to 220°F (−18°C to 110°C). *From National Sanitation Foundation (1980)*

Table 12-4. Timetable for Roasting Beef[a]

Cut	Approximate Weight of Single Roast (lb)	No. of Roasts in Oven	Approximate Total Weight of Roasts (lb)	Oven Temperature (°F)	Interior Temperature of Roast when Removed from Oven (°F)	Minutes per lb Based on One Roast	Minutes per lb Based on Total Weight of Roasts in Oven	Approximate Total Cooking Time
Rib, roast ready, no. 109	20–25			250	130 (rare)	13–15		4½–5 hours
					140 (medium)	15–17		5–6 hours
					150 (well)	17–19		6–6½ hours
Rib, roast ready, no. 109	20–25			300	130 (rare)	10–12		4–4½ hours
					140 (medium)	12–14		4½–5 hours
					150 (well)	14–16		5–5½ hours
Rib, roast ready, no. 109		2	56	300	130 (rare)		5–6	5–5½ hours
					140 (medium)		6	6 hours
					150 (well)		7–8	6–7 hours
Ribeye roll, no. 112 or no. 112A	4–6			350	140 (rare)	18–20		1⅓–1⅔ hours
					160 (medium)	20–22		1½–2 hours
					170 (well)	22–24		1⅔–2¼ hours
Full tenderloin, no. 189 or no. 190	4–6			425	140 (rare)			45–60 minutes
Strip loin, boneless, no. 180	10–12			325	140 (rare)	10		1½–2 hours
Top sirloin butt, no. 184	8			300	140 (rare)	25		3½ hours
Top (inside) round, no. 168	10			300	140 (rare)	18–19		3–3¼ hours
					150 (medium)	22–23		3½–4 hours
Top (inside) round, no. 168	15			300	140 (rare)	15		3½–4 hours
					150 (medium)	17		4–4½ hours
Round, rump and shank off, boneless, tied, special, no. 165B	50			250	140 (medium)	12		10 hours
					155 (well)	14		11–12 hours

[a]From National Live Stock and Meat Board (1977).

Table 12-5. Minimum Internal Temperature for Meat and Poultry Products

Food Item	Temperature (°F)
Beef	130–140
Poultry, poultry stuffing, and stuffed meats	165
Pork and any food containing pork	150

Table 12-6. Temperatures of Seafood Cookery

Type of Seafood	Recommended Cooking Temperature	Approximate Time (min)
Lobster—broiled, split	Broil	10
Lobster and shrimp—steamed, whole	15-lb pressure	3
Fish—deep-fried	350°F–375°F	4
Fish—oven-fried, breaded	450°F–500°F	20–25
Fish—poached	185°F	4–5
Fish—oven-baked, unbreaded fillet	350°F–400°F	15–20

equipment used. Vegetables cooked on the top of a stove in a pot of water take longer than those cooked in low- or high-pressure steamers. In medical foodservice operations, most vegetables are cooked in high-compression steamers for 2 to 3 minutes. The use of progressive cookery method, where small batches are cooked throughout the serving period, is recommended for maximum retention of color, texture, flavor, and nutritive value. Consider the following measures in controlling nutrient losses.

1. Purchase food of high quality. Wilted vegetables will have a lower nutritive value than crisp fresh vegetables because of the evaporation of moisture.
2. Store all foods at the proper temperature and humidity. Undue shrinkage results when the humidity is too low, causing nutrient and weight losses.
3. Use the FIFO system for storing food to avoid excessive storage periods.
4. Avoid excess trimming of vegetables and fruits, since some nutrients such as ascorbic acid are concentrated near the skin.
5. Cook vegetables such as potatoes and carrots with skins on whenever possible.
6. Outer leaves of green vegetables are often higher in vitamins and minerals than the center or core. Avoid excess trimming of vegetables such as cabbage and lettuce. The less tender leaves from cabbage can be cooked first, for a longer period of time, then crisp inner leaves may be added near the end of the cooking cycle.
7. Avoid soaking of vegetables and fruits. Prolonged soaking periods cause loss of nutrients, especially ascorbic acid and thiamine.
8. To prevent solubility of minerals and vitamins, cook vegetables in a steamer without water; if water is used, use as little as possible.
9. Do not add baking soda to green vegetables. The vegetables will retain a bright green color, but the soda will cause a loss of nutrients, such as ascorbic acid.
10. Practice progressive cookery methods, where food is cooked in small batches, as needed.
11. Cook vegetables and fruits whole, when possible. Dicing or cutting into small pieces reduces cooking time, but favors the loss of water-soluble nutrients as a result of greater surface exposure.

Method of Cooking

Food is cooked to make it more digestible, to destroy bacteria, and to increase palatability for some products. The cooking method is determined by a number of factors for different products (Table 12-7). Dry and moist heat methods of cooking, commonly used in medical foodservice operations, are as follows:

Table 12-7. Factors Affecting Cooking Methods for Different Foods

Meat	Poultry	Fish	Fruits and Vegetables
Marbling and fat content	Fat content	Fat content	Texture (cellulose)
Age	Age		Color (green, red, yellow, white)
Connective tissue	Size		Flavor (mild, strong)
Cut			Acidity
Kind of animal			Moisture

1. *Roasting* (dry) involves cooking food uncovered in an oven without added liquids. The term is used interchangeably with baking. For example, ham appears on the menu as "Baked Ham," but it is really cooked by roasting. In addition to meats, poultry, and fish, some vegetables such as potato and squash may be roasted. Oven-baked fish is a popular cooking method for fish fillets or steaks, either breaded or unbreaded. Dry heat methods are suitable for tender cuts of meat. Roasting is a popular method of cooking for poultry, with the exception of young chickens. Because of the lack of fat on young chickens, other methods such as frying may be more appropriate. In common usage, the term *baking* is reserved primarily for desserts, breads, and casseroles.

2. *Pot-roasting* (moist) is not a true roasting method. Since liquid is added to the meat after it is browned and covered during the cooking process, the method is considered a form of braising. The method is popular for less tender cuts of beef.

3. *Broiling* (dry) means cooking by direct heat. The heat source may be above or below the food to be cooked. The method is used for tender cuts of meat such as steaks and chops, fish with high fat content, young poultry, and vegetables and fruits, such as tomatoes, grapefruit, and bananas. Char-broilers (electric or gas) are frequently used because of the distinctive charcoal flavor. When fish or chicken appears on the menu in a medical foodservice operation, the method of preparation is often oven-broiled. Bacon is pan-broiled in the oven by arranging strips of bacon on an 18- × 26-in. sheet pan and baking at a temperature of 400°F for approximately 20 minutes.

4. *Griddling* (dry) involves cooking on a hot, solid surface with or without added fat. For most meats it is not necessary to add fat because of the high fat content already in the meat. Fat is usually added for vegetables such as onions and mushrooms. When fat is added to the griddle, the process is similar to sauteeing. The griddle is frequently located near the service area so that progressive cookery can take place throughout the serving period. Foods that deteriorate in quality when held for long periods, such as eggs, pancakes, and hamburgers are cooked in small batches on a griddle.

5. *Frying* (dry) is a means of cooking in which food is submerged in fat. The method is used less frequently in medical foodservice operations because of the emphasis on reduced fat intake. Frying is especially popular and suitable for breaded products such as fish, shrimp, young chicken, and chops.

·6. *Sauteeing* (dry) is a technique for cooking in a small amount of fat. In medical foodservice, sauteeing is a rarely used method of food preparation.

7. *Steaming* (moist) refers to the process of cooking in steam with or without pressure. Steaming is one of the most popular and versatile methods of preparing food in medical foodservice operations. The method is used for meats, vegetables, and other foods such as hard-cooked and scrambled eggs. Low- and high-pressure steam equipment, along with the tilting skillet have practically eliminated the use of top-of-the-stove cooking on a range.

8. *Braising, swissing, and fricasseeing* (moist) are methods used when meat is dredged in seasoned flour, browned in a small amount of fat, and the cooking process completed by adding a small amount of liquid, covered and cooked in the oven until tender. Popular menu items are "braised short ribs of beef," "swiss steak," and "chicken fricassee."

The use of standardized recipes and the production worksheet can resolve many of the problems associated with food quality. Both time and temperature can be controlled, if cooking tools and equipment are used properly. When the time, temperature, and method of cooking are adhered to, other desirable qualities such as flavor, color, texture, and nutrients are also controlled.

Quantity Control

Quantity control in food production is concerned with minimizing food waste, thereby maximizing expected yield. When the menu is planned, a major factor used in the decision to put a food item on the menu is whether the portion size is within established monetary allowances. When the yield is less than expected because of controllable loss, there is a waste of food and increased cost. Care must be taken to ensure that the portion planned is the amount produced and subsequently served. During the production stage, losses can occur as food is prepared, cooked, and portioned. Quantity losses can be minimized during pre-preparation if an ingredient room is used.

The Ingredient Room

An area where ingredients are measured or weighed and food is pre-prepared for the cooking or final stage of preparation is referred to as an ingredient room. Pre-preparation involves washing, peeling, cubing, slicing, and dicing of fruits and vegetables, as well as weighing, trimming, cubing, dicing, and portioning of meat. There should be a separate room for the pre-preparation of meat or at least a separate area of the room with a sink and counter to be used only for raw meats. This measure is necessary in order to prevent cross contamination of raw fruits and vegetables that require no further cooking.

To be effective, all food should flow directly from storage to the ingredient room, then to the various production areas. Exceptions may be for foods such as dry cereals, instant beverages, commercially baked products, ice cream, milk, and other such items requiring no additional preparation. Ingredient room procedures, in general, are as follows:

1. Using standardized recipes, food is requisitioned from storage for a given meal or for all meals to be served on a given day.
2. All ingredients are measured for each item on the menu. Seasonings are labeled so that cooks can accurately follow the recipe in adding ingredients. All food is washed or prepared in some other manner, as required, at least one day in advance.
3. Food for each menu item is placed on a separate tray and stored dry or refrigerated until ready for use by cooks.
4. On the day of use, trays are issued to cooks for final production.
5. All reusable leftover food is returned to the ingredient room. The food will be reissued as part of a new menu item. This practice prevents cooks from altering recipes by adding extra ingredients at their own discretion.

Cleaned fruits and vegetables may be stored in plastic bags or plastic containers with covers. Potatoes and carrots are usually peeled and stored in containers with enough water to cover the products. The use of sulfiting agents to prevent discoloration of fruits and vegetables is discouraged. The Michigan Department of Public Health, acting under Section 2-101 of the Food Sanitation Code, informed local health departments that fresh fruits, vegetables, and other products served in the raw state, which have been treated with sulfiting agents, may only be served if the customer is informed that such agents have been added. (A memorandum was sent to all local health departments on May 2, 1983.) The recommendation was in response to research indicating that certain individuals, primarily asthmatics, may suffer threatening respiratory distress when exposed to products treated with sulfites. Although cooking reduces the effects of sulfites, some residue may be left.

The ingredient room system promotes quantity control and saves valuable time for highly paid skilled employees. No time is wasted gathering supplies before production can begin. The emphasis on increased productivity and cost control is of concern to some researchers, however, according to Livingston and Chang (1979), the progress made in production controls may well be a step backward in terms of nutrient retention. It is suggested that ingredient preparation should take place as close in time to the cooking and final preparation as possible. Adequate ingredient room facilities should be provided to reduce excessive advance preparation and extended holding of raw ingredients.

Disaster Feeding Plans

As mandated by the Joint Commission on Accreditation of Hospitals (1988), "The dietetic department/service shall be able to meet the nutritional needs of patients and staff during a disaster, consistent with the capabilities of the hospital and community served." In order to fulfill this mandate, the foodservice department must have plans for emergency feeding in the "ready" state at all times.

Disasters may be classified as natural or man-made. Natural disasters include earthquake, fire, flood, hurricane, and tornado. Man-made disasters include chemical, nuclear, and atomic warfare, bombs, and bomb threats. The disaster may be for a short or long period of time. The foodservice department must be able to respond with essential services as soon as possible. Local health authorities must be notified immediately when a disaster occurs that may possibly involve food contamination.

Emergency feeding plans must provide for safe food and water supply. Menu planning should progress from simple, basic food to more complex meals. An initial feeding of a hot beverage and crackers or cookies will have a calming effect on both patient and personnel until food of a more substantial nature can be prepared. It may not be advisable to initially serve uncooked foods such as fruits and vegetables, depending on the amount of available safe water. The first hot meal may consist of a *single-dish* type, such as stew. After full assessment of disaster conditions including available food, water, equipment, refrigeration, and utilities, a full meal can be prepared.

A supply of food and water should be available and stored off-site, in a location convenient to the facility. Depending on resulting conditions such as (1) no refrigeration, (2) no cooking facilities, and (3) no safe water, it may be necessary to rely on canned and packaged foods that can be eaten cold. Suggested food list is as follows:

1. Ready-to-eat cereals
2. Evaporated milk
3. Canned fruits and fruit juice
4. Canned meat and beans
5. Processed cheese, requiring no refrigeration
6. Crackers, cookies, and canned bread
7. Candy, jam, and jelly (individually wrapped)
8. Instant coffee and instant cocoa (if cooking facilities are available)
9. Canned soup and vegetables (if cooking facilities are available)

All bottled, potable water must be from a source that complies with all health laws and must be handled and stored in a way that protects it from contamination. Emergency foods must be inspected and rotated periodically.

The emergency feeding plan should be checked and approved by local health authorities. In some communities, a cooperative emergency feeding plan is in effect. In this type of arrangement, an unaffected facility will prepare and transport food and beverages to the affected facility.

Safety and Sanitation

Producing food under safe and sanitary conditions must be an integral part of the total systems approach. For medical foodservice operations, preventing food-borne illness is a critical task due to the nature of the clients. Patients enter the medical facility under varying physical conditions and are therefore more susceptible to adverse effects from food-borne illness than clients served in other types of foodservice operations. The foodservice director must be aware of the source and cause of food-borne illness and take preventive measures to eliminate hazardous conditions.

Food-Borne Illness

To prevent food-borne illness, food must be protected from filth, pathogenic microorganisms, and toxic chemicals. Bacteria cannot be seen with the naked eye; they are single-cell organisms that are visible with the aid of a microscope. "Sanitary" means that the product or article is free from pathogenic bacteria. It is possible for a product or article to be clean as visually inspected, yet it may not be sanitary. Microorganisms, especially pathogenic bacteria that are capable of causing food-borne illness, are of major concern in producing safe food. Other microorganisms that may cause illness are viruses and trichinae. Hundreds of kinds of germs can cause food poisoning. Most bacteria need warmth, moisture, and food to thrive. Some bacteria need air, whereas others thrive better without air. Bacteria thrive best in *potentially hazardous foods* at temperatures between 45°F and 145°F. A potentially hazardous food has been defined by the U.S. Department of Health and Human Services (1976) as "any food that consists in whole or in part of milk or milk products, eggs, meat, poultry, fish, shellfish, edible crustacea, or other ingredients in a form capable of supporting rapid and progressive growth of infectious or toxigenic microorganisms."

Salmonella, a form of bacteria occurring in the intestinal tract of humans and animals, can cause severe illness (salmonellosis) and even death. One type of salmonella causes typhoid fever. Infected food animals can transmit the disease to humans through contaminated meat, fish, poultry, and other animal products such as eggs and milk. The usual symptoms are fever, diarrhea, and sometimes vomiting. The disease can be dangerous for the very young, very old, and persons already weakened by illness. Salmonella can be destroyed by heat. Pasteurization kills the organism in milk. Certain chemicals also can destroy the organism.

Preventive measures include observing the danger temperature zone for prepared foods by cooking and reheating foods to an internal temperature of 165°F, cleaning and sanitizing work surfaces and utensils used to prepare food of animal origin, establishing and enforcing proper hand-washing procedures for workers, and restricting work by employees suffering from diarrhea, fever, and vomiting.

Staphylococcus aureus is a form of bacteria that produces a toxin causing staphylococcus (staph) food poisoning. Humans carry these organisms on their hands and arms, nose and throat, hairy regions of the body, and in infected boils and abscesses. The usual symptoms of vomiting, diarrhea, and abdominal cramps occur within 3 to 8 hours after eating contaminated food. The toxin is very heat stable and is not destroyed by ordinary cooking methods. The illness is caused by unsanitary work habits in handling protein foods and by exposing such foods to warm temperatures for extended periods of time.

Preventive measures include making sure employees are free of infected lesions and respiratory illness, adhering to proper time-temperature procedures for holding food, and encouraging employees to practice good personal hygiene.

Clostridium botulinum produces a deadly toxin that causes a rare illness known as botulism. The main source of the bacteria is soil and the organism may be found almost any place. In food, the toxin is usually found in underprocessed, nonacid, home-canned products. The toxin can be destroyed by boiling food for 15 minutes. The symptoms are nausea, vomiting, dizziness, and breathing difficulties that may result in death.

Preventive measures include avoiding the use of home-canned foods (or boiling them for 15 minutes), and avoiding the use of commercially canned foods that show signs of spoilage such as bulging, rusting, or leaking.

___ Food Protection Measures ___

Food protection measures are intended to prevent contamination through mishandling and to prevent the rapid and progressive growth of disease-causing organisms that are naturally present in food. The following measures are recommended for preparing food in a sanitary and safe manner.

1. Hot foods should be served hot and cold foods should be served cold. Avoid hazardous food temperatures. The temperature range of 45°F to 140°F is considered the *danger zone* for prepared foods because bacteria growth is rapid if food remains in the zone for 2 or more hours.

2. Prepare potentially hazardous food in small batches to avoid preparation time that requires raw food items to be unrefrigerated for over a 1-hour period.

3. Potentially hazardous foods requiring cooking should be cooked to heat all parts of the food to a temperature of at least 140°F, except:

   a. Poultry, poultry stuffing, stuffed meats, and stuffings containing meat shall be cooked to heat all parts of the food to at least 165°F with no interruption of the cooking process.
   b. Pork and any food containing pork must be cooked to heat all parts of the food to at least 150°F.
   c. Rare roast beef must be cooked to an internal temperature of at least 130°F, and rare beef steaks must be cooked to a temperature of 130°F unless otherwise ordered by the immediate consumer.

4. Potentially hazardous foods requiring refrigeration after preparation must be rapidly cooled to an internal temperature of 45°F or below. Foods prepared in large quantities or of large volume must be rapidly cooled, utilizing such methods as shallow pans, agitation, quick chilling, or water circulation external to the food container.

5. Heat all leftover foods to an internal temperature of 165°F. Holding equipment such as steam tables, thermotainers, and bainmaries are not designed for rapid heating of food.

6. Wash all fresh fruits and vegetables, dried fruits, raw poultry, fish, and variety meats prior to use.

7. Liquid, frozen, dry eggs and egg products are to be used only for cooking and baking purposes.

8. Reconstituted dry milk and dry milk products may be used in instant desserts, whipped products, or for cooking and baking. The product should not be served as a beverage.

9. Avoid the use of home-canned foods in quantity foodservice. Refuse all donations. Underprocessed home-canned food is a frequent source of the deadly toxin of *Clostridium botulinum*.

10. Poultry stuffing should be cooked in a separate pan rather than in the cavity of the bird. Large turkeys that are stuffed are unsafe due to possible lack of heat penetration in the center of cavity.

11. All fillings for sandwiches should be chilled, wrapped for display, and chilled until served. If sandwiches are used in vending machines, the product must show date of preparation.

12. Disposable gloves may be used for food items that must be touched by the hands (check local sanitation codes). Discard gloves after each use. Do not use for more than one task.

13. Defrost food requiring thawing under refrigeration, not to exceed 45°F, or by one of the following:

a. Under potable running water of a temperature of 70°F or below, with sufficient water velocity to agitate and float off loose food particles into the overflow.

b. In a microwave oven only when the food will be immediately transferred to conventional cooking facilities as part of a continuous cooking process or when the entire, uninterrupted cooking process takes place in the microwave oven.

c. As part of the conventional cooking process.

14. The following precautions should be used for wiping cloths.

a. Cloths used for wiping food spills on tableware, such as plates or bowls being served to a consumer, must be clean, dry, and used for no other purpose.

b. Moist cloths or sponges used for wiping food spills on kitchenware and food contact surfaces of equipment must be clean and rinsed frequently in a sanitizing solution and used for no other purpose. These cloths and sponges must be stored in the sanitizing solution between uses.

c. Moist cloths or sponges used for cleaning non–food contact surfaces of equipment such as counters, dining tabletops, and shelves shall be clean and rinsed as specified in (b) above. These cloths and sponges shall be stored in the sanitizing solution between uses.

15. Food containers of food cannot be stored under exposed or unprotected sewer or water lines, except for automatic fire protection piping and sprinkler heads that may be required by law.

16. Equipment, including ice makers and ice storage equipment, cannot be located under exposed or unprotected sewer lines or water lines, open stairwells, or other sources of contamination.

17. Ice for consumer use shall be dispensed by an employee with an approved utensil or through an automatic, self-serve ice-dispensing machine. *Do not use glass containers to scoop ice from ice machine.*

18. A metal stem-type numerically scaled indicating thermometer, accurate to ±2°F, must be used for determining internal temperatures of all potentially hazardous foods (see Fig. 12-6).

19. Where it is impractical to install thermometers on equipment such as bainmaries, steam tables, steam kettles, heat lamps, or insulated food transport carriers, a metal stem product thermometer must be available and used to check internal food temperatures.

20. Containers of food shall be stored a minimum of 6 in. above the floor, except that metal pressurized beverage containers and cased food packaged in cans, glass, or other waterproof containers need not be elevated when the food container is not exposed to floor moisture such as in dry food storage rooms. Containers may be stored on dollies, racks, or cleanable pallets provided that such equipment is easily movable. Food containers *cannot sit directly on the floor* of walk-in coolers.

21. Mollusk shells (snails, clams, etc.) may be used only once as a serving container.

22. Equipment that comes into direct contact with food (choppers, mixers, slicers, etc.) must be dismantled and cleaned after each use.

23. Storage area and equipment used to store clean dishes, silverware, glasses, pots, and pans should be clean in order to avoid recontamination.

24. Discard all chipped or cracked dishes and glasses; they are both unsafe and unsanitary. In addition to the possibility of cuts, the cracks serve as hiding places for bacteria.

25. Canned foods with abnormal odor and color should not be tasted or served. Bulging, rusting, or leaking cans should be discarded.

26. Chemical test strips or chemical test kits for determining concentration of sanitizers in chemical dishwashers and the sanitizing compartment of a three-compartment sink are required in foodservice establishments.

27. Poisonous or toxic materials consist of the following categories:

   a. Insecticides and rodenticides.
   b. Detergents, sanitizers, and related cleaning or drying agents.
   c. Caustics, acids, polishes, and other chemicals.

Each of the above three categories of poisonous or toxic materials must be stored separately from each other. These materials must be stored in cabinets or in a similar physically separate place used for no other purpose. To prevent contamination, poisonous or toxic materials cannot be stored above food, food equipment, utensils, or single-service articles. However, this regulation does not prohibit the convenient availability of detergents or sanitizers stored in identified containers at utensil or dishwashing stations.

28. Personal medications cannot be stored in food storage, service, or preparation areas.

29. Utility sinks should be available and used for cleaning mops and disposal of mop water. Mops used in the foodservice department should not be used in other areas of the facility.

30. In the event of a fire, flood, power outage, or similar event that might result in the contamination of food or that might prevent potentially hazardous food from being held at required temperatures, the local health department should be contacted immediately.

31. Carpeting is prohibited in food preparation, equipment washing, and utensil washing areas where it would be exposed to large amounts of grease or water. Carpeting is also prohibited in food storage areas and toilet rooms where urinals or toilet fixtures are located.

32. All lavatories must be provided with a mixing valve or combination faucet. Self-closing, slow-closing, or metering faucets must provide a flow of water for at least 15 seconds.

33. Adequate lighting is necessary for all areas where inspection for spoilage or cleanliness is required. At least 20 footcandles of light are required in utensil and equipment storage areas, and in lavatory and toilet areas.

34. Dull knives are more dangerous than sharp ones used in food preparation because more pressure is required for cutting. Keep knives sharpened.

35. To avoid cuts, burns, and other accidents, use the following precautions:

- *a.* Place warning tags on all equipment in need of repair.
- *b.* Wash all sharp tools and equipment separately. Never leave sharp instruments in dishwasher. Store sharp tools in proper racks; assemble all sharp equipment immediately after washing.
- *c.* Always cut downward and away from body, using a cutting board for dicing, slicing, and mincing.
- *d.* Before lighting a gas oven, check for leakage.
- *e.* Handle electric equipment with dry hands.
- *f.* Use mittens or dry pot and pan holders to handle hot utensils.
- *g.* Keep passageways and traffic aisles clear; avoid collisions.
- *h.* When lifting, keep back straight. Lift with legs.
- *i.* Use mobile carts to transport food and utensils.
- *j.* Keep floors clean and dry.

36. Train employees in food-handling techniques and the importance of good personal hygiene, such as:

- *a.* Wash hands with soap and warm water before beginning work; before hands touch any food; after using toilet; after touching hair, face, telephone, money; after blowing nose, touching soiled dishes, smoking, or handling garbage and trash; and throughout tour of duty, as necessary.
- *b.* Keep fingernails clean and trimmed. Do not use nail polish.
- *c.* Take a bath daily. Shampoo hair regularly. Use deodorant. Wear a clean, washable uniform.
- *d.* Wear hairnet or head cover to prevent hair from falling into food.
- *e.* Wear well-fitting, low-heel, enclosed shoes in good repair and properly cleaned.
- *f.* Store all personal belongings, including purse, in lockers provided for employees.
- *g.* Refrain from smoking in preparation, service, and food storage areas.
- *h.* Use combs and makeup only in the rest room.
- *i.* Treat all cuts and burns immediately to prevent infection.
- *j.* Do not taste food with the ladle or spoon used in food preparation or service. Utensils used for tasting should be washed between tastes.
- *k.* Keep hands away from face and hair while handling food.
- *l.* Avoid washing hands in sinks where dishes are washed or where food is prepared.
- *m.* Do not lick fingers to pick up menus, diet cards, or napkins.
- *n.* Do not chew gum in preparation and service areas.
- *o.* Do not eat or drink in the food preparation and service areas.
- *p.* Refrain from sitting or leaning on work surfaces.
- *q.* Keep work areas, surfaces, and utensils clean and orderly.

37. Laundry facilities in a foodservice establishment are restricted to the washing and drying of linens, cloths, uniforms, and aprons used in the operation. If such items are laundered on the premises, a gas or electric dryer shall be

used. Separate rooms are required for laundry facilities, except that such operations may be conducted in storage rooms containing only packaged food or packaged single-service articles.

38. Shielding to protect against broken glass falling into food shall be provided for all light fixtures located over, by, or within food storage, preparation, service areas, and display units. Facilities where utensils and equipment are cleaned and stored shall also be protected.

39. Infrared or other heat lamps shall be protected against breakage by a shield surrounding and extending beyond the bulb exposed.

The establishment of an in-service training program, incorporating the above recommendations, is an effective way of keeping employees informed. The program should be ongoing, with topics repeated as often as necessary.

Computer Assistance in Food Production

Food production has many important facets that can be made easier, more accurate, and less time-consuming by use of a computer. Delegating, timing, assigning tasks, and supervising food preparation are all part of the process of preparing food for patients and personnel. These processes can be simplified and made more orderly by standardizing individual tasks using a computer. Better working conditions can be realized when employees know what they are to do, when they are to do it, and how much time is allotted for the task.

A computer program can be designed to print a procedure standardization each day for each worker. The program would need an input of recipes with time analysis included to be used for the day (Maloff & Zears 1979). Mealtimes would be entered, and forecasted servings extended, when appropriate. In turn, the computer would print a list of timed instructions describing each task and the time it takes to perform it. The report would include the menu for the meal, number of servings, and complete instructions for preparing each meal. The manager's input in the system would consist of a recipe code, number of servings, and time the meal is to be served. In turn, the program would locate the recipes and instructions. Having received the number of servings needed, the program would determine the exact amounts needed of each ingredient and preparation time. Working backward from serving time, the program computes the time schedule for preparation of the recipe.

Computing a time schedule for recipe preparation is more difficult than the other processes in this program. Although extending ingredients to meet a certain number of servings is an uncomplicated maneuver, it does not always take the same amount of time to prepare for larger numbers. For example, making beef stew for 400 may take very little more time than preparing the same item for 200. The system must be programmed to readjust times to amounts needed. Some tasks vary directly with amount and some do not vary at all. Special mathematical formulas need to be designed to account for increase or decrease in servings, as related to time to prepare a food item.

Since standardization and materials control are required components for a computer-assisted system in food production, an ingredient room should be introduced if one does not already exist. With an ingredient room, ingredient lists can be compiled by the computer into a storeroom requisition one day prior to production. Ingredient amounts are subtracted from the inventory and the list is automatically issued to the ingredient room. The ingredient room employee weighs and assembles the ingredients according to the updated census and as specified for each recipe. This system of ingredient control is cost-efficient in that the computer combines the amounts of each ingredient needed from all recipes and presents the total amount required and the total cost of each ingredient. The difference is returned to the storeroom rather than left in the preparation area to be added to a recipe or wasted. A food cost savings can be realized, and a better product is produced.

Computer assistance can work well only in a well-organized facility. Standardized recipes and effective purchasing and storeroom controls are necessary to provide accurate data. According to Andrews and Tuthill (1968), increased efficiency of managerial resources suggests a need to change from the present method of intuitive decision making to a more objective, scientific method of management.

Energy Conservation in Food Production

More energy is consumed in the production of food than for any other activity in the foodservice system. To comply with energy conservation measures, the foodservice director needs the understanding and cooperation of all employees in the area. To reduce the amount of energy used, the following recommendations are offered:

1. Refrain from turning on all equipment and lights at the beginning of the work shift. Enforce this practice. Most morning cooks will turn on all stoves, ovens, and other equipment requiring preheat time whether the equipment is to be used or not. Also, all cafeteria lights often are turned on even though the service in the cafeteria may not begin for another hour. Do not tolerate these practices.

2. Label all equipment with preheat time instructions. Preheat times vary, depending on the particular piece of equipment. For example, less time is required to preheat convection ovens than deck ovens. Setting the thermostat higher will not reduce preheat time; it will only waste energy.

3. Observe that low temperatures for roasting meats results in reduced energy, higher yield, and a more tender and juicy product.

4. Programmed use and care procedures reduce fuel cost. Load ovens to full capacity and take advantage of receding heat. Use correct size cooking utensils as much as possible. Unused space that must be heated is a waste of fuel.

5. Maintain equipment in good working order. Post cleaning instructions on all major equipment. Tag all equipment in need of repair.

6. Clean equipment regularly. Establish a cleaning schedule, indicating when the equipment is to be cleaned and who is responsible for the task.

7. Avoid overloading fryers. Overloaded baskets increase cooking time, waste energy, and produce a less desirable product. Never use temperatures higher than 357°F.

8. Conduct an ongoing employee training program on the following:

   a. How to use all major equipment.
   b. How to clean all major equipment.
   c. How to maintain equipment.
   d. How to conserve energy. (See Chapter 15 for information on establishing an energy management program).

References

Andrews, J. T., and Tuthill, B. H. (1968). Computer-Based Management of Dietary Departments. *Hospitals 42*(14), 117–123.

Anon. (1977). Reed's Semi-Automatic Food Service: Moving Beyond the Kitchen. *Stripe 33*(38), 16–17. (Special service edition of newspaper published for patients and staff at Walter Reed Medical Center.)

Bjorkman, A., and Delphin, K. A. (1966). Sweden's Nacka Hospital Food System Centralizes Preparation and Distribution. *Cornell H.R.A. Quart. 7*(3), 84–87.

Bobeng, B. J., and David, B. D. (1978). HACCP Models for Quality Control of Entree Production in Hospital Foodservice Systems. *J. Am. Diet. Assoc. 73*, Nov., 524–529.

Federal Register. (1978). *Alternative Processing Procedures for Preparing Cooked Beef. 43*(85), Sept. 2, 18681–18682.

Joint Commission on Accreditation of Hospitals. (1988). *Accreditation Manual for Hospitals.* Chicago: JCAH.

Kaud, F. A. (1972). Implementing the Chilled Food Concept. *Hospitals 46*(15), 97–100.

Livingston, G. E., and Chang, C. M. (1979). Food Service Operation Design for Nutrient Retention in Foods. *Food Tech. 33*(3), 32–37, 42.

MacLennan, H. A. (1968). Ready Foods. *Cornell H.R.A. Quart. 8*(4), 56–58.

Maloff, C., and Zears, R. W. (1979). *Computers in Nutrition.* Dedham, MA: Artech Publishing.

McGuckian, A. T. (1969). The A.G.S. Food System: Chilled Pasteurized Foods. *Cornell H.R.A. Quart. 10*(1), 87–92.

McIver, C. (1970). Batch Cooking. *Hospitals 44*(20), 84–85.

National Sanitation Foundation. (1980). *Instructional Guide: Temperature Control in Food Service.* Ann Arbor, MI: NSF.

National Live Stock and Meat Board. (1977). *Meat in the Foodservice Industry.* Chicago: NLSMB.

Rinke, W. J. (1976). Three Major Systems Reviewed and Evaluated. *Hospitals 50*(4), 73–78.

Simler, S. (1978). Walter Reed Gears Up Fancy Kitchen. *Mod. Healthcare 8*(10), 32–33.

U.S. Department of Health and Human Services. (1976). *Food Service Sanitation Manual.* Washington, DC: USDHHS, Public Health Service, Food and Drug Administration.

Chapter 13

Subsystem for Distribution and Service

Service of food is the stage in the foodservice system where the output (prepared food product) is evaluated by the consumer. As discussed in Chapter 1, if the outcome is unacceptable, mechanisms must be available for corrective actions. In most facilities both the patients and personnel are serviced simultaneously, a situation that accounts for the peak periods of operation experienced in medical foodservice and the complexities involved in service.

Patient Foodservice

Food served to patients is based on the menu selections by individual patients or as prescribed by the physician, under the supervision of a Registered Dietitian. Standard operation procedures should be in effect for determining the type and amount of food served to patients. The procedure used for diet ordering and menu selection vary, depending on the type of facility.

Diet Ordering

Methods of diet ordering will vary, but most procedures will consist of the following:

1. Obtain the physician's diet order (usually given on diet request sheet prepared by nursing personnel).
2. Interview all patients prior to diet preparation to ascertain preferences.
3. Record necessary information on patient's chart and on master diet card maintained in the foodservice department.
4. Plan menu according to established patterns, taking into consideration patient preferences.
5. Translate diet order for meal service (special preparation notes, etc.)
6. Serve meals to patients as needed.

There should be certain policies established within the department regarding diet orders, such as:

1. Effective time for order.
2. Changes in diet order.
3. Request for special foods.
4. New admissions.
5. Delayed trays.

		Type of Diet If diabetic, include insulin order. If restricted, indicate level.
Room No.	Patient's Name	

Ward _____   Date _____

Figure 13-1. Sample patient census sheet.

6. Orders for diets not listed in the manual.
7. Patient diet instructions for use after the patient leaves the hospital.

In nursing homes, where the length of stay is for an extended period of time, the patient census sheet is changed less frequently than in acute care facilities. A new census sheet may be written once a week, with written instructions for additions or deletions as patients are admitted or discharged during the week. In hospitals, a new census sheet (Fig. 13-1) is prepared by nursing personnel on a daily basis, and is available to foodservice personnel prior to service of the breakfast meal. When tray setup is accomplished the day before service, the new census sheet is used to make any necessary changes. Prior to each meal, a diet change sheet (Fig. 13-2) is prepared by nursing personnel and forwarded to the foodservice department. The practice of making diet changes by telephone should be discouraged since there is no authorized documentation of changes made. In addition, the possibility of error is increased when diet orders are issued verbally. The foodservice department should have a copy of diet changes at least ½ hour prior to tray assembly. Timely communication is important for promoting patient satisfaction.

Menu Selection

Patients on regular and modified diets have an opportunity to choose their own food when selective menus are used. The selective menu may be of the restaurant type, as shown in Figure 13–3, with a separate sheet used for making selections. All patients are encouraged to select foods that will provide a nutri-

Room and Bed	Patient's Name	N.P.O.	Delay Next Meal Only	Omit Next Meal Only	Special Meal (Test)	Change in Diet	Isolation— Protection	Admission	Discharge	Transfer to:	Ward _____ Date _____ Time _____
											Type of Diet If diabetic, include insulin order. If restricted, indicate level.

Signature of Charge Nurse Must Appear Below:

6:00 A.M. _____   10:00 A.M. _____

2:00 P.M. _____   5:00 A.M. _____

Figure 13-2. Sample diet change sheet.

tionally balanced diet. The patient on a regular diet has a choice of 153 food items from which to make a selection for the day. The choices made by the patient are monitored by the dietitian for nutritional adequacy. The reverse side of the menu (Fig. 13-4) provides a guide to good eating and instructions on how to complete the menu selection sheet. In some operations, a different menu is used each day. A selective menu, as shown in Figure 13-5, is used only once. After the tray is served, the selection sheet is discarded. The menus in this system are planned on a 10-day rotation, and are numbered 1 through 10. In addition to the selective menus, there are two menus used exclusively for Sundays. The reverse side of the menu provides general introduction remarks about the department, dietetic services, and information on the Basic Four food groups (Fig. 13-6).

To the extent possible, the selective menu for patients on modified diets provides the same foods as those served on the regular diet. Patients are visited by the Registered Dietitian and instructed on principles of the prescribed diet prior to menu selection. Sample menus for two modified diets are given in Figures 13-7 and 13-8. Follow-up diet instructions are given throughout the patient's stay in the hospital. The selective menus are distributed, collected, and tabulated by dietary aides or volunteer workers. The dietary aide or volunteer may also assist patients who need help in completing the selective menu.

When nonselective menus are used, the decision on food choices is made by foodservice personnel. The amount of input from patients varies from one facility to another. One method of promoting patient satisfaction is to conduct a

BREAKFAST MENU

FRUITS AND JUICES

1. Sunsweetened Pineapple Juice
2. Tangy Grapefruit Juice
3. Sunshine Orange Juice
4. Mellow Apple Juice
5. Special Blended Juice
6. Fresh Banana
7. Choice Pineapple Chunks
8. Tropical Fruit Sections
9. Tree Ripened Applesauce
10. Sun Ripened Stewed Prunes

HOT CEREALS

25. Oatmeal
26. Malt-O-Meal
27. Cream of Wheat

COLD CEREALS

28. Crispy Cornflakes
29. Snappy Rice Krispies
30. Puffed Wheat
31. Puffed Rice
32. Krunchy Special K
33. Cheerios
34. 40% Bran Flakes

HOT BREAKFAST ENTREES

36. Softly Scrambled Eggs (2)
38. Golden Cheese Omelet/with Ham Slice
40. Sausage Patty
41. Country Style Pancakes with Butter/Syrup and Pork Sausage Links
42. Egg Rich French Toast Lightly Browned served with Butter/Syrup and a Baked Spiced Peach Half
44. Tender Pork Sausage Links (2)

LUNCHEON AND DINNER FINE FOODS MENU

APPETIZERS

2. Chilled Grapefruit Juice
4. Chilled Apple Juice
11. Chilled Prune Juice
13. Chilled Garden Vegetable Juice V-8
16. Beef Consomme
17. Golden Chicken Consomme
18. Fancy Cream of Mushroom Soup
20. Home Style Vegetable Soup
21. Hearty Split Pea Soup
22. Vegetarian Bouillon

SALADS

120. Crisp Lettuce Salad
121. Three Bean Salad
122. Carrot and Raisin Salad
123. Coleslaw
124. Assorted Relish Plate
125. Cottage Cheese Salad
126. Potato Salad
127. Tossed Vegetable Salad
128. Jello Fruit Mold

SALAD DRESSINGS

129. French Dressing
130. Italian Dressing
131. Thousand Island Dressing
132. Blue Cheese Dressing

FAMOUS COLD MAIN DISH ENTREES

45. MAURICE SALAD BOWL
Tender Strips of Turkey, Ham and Swiss Cheese served with Club Crackers. Please order dressing and specify if you would like a small serving.

46. THE AMBASSADOR SALAD PLATE
Tasty Chicken Salad on Lettuce with Tender Sliced Tomatoes. Served with Crackers.

47. MEDICAL CENTER COLD PLATE
Thin Slices of Choice Meats and Cheese with Tender Sliced Tomatoes. Served with Crackers.

48. THE STATE FAIR
Weight Watcher's Special. Crisp Iceberg Lettuce filled with Fresh Fruit in Season and Cottage Cheese. Served with Nut Bread.

FAMOUS COLD SANDWICH ENTREES

49. SPIRIT OF DETROIT
Special Club Sandwich. A Triple Decker ... Tender Sliced Ham and Turkey, Tomato and Cheese, with Lettuce on White and Whole Wheat Bread.

50. THE RIVERFRONT SPECIAL
The Delicacy of Tuna with Mayonnaise and Crisp Lettuce on Whole Wheat Bread, served with Dill Pickle and Corn Chips.

51. THE RENAISSANCE
Combination of Ham and Swiss Cheese served on Rye Bread with Crisp Potato Chips.

52. THE MOTOWN
Mounds of Tender Shaved Roast Beef served on Freshly Baked Kaiser Roll with Potato Chips and Dill Pickle Slices.

ALL AMERICAN HOT SANDWICH ENTREES

54. GRILLED HAMBURGER PLATE
Choice Ground Beef on Bun, served with a thick Slice of Onion, Tender Tomato Slice and Crisp Lettuce. Served with Potato Chips.

55. TOASTED REUBEN SANDWICH
Shaved Corned Beef, Swiss Cheese and Sauerkraut on Rye Bread. Served with Fresh Potato Chips and Pickle.

56. BALL PARK SPECIAL
Juicy Steamy Hot Dog on Bun with Chopped Onions and Relish. Served with American Potato Sticks.

57. TOASTED CHEESE SANDWICH
Tasty American Cheese on Toasted White Bread with Dill Pickle Slices. Served with Corn Chips.

HOT MAIN DISH ENTREES

63. TENDER BAKED PORK CHOPS
Served with Mashed Potatoes and Gravy.

64. CHOICE ROAST BEEF
Served with Mashed Potatoes and Gravy.

65. CHOPPED SIRLOIN
Quickly broiled to seal in flavor. Served with Mashed Potatoes and Gravy.

67. TURKEY A LA KING
Served on Holland Rusk.

70. IRISH BEEF STEW
Tender pieces of Beef slowly simmered with Fresh Garden Vegetables. **Served with a Buttermilk Buscuit**

HOT MAIN DISH ENTREES

68. TOMATO BEEF NOODLE CASSEROLE
Combination of delicately stewed Tomatoes, Choice Ground Beef and Tender Macaroni Noodles, gently seasoned.

69. ITALIAN SPAGHETTI WITH MEAT SAUCE
A deliciously authentic sauce made from Choice Ground Beef, Tomatoes and Select Seasonings. Served with Parmesan Cheese.

71. BAKED MACARONI AND CHEESE CASSEROLE
This favorite is topped with Aged Cheddar Cheese and baked to perfection.

72. ROAST TURKEY
Stuffed with Sage Dressing, served with Baked Sweet Potatoes and Creamy Gravy, garnished with Cranberry Sauce.

73. MARYLAND BAKED CHICKEN
House Specialty served with Gravy and Herbed Rice

74. BAKED HAM
Glazed with Orange Sauce and served with Sweet Potatoes.

75. SUCCULENT BRAISED BEEF SHORT RIBS
In Gravy served with Buttered Rice.

76. FILET OF HADDOCK
Baked in Lemon Butter Sauce and served with Au Gratin Potatoes.

77. BAKED FRENCH MEATLOAF
Served with Mild Tomato Sauce and Au Gratin Potatoes.

VEGETABLE SELECTIONS

106. Green Beans with Buttersauce
107. Parslied Carrot Coins
108. Chopped Collard Greens
109. Broccoli Spears
110. Mixed Vegetable Medley
111. Whole Kernel Corn
112. Mashed Winter Squash
113. New Green Peas
114. Cauliflower
115. Harvard Beets
116. Leaf Spinach
117. Stewed Tomatoes

DESSERTS

135. Sugar Cookie
136. Baked Custard
137. Vanilla Ice Cream Cup
138. Sherbet
139. Rice Pudding
140. Butterscotch Pudding
141. Cherry Crisp
142. Chocolate Brownies
143. Jello Cubes
144. Banana Cake
145. Lemon Tart
146. Yellow Cake, Chocolate Frosting
147. Apple Pie
148. Cling Peaches
149. Bartlett Pears
150. Fresh Fruit
153. Apple Crisp

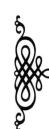

Figure 13-3. Restaurant-type selective menu for regular diet. *From Detroit Receiving Hospital*

MENU

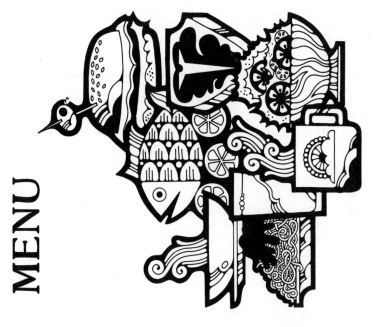

Detroit Receiving Hospital
A Member Institution
of the Detroit Medical Center

A Guide to Good Eating has been included to assist you in selecting menu items for a nutritious healthful diet.

Milk Group

2 Servings/Adults
4 Servings/Teenagers
3 Servings/Children

Calcium
Riboflavin (B₂)
Protein

Foods made from milk contribute part of the nutrients supplied by a serving of milk.

Meat Group

2 Servings

Protein
Niacin
Iron
Thiamine (B₂)

Dry beans and peas, soy extenders, and nuts combined with animal protein (meat, fish, poultry, eggs, milk, cheese) or grain protein can be substituted for a serving of meat.

Fruit-Vegetable Group

4 Servings

Vitamins A and C

Dark green, leafy or orange vegetables and fruit are recommended 3 or 4 times weekly for vitamin A. Citrus fruit is recommended daily for vitamin C.

Grain Group

4 Servings

Carbohydrate
Thiamine (B₂)
Iron
Niacin

Whole grain, fortified or enriched grain products are recommended.

YOUR MENU

Detroit Receiving Hospital is happy to offer you a Personal Menu designed to provide a broad selection of delicious, nourishing foods for breakfast, lunch and dinner. We have provided this menu for you which follows the Diet prescribed by your Doctor. Your menu selections are prepared in our modern kitchen by a Professional Dietary Staff.

HOW TO ORDER

When you arrive at Detroit Receiving Hospital, and each day during your stay, you will receive a Menu Selection Sheet. Let's assume you want to order a breakfast consisting of:

Orange Juice (No. 3)   White Toast
Oatmeal (No. 25)   Coffee, Cream, Sugar
Scrambled Egg (No. 36)   Milk, Jelly

Your menu should look like this:

NAME SMITH
ROOM 4N-5
CIRCLE DAY: Sun Mon Tues Wed Thurs Fri Sat

REGULAR DIET

[3] FRUIT OR JUICE
[25] CEREAL
[36] ENTREE

Check ☑ Selections Below

☑ Buttered White Toast
☐ Buttered Wheat Toast
☐ Buttered Rye Toast
☐ Danish Pastry (97)   ☐ Doughnut (96)
☐ Coffee   ☐ Hot Chocolate   ☐ Decaffeinated Coffee
☐ Tea
☑ Milk   ☑ Butter   ☑ Cream
☐ Skim Milk
☐ Margarine   ☐ Lemon Wedge
☑ Jelly
☑ Sugar   ☐ Artificial Sweetener

BREAKFAST

NAME SMITH
ROOM 4N-5
CIRCLE DAY: Sun Mon Tues Wed Thurs Fri Sat

REGULAR DIET

☐ APPETIZER
☐ ENTREE
☐ STARCH OR SUBSTITUTE
☐ VEGETABLE
☐ SALAD
☑ SALAD DRESSING
☐ DESSERT

Check ☑ Selections Below

☐ White Bread   ☐ Butter
☐ Wheat Bread   ☐ Margarine
☐ Rye Bread   ☐ Jelly
☐ Dinner Roll   ☐ Crackers
☐ Coffee   ☐ Decaffeinated Coffee
☐ Tea   ☐ Buttermilk
☐ Milk   ☐ Chocolate Milk
☐ Skim Milk   ☐ Lemon Wedge
☐ Cream
☐ Sour Cream   ☐ Mustard
☐ Mayonnaise   ☐ Vinegar
☐ Catsup   ☐ Artificial Sweetener
☐ Sugar

LUNCHEON

NAME SMITH
ROOM 4N-5
CIRCLE DAY: Sun Mon Tues Wed Thurs Fri Sat

REGULAR DIET

☐ APPETIZER
☐ ENTREE
☐ STARCH OR SUBSTITUTE
☐ VEGETABLE
☐ SALAD
☐ SALAD DRESSING
☐ DESSERT

Check ☑ Selections Below

☐ White Bread   ☐ Butter
☐ Wheat Bread   ☐ Margarine
☐ Rye Bread   ☐ Jelly
☐ Dinner Roll   ☐ Crackers
☐ Coffee   ☐ Decaffenated Coffee
☐ Tea   ☐ Iced Tea (95)
☐ Milk   ☐ Buttermilk
☐ Skim Milk   ☐ Chocolate Milk
☐ Cream   ☐ Lemon Wedge
☐ Sour Cream   ☐ Mustard
☐ Mayonnaise   ☐ Vinegar
☐ Catsup   ☐ Artificial Sweetener
☐ Sugar

DINNER

A representative from the Dietary Department will visit you to answer your questions. Please complete your menu selections as soon as possible as menus not turned in by 11:30 a.m. cannot be honored for the following day.

Figure 13-4. Tri-fold menu cover for restaurant type regular diet. *From Detroit Receiving Hospital*

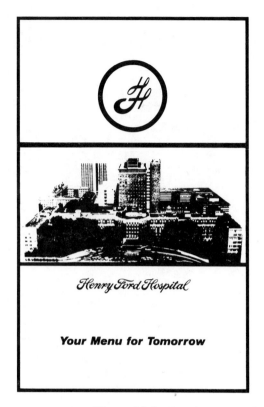

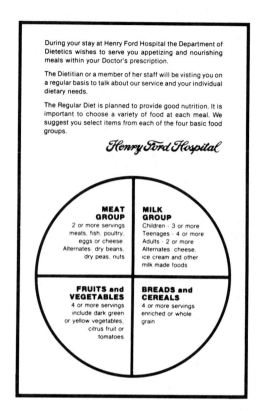

Figure 13-5. Rotation-type selective menu for regular diet. *From Henry Ford Hospital, Detroit*

survey of patient's food preferences. A food preference survey (Fig. 13-9) may be used with both the selective and nonselective menu system, but it is especially helpful when patients have no choice in the type of food served. It is not enough to determine the likes and dislikes; there must be follow-through. For example, if a patient indicates a dislike for liver, there should be a mechanism established to ensure that the patient is not served that particular food item. The information should be recorded for use by dietary personnel responsible for tray assembly and also communicated to food preparation personnel so that an alternate food item is prepared and ready for service. The dietitian will lose credibility if the patient's food preferences are ignored. A cardex-type card, as shown in Figure 13-10, can be used to record likes and dislikes and other patient-related information and data.

── Tray Assembly ──

Tray assembly may be a continuous process, depending on the type of food production used. In facilities where food is prepared in advance (cook-freeze or cook-chill), there is no delay in tray assembly. As soon as one meal is assembled and served, the process begins for the next meal. Tray assembly may also depend on whether the tray service is centralized or decentralized. In a *centralized tray service,* all trays are assembled in one location near the production area. With the aid of a patient menu selection sheet or a patient meal pattern card, individual trays are assembled, checked for accuracy, and loaded on food carts or other equipment used for distribution. In most operations, food serving tables for hot and cold foods, and other equipment, such as toasters and coffee urns, are conveniently arranged alongside a conveyor belt. Food items are dished, if not preplated, and placed on the trays, which are carried down the line

Your Menu for Tomorrow

NAME _____ ROOM NO _____

DIET ORDER _____

PLEASE **CIRCLE** SELECTIONS

FRUITS AND JUICES
Orange Juice
Grapefruit Juice
Pineapple Juice
Prune Juice

BREAKFAST ENTREES
Scrambled Egg
Sausage Links
Pancakes with Syrup

CEREALS
Grits
Oatmeal
Cornflakes
Special K
Branflakes
Shredded Wheat
Puffed Rice
Frosted Flakes
Cheerios

BEVERAGES
Coffee
Decaffeinated Coffee
Hot Tea
Lemon Wedge
Hot Cocoa
Non-dairy Creamer
Whole Milk
Low Fat Milk
Skim Milk
Buttermilk
Chocolate Milk

BREADS
Wheat Toast
White Toast
Coffee Cake
Margarine
Jelly
Honey

SEASONINGS
Sugar   Herb Seasoning   Salt   Pepper   Artificial Sweetener

BREAKFAST   REGULAR

1

63-36-1 (11-82)

Your Menu for Tomorrow

NAME _____ ROOM NO _____

DIET ORDER _____

PLEASE **CIRCLE** SELECTIONS

SOUP
Manhattan Clam Chowder
Chicken Bouillon

ENTREES (Select One)
Barbequed Ribs
Baked Chicken
Fried Chicken
Cheese Omelet
Maurice Salad

VEGETABLES
Whipped Potato
Gravy
Spinach
Yellow Squash

SALAD AND JUICE
Tossed Salad
Cottage Cheese
Potato Salad
Blended Juice

DESSERTS (Select One)
Orange Cake
Chocolate Pudding
Pear Halves
Ice Cream
Sherbet
Gelatin Cubes
  with Whipped Topping
Fresh Fruit in Season

BEVERAGES
Coffee
Decaffeinated Coffee
Hot Tea
Lemon Wedge
Hot Cocoa
Non-dairy Creamer
Whole Milk
Low Fat Milk
Skim Milk
Buttermilk
Chocolate Milk

BREADS
Cornbread
Wheat Bread
White Bread
Dinner Roll
Melba Toast
Saltines
Margarine
Jelly
Honey

ACCOMPANIMENT
French Dressing
Italian Dressing
1000 Island Dressing
Bleu Cheese Dressing
Mayonnaise
Catsup
Mustard
Relish

SEASONINGS
Sugar   Herb Seasoning   Salt   Pepper   Artificial Sweetener

LUNCHEON   REGULAR

1

Your Menu for Tomorrow

NAME _____ ROOM NO _____

DIET ORDER _____

PLEASE **CIRCLE** SELECTIONS

SOUP
Vegetable Soup
Beef Bouillon

ENTREES (Select One)
Baked Fish
  with Lemon Wedge/Tartar Sauce
Pepper Steak on Rice
Hamburger on Bun
Cottage Cheese Fruit Plate

VEGETABLES
White Rice
Whipped potato
Gravy
Wax Beans
Baby Whole Carrots

SALAD AND JUICE
Tossed Salad
Cottage Cheese
Marinated Vegetable Medley
Tomato Juice
Lettuce/Tomato/Onion

DESSERTS (Select One)
Blueberry Pie
Vanilla Pudding
Chilled Apricots
Ice Cream
Sherbet
Gelatin Cubes
  with Whipped Topping
Fresh Fruit in Season

BEVERAGES
Coffee
Decaffeinated Coffee
Hot Tea
Lemon Wedge
Hot Cocoa
Non-dairy Creamer
Whole Milk
Low Fat Milk
Skim Milk
Buttermilk
Chocolate Milk

BREADS
Wheat Bread
White Bread
Dinner Roll
Melba Toast
Saltines
Margarine
Jelly
Honey

ACCOMPANIMENT
French Dressing
Italian Dressing
1000 Island Dressing
Bleu Cheese Dressing
Mayonnaise
Catsup
Mustard
Relish

SEASONINGS
Sugar   Herb Seasoning   Salt   Pepper   Artificial Sweetener

DINNER   REGULAR

1

Figure 13-6. Tri-fold menu cover for rotation type selective menu. *From Henry Ford Hospital, Detroit*

BREAKFAST MENU

FRUITS AND JUICES

(1 Fruit Exchange)

1. Sunsweetened Pineapple Juice ..... ⅓ c.
2. Tangy Grapefruit Juice .... ½ c.
3. Sunshine Orange Juice .... ½ c.
4. Mellow Apple Juice .... ⅓ c.
6. Fresh Banana .... ½ small
7. Choice Pineapple Chunks ....½ c.
8. Tropical Fruit Sections .... ½ c.
9. Tree Ripened Applesauce .... ½ c.
10. Sun Ripened Prunes 2
15. Select Apricot Halves 4

HOT CEREALS / COLD CEREALS

(1 Bread exchange)

25. Oatmeal .... ½ c.
26. Malt-O-Meal .... ½ c.
27. Cream of Wheat .... ½ c.
28. Crispy Cornflakes .... ¾ c.
29. Snappy Rice Krispies .... ¾ c.
32. Krunchy Special K .... ¾ c.
31. Puffed Rice .... 1 c.
30. Puffed Wheat .... 1 c.
33. Cheerios .... ¾ c.
34. 40% Bran Flakes .... ½ c.

HOT BREAKFAST ENTREES

24. Egg Beaters

LUNCHEON AND DINNER FINE FOODS MENU

APPETIZERS

2. Chilled Grapefruit Juice............... 1 fruit exchange; ½ c.
3. Chilled Orange Juice.................. 1 fruit exchange; ½ c.
4. Chilled Apple Juice..................... 1 fruit exchange; ⅓ c.
11. Chilled Prune Juice.................... 1 fruit exchange; ¼ c.
13. Chilled Tomato Juice............ 1 vegetable exchange; ½ c.
16. Beef Consomme......................... free exchange; ½ c.
17. Golden Chicken Consomme............. free exchange; ½ c.
22. Vegetarian Bouillon..................... free exchange; ½ c.

SALADS

120. Crisp Lettuce Salad .... free exchange; ½ c.
123. Coleslaw Salad .... 1 vegetable exchange; ½ c.
124. Assorted Relish Salad .... 1 vegetable exchange; ½ c.
127. Tossed Vegetable Salad .... 1 vegetable exchange; 1 c.
128. Molded Fruit Salad ....1 fruit exchange; ½ c.

SALAD DRESSING

129. Lo-Cal French Dressing ....1 fat exchange; 2 Tbsp.
130. Lo-Cal Italian Dressing .... free exchange; 1 Tbsp.
133. Lo-Cal Green Goddess Dressing ..... 1 fat exchange; 2 Tbsp.

FAMOUS COLD MAIN DISH ENTREES

46. CHICKEN SALAD PLATE - Tasty Sliced Chicken Lettuce with Tender Sliced Tomatoes .... 2 oz. meat, 1 vegetable exchange; .... 2 oz. chicken, ½ c. tomato

47. COLD SALAD AND MEAT PLATE - Thin Slices of Choice Meats with Fresh Vegetables.....................2 meat, 1 vegetable exchange; .... 2 oz. meat, ½ c. vegetable

48. FRUIT SALAD PLATE - Crisp Iceberg Lettuce filled with Fruit and Cottage Cheese .... 2 meat, 1 fruit exchange; .... ½ c. cottage cheese, ½ c. fruit

FAMOUS COLD SANDWICH ENTREES

50. TUNA SALAD SANDWICH - Fresh Tuna Salad served on Whole Wheat Bread................................ 2 meat, 2 bread, 1 fat exchange

52. ROAST BEEF SANDWICH - Tender Shaved Roast Beef served on Whole Wheat Bread ....2 meat, 2 bread exchanges; .... 2 oz. meat

58. SLICED TURKEY SANDWICH - Tender Turkey and Crisp Lettuce on White Bread .... 2 meat, 2 bread exchanges; 2 oz. meat

ALL AMERICAN HOT SANDWICH ENTREES

54. GRILLED HAMBURGER - Choice Ground Beef on Bun served with Tender Tomato Slice and Crisp Lettuce..... ....3 meat, 2 bread .... 3 oz. meat

HOT MAIN DISH ENTREES

64. CHOICE ROAST BEEF ....3 meat exchanges; 3 oz. meat

65. BROILED CHOPPED SIRLOIN ....3 meat exchanges; 3 oz. meat

69. ITALIAN SPAGHETTI WITH MEAT SAUCE..................2 meat, 1 bread exchange

72. ROAST TURKEY ....3 meat exchanges; 3 oz. meat

73. GOLDEN BAKED CHICKEN ....3 meat exchanges; 3 oz. meat

76. BAKED FILET OF HADDOCK ....3 meat exchange; 3 oz. fish

77. BAKED FRENCH MEATLOAF ....3 meat exchanges; 3 oz. meat

STARCH OR STARCH SUBSTITUTE

(1 Bread Exchange)

100. Mashed Potatoes............... ½ c.
101. Fluffy Rice...................... ½ c.
102. Noodles......................... ½ c.
104. Bread Dressing.. 1 fat exchange; ⅓ c.
105. Baked Sweet Potatoes.......... ¼ c.
111. Whole Kernel Corn.............. ⅓ c.
112. Mashed Winter Squash.......... ½ c.
113. New Green Peas................ ½ c.

VEGETABLE SELECTION

(1 Vegetable Exchange)

106. Green Beans.................... ½ c.
107. Parslied Carrot Coins........... ½ c.
109. Broccoli Spears................. ½ c.
110. Mixed Vegetable Medley......... ⅓ c.
114. Cauliflower..................... ½ c.
115. Beets........................... ½ c.
116. Leaf Spinach................... ½ c.
117. Stewed Tomatoes............... ½ c.

DESSERTS

9. Unsweetened Applesauce .... 1 fruit exchange; ½ c.
143. Cubed Jello Jewels .... D'Zerta ....free exchange; ½ c.
148. Unsweetened Peach Halves ....1 fruit exchange; ½ c.
149. Unsweetened Pear Halves ....1 fruit exchange; ½ c.
150. Fresh Fruit in Season ....1 fruit exchange
151. Unsweetened Fruit Cocktail ....1 fruit exchange; ½ c.
152. Unsweetened Bing Cherries ....1 fruit exchange; ½ c.

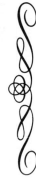

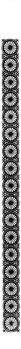

Figure 13-7. Restaurant-type selective menu for calorie-controlled, cholesterol-restricted diet. *From Detroit Receiving Hospital*

BREAKFAST Menu

Your Menu for Tomorrow

NAME _____ ROOM NO _____
DIET ORDER _____

PLEASE **CIRCLE** SELECTIONS

FRUIT
Applesauce
  K65 P5

BREAKFAST ENTREES
Scrambled Egg
  K70 P98
*Low Cholesterol Scrambled Egg
  K123 P43
Pancakes/Syrup
  K42 P70

CEREALS
++Grits
  K11 P10
++Oatmeal
  K65 P84
Cornflakes
  K40 P16
Puffed Rice
  K50 P13
Frosted Flakes
  K40 P16

BEVERAGES
Coffee
Decaffeinated Coffee
Hot Tea
Lemon Wedge
Non-dairy Creamer
  K39 P26
Whole Milk (50cc)
  K71 P46

BREADS
Wheat Toast
  K63 P52
White Toast
  K25 P22
Plain Muffin
  K42 P50
Coffee Cake
  K39 P58
++Margarine
Jelly
Honey

SEASONINGS
Sugar Pepper Herb Seasoning

*Special fat controlled product
++Special sodium controlled product

1   **BREAKFAST**   REGULAR

63-36-1 (11-82)

LUNCHEON Menu

Your Menu for Tomorrow

NAME _____ ROOM NO _____
DIET ORDER _____

PLEASE **CIRCLE** SELECTIONS

ENTREES (Select One)
Baked Chicken
  K121 P46
*Low Cholesterol Omelet
  K123 P43

VEGETABLES
Whipped Potato (No Milk)
  K250 P48
Spinach
  K291 P33
Yellow Squash
  K207 P32

SALAD
Shredded Lettuce
  K58 P12

DESSERTS
Vanilla Wafers
  K8 P7
Chilled Pear Halves (Drained)
  K84 P7
Sherbet (70cc)
  K22 P13
Low Protein Cookies

BEVERAGES
Coffee
Decaffeinated Coffee
Hot Tea
Lemon Wedge
Non-dairy Creamer
  K39 P26
Whole Milk (50cc)
  K71 P46

BREADS
Wheat Bread
  K63 P52
White Bread
  K25 P22
Dinner Roll
  K41 P36
++Margarine
Jelly
Honey

MISCELLANEOUS
Hard Candy
Jelly Beans
Gum Drops

SEASONINGS
Sugar Pepper Herb Seasoning

*Special fat controlled product
++Special sodium controlled product

1   **LUNCHEON**   REGULAR

DINNER Menu

Your Menu for Tomorrow

NAME _____ ROOM NO _____
DIET ORDER _____

PLEASE **CIRCLE** SELECTIONS

ENTREES (Select One)
Baked Fish with Lemon Wedge
  K90 P81
++Pepper Steak
  K423 P125
Hamburger on Bun
  K112 P57 K50 P44

VEGETABLES
White Rice
  K50 P40
Baby Whole Carrots
  K120 P22
Wax Beans (Drained)
  K151 P37

SALAD
++Marinated Vegetable Medley
  K190 P50

DESSERTS
Blueberry Pie
  K104 P37
Pineapple Rings (Drained)
  K96 P6
Sherbet (70cc)
  K22 P13
Low Protein Cookies

BEVERAGES
Coffee
Decaffeinated Coffee
Hot Tea
Lemon Wedge
Non-dairy Creamer
  K39 P26
Whole Milk (50cc)
  K71 P46

BREADS
Wheat Bread
  K63 P52
White Bread
  K25 P22
Dinner Roll
  K41 P36
++Margarine
Jelly
Honey

MISCELLANEOUS
Hard Candy
Jelly Beans
Gum Drops

SEASONINGS
Sugar Pepper Herb Seasoning

*Special fat controlled product
++Special sodium controlled product

1   **DINNER**   REGULAR

Figure 13-8. Rotation-type selective menu for renal diet. *From Henry Ford Hospital, Detroit*

	Room &		Date of	
Name _____	bed no. _____		admission _____	

☐ Check here if you have *no* food dislikes.

In Column I, check only your *likes* next to the food items listed.

In Column II, check only your *dislikes* next to the food items listed.

Col. I Likes	Col.II Dislikes	Foods	Col. I Likes	Col. II Dislikes	Foods
Breakfast			**Lunch and Dinner**		
		Fruit			Roll at Lunch
		Juice			Melba Toast
		Dry Cereal			Soup
		Hot Cereal			Juice
		White Bread			Beef
		Whole Wheat Bread			Lamb
		Rye Bread			Veal
		Marmalade			Pork
		Jelly			Liver
		Honey			Corned Beef
		Maple Syrup			Stews
		Apple Butter			Hash
		Milk			Casserole Dishes

Col. I Likes	Col. II Dislikes	Foods	Col. 1 Likes	Col. II Dislikes	Foods
Lunch and Dinner			**Lunch and Dinner**		
		Smoked Tongue			Noodles
		Chicken			Aspics
		Turkey			Molded Salads
		Canned Fish			Cooked Vegetables
		Frozen Fish			Raw Vegetables
		Fresh Fish			Fresh Fruit
		Eggs			Stewed Fruit
		Croquettes			Canned Fruit
		Omelettes			Fruit Cocktails
		Shrimp			Pie
		Scallops			Cake
		Clams			Cookies
		Sliced Cheese			Pudding
		Cottage Cheese			Pastries
		Potatoes			Jello
		Rice			Custard
		Macaroni			Ice Cream
		Spaghetti			Sherbets

Circle any style of preparation you dislike:

Boiled   Broiled   Baked   Fried   Stewed   Steamed   Sauteed

Figure 13-9. Food preference survey. *From Detroit-Macomb Hospital Corporation*

Meal Pattern				Date	Diet Prescription Changes
Bev: B_____ L_____ D_____					
A.M.	P.M.	HS			

Likes:			Patient Profile		
				Yes	No
			Difficulty chewing		
			Difficulty swallowing		
Dislikes:			Needs help eating		
			Needs help with menu selection		
Allergies:					
Room	Name	Nourishments	Current Diet Prescription		

Figure 13-10. Patient record (cardex type).

on the belt. With the cook-serve production system, assembled trays are transported to the wards and served immediately. For other production systems, food is preplated in a cold state, assembled, transported to a floor pantry or galley, and rethermalized at time of service. Trays are assembled according to room numbers, as listed on the patient census sheet, not according to type of diet.

When prepared food is transported to the floor pantry in the bulk form, the system is known as a *decentralized tray service*. The pantry is equipped with hot and cold holding equipment, plus dishwashing facilities. Empty pans are returned to the kitchen for cleaning. The decentralized tray service is not used on a large scale in medical foodservice today because of technological advances in equipment, layout, and design of facilities. Major problems associated with decentralized service are as follows:

1. *High labor costs.* Employees must be assigned to each service area for tray assembly, distribution, and cleanup.
2. *Lack of adequate supervision.* The manager loses control over the amount of food served since a supervisor cannot be in all floor pantries at the same time to observe tray assembly.

3. *Excessive equipment cost.* Duplication of equipment occurs since each pantry must be fully equipped.

4. *Undesirable environmental factors.* Undesirable factors—such as excessive noise generated in pantries from dishwashing and other cleanup duties and food odors close to patient areas—are a problem.

In a centralized system a tray line is usually in operation. The following procedures should be followed for the tray assembly system:

1. Assembly should be standardized for speed and accuracy. A diagram of a completed tray should be available so that employees will know exactly where to place each food item on the tray. The diagram provides for ease of checking by the line supervisor prior to loading trays onto tray carts.

2. Modified diets should be included in the regular tray assembly so that all trays in a particular unit may be served at the same time.

3. In facilities where an automatic tray line is not used, it may be necessary to assemble trays in two phases. The cold food is put on the tray in advance of serving time, and the hot food is assembled just prior to service. This procedure results in double work because the trays are handled twice.

4. Each tray should be checked for accuracy before it leaves the assembly area.

Tray Identification

Tray identification is simply a method of designating the correct food tray for each patient. Color coding is often used to identify the various modified diets. For patients using selective menus to indicate desired foods, the same menu is used for tray identification. For a nonselective menu system, the individual diet pattern must be written on color-coded cards.

Food Transport

The assembled trays must be transported to the various units for either immediate service to patients or rethermalizing prior to patient service. Types of equipment used for transport are described below.

MATCH-A-TRAY This type of food cart is appropriate for a cook-serve production system. The cart has cold holding space for 20 trays and the hot section has space for 20 plates and 20 soup bowls. A coffee urn is built in on top of the hot food section, and freezer space for ice cream and other frozen desserts is on top of the cold section. For distribution and service, the hot food must be removed and placed on the tray with cold food. Careful attention is required in matching the hot food plate to the proper tray.

UNI-TRAY This cart is used for a cook-serve production system. All menu selections are placed on a single tray that is divided by a hard rubber seal to separate the cold and hot foods. The advantage of using this equipment is that the tray assembly is complete when the cart leaves the production area. No further assembly or handling is required prior to service to the patient.

INTEGRAL HEATING SYSTEM This equipment is appropriate for assembly-serve, cook-freeze-serve, and cook-chill-serve production systems. Electrical energy is converted to heat through the use of resistors fused to the bottom of the dishes. The dishes used to heat the prepared frozen or chilled food are also used for service. Preplated trays are delivered to the floor pantry in refrigerated carts. The dishes, requiring heat, are placed in a heating cabinet that has an electronic memory unit, designed for variable programming. A variety of food items requiring different heating times can be rethermalized in the same cabinet at the same time. Cabinets may be placed in the floor pantry or transported to any patient area for use and service.

CHILL-THERM This system is appropriate for assembly-serve, cook-freeze-serve, and cook-chill-serve production systems. The transport units are designed to refrigerate and cook foods simultaneously in dishes on fully assembled trays. The carts contain stainless steel shelves, with fine dish-sized heating elements for each shelf. All foods, including cold beverages, are placed on the patient tray. Trays are loaded on the carts that are transported to patient areas by monorail, where they are attached to wall units that provide refrigerated air and electric power for hot plates. The carts remain refrigerated until the heating cycle begins. Each of the five heating elements is separately controlled and timed. Instructions for each tray are electronically coded at the tray assembly line, allowing each heater to turn on and off during the heating cycle, ensuring that each food item reaches and remains at the desired temperature. Delayed meals are individually programmed and controlled to coincide with the patient's schedule (Riggs 1981).

AMSCAR The AMSCAR transport system is appropriate for assembly-serve, cook-freeze-serve and cook-chill-serve production systems. Chilled or frozen food that has been preplated is assembled on patient trays according to menu selection and loaded on refrigerated carts. Programmed for a specific destination, the battery-operated carts travel hospital corridors at a 1-mile-an-hour speed. The carts follow electronic signals generated from wires located within the corridor floors. The units can be programmed to wait at hallway intersections for clearance before proceeding, enter and leave elevators, travel through tunnels, and stop upon contact with people and other machinery. It was reported in 1982 that the cost of each cart was $11,000 to $12,000; however, they are capable of reducing "portering" hours by 80% to 90% (Anon. 1982). When the AMSCAR reaches the floor pantry, the entire inside unit can be removed and transferred to a refrigerated unit until it is time to rethermalize food items requiring heat. The AMSCAR is programmed to return to the foodservice department, where it goes through an automatic cart wash, then to tray assembly area for reloading. A microwave or some other type of oven is used in the floor pantry to rethermalize food prior to service.

UNITIZED BASE This unit is appropriate for the cook-serve production system. All food items are placed on one tray. The entree plate (either square or round) is placed on a preheated unitized base, and covered with a dome-type cover. A suction lifter is used to remove the heated base from a lowerator. Insulated soup and coffee mugs, with disposable lids, are filled and placed on the tray. Square dishes are used for salads and desserts and may be left uncovered if trays are transported in enclosed carts. Tray assembly is completed in the central area, and thus the tray is ready for service when it reaches the floor pantry or patient corridor area.

PELLET SYSTEM This system is similar to the unitized base except that a metal disk (pellet) is heated in a pellet machine, designed to lower one pellet at a time onto a metal base. The plate, with hot foods, is placed directly onto the hot pellet and covered with a dome-type cover. Insulated servers are used for other hot foods. Cold foods may be left uncovered if trays are transported in closed carts.

INSULATED COMPONENT This type of service is appropriate for the cook-serve production system. The unit is composed of a bottom plastic tray with modular-shaped grooves to accommodate specially designed disposable service-ware. After filled containers are placed on the tray in the proper section, the tray is covered with a tight-fitting plastic cover. The grooves in the top covers match the grooves in the bottom tray, thereby providing the necessary insulation. Trays can be stacked one on top of another and transported to patients on an open cart. Initial food temperatures are maintained for over a 2-hour period. The completely assembled tray is removed from the cart and served to the patient.

Food Distribution and Service

The distribution and service of patient trays may be performed by foodservice or nursing personnel. The task is less difficult when the patient's tray is completely assembled in the central area, requiring no further handling by service personnel. When food requiring heat must be thermalized in the floor pantry, the task becomes more difficult. Considering the amount of time and effort expended in presenting an acceptable product to the patient, controls during final process of service should not be left to untrained persons with little interest in how the task is to be performed. Foodservice personnel responsible for distribution and service have been oriented and trained on the objectives, policies and procedures, and standards related to patient foodservice. When the task is performed by nursing personnel, the foodservice director should require a similar orientation and training for nurse's aides or other persons assigned to distribute and serve food to patients. Since nurse's aides are not directly responsible to the foodservice director, the training program requires the cooperation and input of nursing personnel. The training may require instruction on how to rethermalize food items in facilities using the assembly-serve, cook-freeze-serve, and cook-chill-serve production systems. An overcooked or undercooked entree can ruin an entire meal.

Tray Presentation

In presenting the food tray to patients, the following recommendations are offered.

1. Every effort should be made to make mealtime a pleasant experience for the patient. The patient should be prepared for meals with an adjustment of bed and/or tray stand. (Dietary personnel must not adjust beds.) An announcement should be made that the meal is about to be served.
2. The tray must be attractive in appearance, with food items conveniently and neatly arranged. The tray cover should be clean and free from spills from soup, coffee, or other beverages.
3. A final check of food trays for accuracy should be made.
4. When the tray reaches the patient, hot foods should be hot and cold foods should be cold. If necessary, the patient should receive assistance with removing covers and lids from containers.

Personnel and Guest Service

In most medical foodservice operations, cafeteria service is provided for employees and guests. Additional services may include a physicians' dining room, administrative dining room, coffee shop, and vending machines.

Cafeteria Service

The cafeteria should be a convenient, clean, comfortable place for employees to eat at reasonable cost. Most employees have only a ½-hour meal period and would prefer to eat in the cafeteria rather than going to an outside food establishment. The serving of appetizing, high-quality food will attract enough employees to the cafeteria that the foodservice operation can break even or even make a small profit.

MENUS The cafeteria menu should be an extension of the menu planned for patients, with additional food items added for variety. The practice of using the same menu for the patients and personnel reduces materials handling for purchasing and production employees and eliminates the perception that more attention is given to the feeding of personnel than to patients. A 4-week cycle menu, even for those persons who eat in the cafeteria on a regular basis, offers enough variety to prevent menu boredom. As shown in Figure 13-11, the cycle menu has been precosted to indicate the selling price of each food item. The lower price is the amount paid by hospital employees; the higher price is paid by guests. To attract customers, *specials of the day* may be offered at a reduced price, daily menus may be posted on bulletin boards throughout the facility, and an attractive, up-to-date menu board may be displayed near the cafeteria entrance.

SERVICE The design of the service area should promote speed so that employees can make food selection, eat, and return to work in the time allowed for meals. The conventional design is a *straight-line* type of service. Customers enter at one end of the line, and remain in line until all food is selected and paid for at the other end. The order of the line is cold entrees, salads, desserts, hot entrees, bread, and beverages. All self-serve foods, such as salads and desserts, should be clearly marked with the selling price to avoid return of food items to the counter once it has been handled by the customer. Service may be slow, depending on the speed of the servers, the variety of food items, and the number and speed of cashiers. The straight service is frequently designed with space for a tray slide and space to bypass certain areas of service if no selection is desired. Yet most customers will stand in line just to purchase one or two food items, rather than cut in line in front of another person. In facilities where it is impossible to rearrange the service counters, there are some measures that management can take to reduce bottlenecks, such as:

1. Removing from the counter all services that can be provided in a remote location, such as toaster, condiments, water dispenser and glasses, cutlery, and napkins.
2. Providing a *fan-type* cashier area during peak periods. When customers reach a certain point in the serving line, they may form two or more lines to pay for selected items.
3. Training employees to work efficiently, avoiding delays by keeping the service counters replenished at all times.

An alternate type of service is the *scatter system*, also referred to as scramble, freeflow, and hollow square. Instead of following a straight line, customers enter the service area and proceed to the service counter of their choice. Depending on the size of the area and the variety of menu offerings, there may be eight or ten different service stations. Each service station is clearly marked to indicate the type of foods available such as "Soups," "Hot Sandwiches," "Cold Sandwiches," "Hot Vegetables," and "Hot Entrees." The customers are free to leave the service area without delay by paying for selections as they exit. The scatter system provides flexibility for persons selecting a full-course meal, and especially for those customers desiring only one or two food items.

Days	Sunday	Monday	Tuesday	Wednesday	Thursday	Friday	Saturday
Entrees	$1.20 $1.80 Hot Beef Sandwich $1.10 $1.65 Fried Pork Chops with Spiced Apples	$1.95 $2.60 Shrimp Fried Rice $1.20 $1.80 Roast Pork with Dressing and Crabapple Garnish $1.75 $2.65 Lamb Shanks and Potatoes	$1.90 $2.85 Spud Bar Turkey à la King Stroganoff Seafood Newburg $1.15 $1.75 Baked Chicken	$1.25 $1.90 Spaghetti with Meatballs $1.15 $1.75 Baked Haddock $1.00 $1.50 Beef Pastry	$1.15 $1.75 Liver and Onions $1.00 $1.50 Macaroni and Cheese $1.50 $2.25 Stir Fried Turkey with Broccoli and Rice	$2.00 $3.00 Roast Duck à l'Orange $1.20 $1.80 Hot Beef Sandwich $2.70 $3.25* Fried Pickerel Cole Slaw* Roll*	$1.05 $1.60 Meatloaf $1.15 $1.75 Breaded Veal with Mushroom Gravy
Starch	$0.30 $0.40 Whipped Potatoes	$0.40 $0.60 Oven-Browned Potato	$1.00 $1.25 Baked Potato $0.30 $0.40 Noodles	$0.45 $0.70 Au Gratin Potato	$0.30 $0.40 Rice	$0.30 $0.40 Mashed Potatoes	$0.30 $0.40 Whipped Potatoes
Vegetable	$0.35 $0.55 Corn $0.35 $0.55 Stewed Tomatoes	$0.60 $0.90 Ratatouille $0.35 $0.55 Green Beans	$0.35 $0.55 Leaf Spinach $0.35 $0.55 Cauliflower	$0.35 $0.55 Green Peas $0.50 $0.75 Fried Eggplant	$0.40 $0.60 Zucchini and Tomatoes $0.40 $0.60 Asparagus	$0.35 $0.55 Whole Baby Carrots $0.65 $1.00 Corn on Cob	$0.35 $0.55 Mixed Vegetables $0.35 $0.55 Broccoli
Soup	$0.35 $0.55 French Onion	$0.60 $0.90 Nacho Bean	$0.35 $0.55 Chicken Gumbo	$0.35 $0.55 Cream of Asparagus	$0.35 $0.55 Turkey Noodle	$0.60 $0.90 Potato Leek	$0.35 $0.55 Chicken Rice
Grill	$1.25 $1.90 Knockwurst on Sub	$1.25 $1.90 Slim Jim	$1.35 $2.05 Gyros	$1.95 $2.25 Filet of Chicken	$1.25 $1.90 Chopped Sirloin	$1.05 $1.60 BLT	$2.25 $3.40 Pastrami, Deli Onion
Specials				$1.55 $2.40 Baked Haddock with Potatoes	$1.40 $2.10 Liver and Onions with Rice	$1.45 $2.15 Hot Roast Beef Sandwich with Potatoes	

Figure 13-11. Week 1 cycle menu for cafeteria giving selling price of food items. The higher price is the amount charged to guests; the lower price is charged to employees. In Friday's entrees, starred items are included in the starred price. *From Detroit Receiving Hospital*

276

An innovative and relatively new type of cafeteria service system is the *circular counter*. This system, used primarily in commercial operations, eliminates all personal contact between the customer and service employees. Food is arranged in serving dishes on a circular counter that revolves slowly through the production and service areas. Tiers are provided for the separation of hot and chilled food items. As the counter revolves through the production area, counters are replenished with fresh hot and chilled food items. Hot food temperatures are maintained by means of infrared food warmers. Customers make their selections as the food counter slowly revolves from production to service. Labor cost is reduced, yet customers receive fast, efficient service.

CASHIER'S STATION Delays may occur at the cashier's station in both the straight-line and scatter systems. The cashier must be familiar with all food prices; able to quickly scan food selection on each tray; able to read scales accurately, if food price is based on weight; able to discern whether the food item is a single or double portion; and able to handle cash quickly and accurately. In medical foodservice operations, select groups of individuals are authorized to charge purchases, other individuals receive a free meal as part of fringe benefits. All food served must be accounted for either in cash or by signed receipts. The use of computerized cash registers at the point of sales can eliminate many of the problems associated with cash accountability by providing the following information: (1) food item description, (2) quantity sold, (3) price of each food item, (4) employee sales, (5) nonemployee sales, (6) cash sales, (7) charge sales, (8) free employee meal, (9) total sales, (10) total tax collected, (11) total voids, and (12) grand total.

Quantity Control

The number of portions available for service should be the same as the amount planned for at the time of purchase. Assuming that quantity was controlled at all critical points, final control measures rest with the server. All employees responsible for dishing, cutting, weighing, and slicing of prepared food should be thoroughly trained in portion control.

── Portions ──

Standardized portions should be established for all food items. The use of scoops, ladles, serving spoons, and certain dishes can serve as dependable measures for portion portioning (Table 13-1). *Scoops* may be used for portioning such foods as drop cookies, muffins, meatballs and patties, some vegetables such as mashed potatoes, and some salads such as coleslaw, potato salad, and other similar foods. The number of the scoop indicates the number of scoopfuls to make 1 quart. *Ladles* may be used to serve gravies, sauces, soups, stews, cream dishes, vegetables of thin consistency, and batters such as waffle and pancake. The ladles are labeled *ounces* (Table 13-2); these are actually *fluid ounces*, which is a volume, not a weight measurement. Solid or perforated *serving spoons* may be used instead of a scoop or ladle. Since these spoons are not identified by number, it is necessary to measure or weigh the quantity of food from the various sizes of spoons used, to obtain the number of spoonfuls needed for the required serving size. *Automatic slicers* are available that can weigh slices of meat as sliced for service. The equipment aids portion control of sliced meat for sandwiches. *Scales* may be used at the cashier's stand for weighing food priced by weight, such as self-serve salad bars.

Table 13-1. Scoop Numbers and Approximate Measures[a]

Scoop or Disher No.	Level Measure
6	2/3 cup
8	1/2 cup
10	3/8 cup
12	1/3 cup
16	1/4 cup
20	3 1/5 Tbsp
24	2 2/3 Tbsp
30	2 1/5 Tbsp
40	1 3/5 Tbsp
50	3 4/5 Tbsp
60	1 Tbsp

[a] From Food Buying Guide for School Food Service (USDA, 1980).

Table 13-2. Ladle Numbers and Approximate Measures[a]

No. on ladle (oz)	Approx. measure (cup)
1	1/8
2	1/4
4	1/2
6	3/4
8	1
12	1 1/2

[a] From Food Buying Guide for School Food Service (USDA, 1980).

The shift supervisor or head cook must make sure that employees on each shift are familiar with portion sizes, proper utensils, and dishes to use for all food served. Information pertaining to portion sizes can be written on the production worksheet under instructions. The serving of carved meats, such as beef rounds and ham, should be performed by an individual who can make a fair estimate of weight by looking at the size and thickness of a cut or by using portion scales that are concealed from public view. The importance of portion control cannot be overemphasized, but it is not necessary to remind the customer constantly that every portion has been weighed or measured.

Leftovers

With accurate forecasting, leftovers can be eliminated or at least reduced to a minimum. The disposition of leftovers should be recorded on the production worksheet at the end of service. If the leftover food is to be served at the next meal, it should be chill stored until time for reheating. Leftover food should never be left in a food warmer or on the cook's table until the next meal; nor should it be served in the same form for the next meal. Normally, personnel will not complain about leftover food if is served as an added menu selection. The practice of using leftovers after the planned menu selections have been served should be discouraged.

Quality Control

Standards of quality for prepared food are maintained when standardized recipes are used properly. Precautions must be taken to preserve quality until the food is consumed.

Temperature

The texture, flavor, and appearance of prepared food quickly deteriorate when improper temperatures are used for holding and serving. All hot food should be served hot, above 140°F; and all cold food should be served cold, below 45°F. Some prepared foods require a higher temperature than the minimum 140°F for improved palpability. The holding and serving temperatures of hot beverages, soups, and gravies should be at least 180°F; for hot cereals and casseroles, at least 150°F. A serving temperature should be established and maintained for all items served. Policies and procedures should require quality checks for temperature with a probe thermometer during assembly and prior to patient service. If temperatures fail to meet prescribed standards, corrective action should be taken.

Food Acceptance

It is important for management to know whether the food served to patients and personnel is of acceptable quality. Mechanisms should be established to provide both positive and negative feedback, with plans on how to take corrective action. For personnel and guests eating in the cafeteria, the placing of suggestion boxes in prominent places throughout the area may be sufficient to determine food acceptance. All foodservice personnel should have a general knowledge of menu items, such as major ingredients used in the preparation techniques. Informed employees can answer questions from customers immediately, thus reducing the number of written complaints. All comments should be brought to the attention of supervisory personnel. Supervisors should review, analyze, and act on written comments in a systematic manner, at regularly scheduled intervals.

To evaluate the level of patient satisfaction with foodservice and nutritional care, a survey (Fig. 13-12) can be administered on a regular basis. The survey should be conducted by clinical dietitians and reviewed and analyzed by both administrative and clinical personnel. Results of the analysis will dictate the action plan to take. A more objective tool is a record of food acceptance as observed by the amount of food consumed by patients. Menus are carefully planned to meet the nutritional needs of patients. When food is not consumed, the objective is not met. As part of the nutritional care plan, the clinical dietitian must make notations in patients' records on the acceptance of food, as prescribed. The charting of "appetite is good, fair, or poor" is meaningless; more concrete data are required. A record of food acceptance, as shown in Figure 13-13, can be used to collect data from patients on regular and modified diets. In most health care facilities, the majority of the nutritional care planning is done on modified diets. However, teaching the protective value of following a nutritionally adequate, well-balanced diet can be beneficial for all patients and should be routinely practiced by the clinical dietitians. The monitoring of food choices and consumption can point out the need for individual counseling.

The clinical dietitian, with direct patient contact, represents the foodservice department. The individual must be knowledgeable of the administrative functions involved in providing nutritional care. In making ward rounds, the dietitian should be able to answer general questions on major ingredients used in menu food items and the preparation procedure. A reply such as "I do not have anything to do with the preparation of food" is inadequate. The dietitian should respond as intelligently as possible without shifting the blame to any individual or area within the department. All patients should be visited within 24 hours after admission, with follow-up visits on a daily basis.

Quality Assurance

Quality assurance, as related to dietetic services, can be defined as a systematic approach to verifying that optimal nutrition care is provided on a continuous

		Breakfast	Lunch	Supper

Food Questionnaire

1. Name _____ Room number _____ Date _____
2. What type of diet?
   Regular _____ or Modified diet (type) _____
3. How long have you been in the hospital? _____ days
4. Have you been visited by a dietitian to discuss your diet? Yes _____ No _____
5. Were there items missing from your tray which had been ordered? Yes _____
   No _____
   If *yes*, which item(s) _____
   _____
   If *yes*, was it explained why these items were missing? Yes _____ No _____
6. How would you rate our food and service? Please check the appropriate box.

		Breakfast	Lunch	Supper
6a.	Appearance of food on tray Excellent			
	Good			
	Satisfactory			
	Poor			
6b.	Taste of main course Excellent			
	Good			
	Satisfactory			
	Poor			
6c.	Taste of other items Excellent			
	Good			
	Satisfactory			
	Poor			
6d.	Size of portions Excellent			
	Good			
	Satisfactory			
	Poor			
6e.	Menu variety Excellent			
	Good			
	Satisfactory			
	Poor			
6f.	Temperature of food Excellent			
	Good			
	Satisfactory			
	Poor			
6g.	Temperature of beverages Excellent			
	Good			
	Satisfactory			
	Poor			
6h.	Coffee or tea Excellent			
	Good			
	Satisfactory			
	Poor			
6i.	Courtesy of serving staff Excellent			
	Good			
	Satisfactory			
	Poor			
Additional comments or suggestions:				

Figure 13-12. Sample patient food questionnaire.

Record of Food Acceptance

Patient _____

Room no. _____

Weight (lb) _____

Height (in.) _____

Diet _____

Diagnosis _____

Age (yr) _____

Date: _____ To: _____

Days	Meat/Egg			Cereal/Potato			Bread			Fruit			Vegetable			Milk			Initials
	B	D	S	B	D	S	B	D	S	B	D	S	B	D	S	B	D	S	
Monday																			
Tuesday																			
Wednesday																			
Thursday																			
Friday																			
Saturday																			
Sunday																			

Use the following symbols:

A   All food eaten.

T   Takes feeding given.

U   Unable to eat.

R   Refused to eat.

$^1/_2$, $^1/_4$, or $^3/_4$ Amount of food eaten.

S   Substitution. (Record date, food substituted, and amounts on back of sheet.)

Figure 13-13. Sample record of food acceptance.

basis. In order to assure quality, the foodservice director must first develop and implement quality control standards. In medical foodservice, acceptable criteria should be 100% for all patient-related tasks. Let us suppose that trays were set up and served to patients on 9 of the 10 wards; hence the service was 90% correct. Is this acceptable quality? Suppose the dietitian conducts an initial assessment on 75% of patients admitted to facility. Is this situation acceptable? The answer to both questions is no. When quality is less than 100%, the impact on patient outcome has a negative effect.

According to the Joint Commission of Accreditation of Hospitals (1988), the dietetic department must have a planned and systematic process for monitoring and evaluating the quality and appropriateness of patient care (see Appendix I). Although the process must be expressed in writing, it need not involve excessive paperwork in order to be efficient and effective. After policies and procedures are established by the quality assurance committee, a one-sheet form can be used to document actions taken. The form should include space to document the following:

- Date problem was identified
- Date problem was resolved
- Signature of person conducting quality assurance audit
- Identified problem
- Source of problem (patient or employee complaint, routine quality check)
- Findings
- Resolution of problem
- Implementation of corrective action
- Results of monitoring and evaluation
- Impact on patient care

The program should be ongoing; records should be maintained and filed for future reference. From a managerial perspective, problems should be resolved at the departmental level to the extent possible. Be prepared to report results at Hospital Quality Assurance Committee meetings.

Sanitation

Policies and procedures on the display, service, and transport of food, the return of soiled dishes, and dishwashing should be an integral part of any sanitation program designed to protect food from external contamination and the rapid, progressive growth of microorganisms.

Display of Service of Food

Any lapse in sanitary procedures during display and service can negate all the effort of buying, storing, and preparing quality products that are safe for human consumption. The following practices should be observed:

1. Potentially hazardous foods should be kept at an internal temperature of 45°F or below, or at an internal temperature of 140°F or above during display and service, except that rare roast beef may be held for service at a temperature of at least 130°F.

2. Milk and milk products for drinking should be served in an unopened, commercially filled package, or drawn from a commercially filled container stored in a mechanically refrigerated bulk milk dispenser. Where a bulk dis-

penser is not available and portions of less than ½ pint are required, milk products may be poured from a commercially filled container of not more than ½-gallon capacity.

3. Cream, half-and-half, and nondairy cream should be served in individual containers, protected pour-type pitchers, or drawn from a refrigerated dispenser designed for such service.

4. Condiments, seasonings, and dressings for self-service use should be provided in individual packages, from a dispenser or containers, or from a serving line or a salad bar with protector devices.

5. Condiments provided for table or counter use should be individually portioned except that catsup and other sauces may be served in the original container or pour-type dispenser. Sugar should be in individual packages or in pour-type containers.

6. Ice for consumer use should be dispensed only by employees with scoops, tongs, or other ice-dispensing utensils or through automatic self-service ice-dispensing equipment. Ice-dispensing utensils should be stored on a clean surface or in the ice with the utensil's handle extended out of the ice. Between uses, ice transfer receptacles should be stored to protect them from contaminations.

7. Wiping cloths used for wiping food spills on tableware, such as plates or bowls being served to a customer should be clean, dry, and used for no other purpose. Cloths used for wiping food spills on kitchenware and food contact surfaces of equipment should be cleaned and rinsed frequently in a sanitizing solution and used for no other purpose. These cloths and sponges should be stored in the sanitizing solution between uses. Moist cloths or sponges used for cleaning nonfood contact surfaces of equipment such as counters and dining tabletops should be cleaned and rinsed in a sanitizing solution.

8. The reuse of soiled tableware by employees or self-serving customers returning for additional food at a buffet table or salad bar is prohibited. Clean tableware must be provided and used for additional food servings. Glasses and beverage cups are exempt from these requirements.

9. Liners are not allowed for use in covering food, except for lining a basket or covering bread or rolls to be served to the customer.

10. Between use and during service, food-dispensing utensils such as scoops and ladles should be stored either in the food with the handle extending out of the food (the handle must be clean and dry) or in a running-water dipper well.

11. Food on display should be protected from customer contamination by the use of packaging or by counter, serving line, or salad bar protecting devices.

12. No animals should be kept or allowed in any room in which food or drink is prepared, stored, or served. Check local regulations on exemption of leader dogs used by legally blind customers.

13. Ice cream should be purchased in single-service containers. If the ice cream is dipped, the scoop should be stored under running water.

14. Train employees in the following:

a. Washing hands before starting work, after using toilet, blowing nose, handling dirty dishes, smoking, or touching face or hair.

b. Wear clean clothing and appropriate head covering.

c. Refrain from licking fingers to pick up diet cards, napkins, or paper placemats. Fingers should not touch food contact surfaces of glasses, cups, bowls, or eating ends of knives, forks, and spoons.

d. Fingernails should be clean, properly trimmed, and unpolished. Avoid excessive jewelry.

   e. Food should be served with a minimum amount of handling. Use appropriate tools for handling food.

   f. Avoid sitting or leaning on work surfaces.

   g. In cleaning the dining area, chairs should not be stacked so that seat of the chair is in contact with the tabletop.

Food Transport

Protection from contamination and proper temperatures are critical for the safety and quality of transported food. During transportation, food and food utensils should be kept in covered containers or completely wrapped or packaged to be protected from contamination. Foods in original individual packages do not need to be overwrapped if the original package has not been torn or broken. During transportation, food should meet the requirements relating to food protection and food storage.

Return of Soiled Dishes

Trays should be collected from the patient areas and returned to the foodservice department approximately 45 minutes after trays have been served. Employees responsible for removing food trays from patient areas should be trained to look for and save all tray identification cards that may contain written comments from the patients. The comments should be given to supervisory personnel for analysis and corrective action, if necessary. Soiled disposable trays from isolated patient areas are double-bagged by nursing personnel and destroyed. Soiled isolated tray service should not be returned to the foodservice department. The food cart used to return soiled trays should be washed and sanitized prior to further use.

Dishwashing

To prevent cross contamination, tableware and kitchenware should be washed, rinsed, and sanitized after each use and following any interruptions of operations during which time contamination may have occurred. The following procedures are recommended:

1. A three-compartment sink should be used for manual cleaning and sanitizing of utensils and equipment.
2. For manual cleaning, all equipment and utensils should be sanitized by:
      a. Immersion for at least ½ minute in clean hot water at a temperature of 170°F or
      b. Immersion for at least 1 minute in a clean solution containing at least 50 parts per million of available chlorine such as a hypochlorine and at a temperature of at least 75°F or
      c. Immersion for at least 1 minute in a clean solution containing at least 12.5 parts per million of available iodine and having a pH not higher than 5.0 and at a temperature of at least 75°F.
3. Temperatures for mechanical cleaning and sanitizing of equipment and utensils should be at least 140°F for wash, 160°F for rinse, and 180°F for final rinse.
4. Clean and sanitized silverware should be touched only by the handles. This applies also to the practice of bagging or wrapping silverware for tray assembly.
5. Clean and sanitized cups, glasses, bowls, plates, and similar items should be handled without contact with inside surfaces or surfaces that touch the user's mouth.

6. Clean and sanitized utensils and equipment should be stored at least 6 inches above the floor in a clean, dry location, protected from contamination by splashing, dust, or other contaminants.
7. Utensils should be air-dried before being stored or should be stored in a self-draining position.
8. Glasses and cups should be stored inverted.
9. Silverware in containers should be stored so that the handle is presented to the customer.

Computer-Assisted Foodservice Distribution

Development of a computerized foodservice distribution system takes a great deal of time and effort. As described by McLaren (1982), the computerized system at Community Hospital in Indianapolis was 10 years in the making. In this program all previously discussed systems (menu planning, purchasing, and production) are interrelated. Community Hospital's system is designed with five modules, each one handling a separate function.

The first module involves all the processes of procuring food, the second handles food production (worksheets and recipes) and the third handles food distribution (forecast and destination sheets). Clinical dietetics records and fiscal reports are contained in the other modules. The following discussion centers on the distribution aspect of their program.

At Community Hospital in Indianapolis, distribution of food involves forecasting the amounts and destination of food requirements. Patient forecasts are automatically updated because the computer stores patient data from the tray assembly at each meal. This information is then communicated to the forecast file for the next time the menu is used. Therefore, menu forecasts are based on usage information entered during each menu cycle. In the future, cafeteria cash registers will be used to update nonpatient forecasting.

The next step in the process is the collection of patients' marked menus, which are stacked in a central office on electronic tabbing units. Menu data are stored for use later in assembling meal trays. The computer, when asked, will produce a complete and accurate listing of required food items. At mealtime the tray assembly line is started. This line has a conveyor belt, serving stations and a checking station. As trays are released by the computer in a predetermined sequence on the line, light-emitting diodes (LEDs) designate which foods go on each patient tray, and workers find the right item and place it on the tray.

At the checker's station there is a television-like screen, a cathode-ray tube (CRT), where one can receive or enter data, and a printer. The CRT flashes all pertinent information about the patient and food items that should be on the tray. The printer produces a hard copy of this information. As the checker verifies accuracy of tray items she or he tears off the printout and puts it on the tray. The numbers of portions actually served are stored in the program and used in the forecasting file for the next time this menu is used. This system has saved money by eliminating tray line mistakes and reducing labor hours by 30 each week.

As reported by Nicolaus (1970), an electronically controlled food distribution system used in several hospitals in Europe was developed by Vosowerke in Hannover, Germany. This system offers rapid distribution of 920 meals per hour and includes various data processing programs for various functions. The most favorable method of cooking foods was researched by the group. Then, after extensive investigation and testing as to proper cooking methods, correct timing, and efficient use of energy, equipment was developed to prepare food in a continuous-flow system. The whole process is programmed by automatic devices on a computer.

Working units are given specific directions and automatically dispensed on a moving belt. The same container is used from beginning to end. It travels through both the preparation and distribution areas, reducing handling to a minimum. The container is emptied at the tray service table and automatically moved to dishwashing and then carried back to the container area, producing a continuous flow and transport of food. Tray assembly has been computerized in some foodservices by using two employees: One runs a console, which electronically released food items previously stored in magazines; the second employee loads the food onto the patients' trays.

"Robots" have also been used for food and tray delivery in many foodservices (Anon. 1982) and have sometimes been known to get off the track and been found wandering around the laundry room with the laundry robots. It will take money, research, and time to perfect computer-assigned delivery systems but it will probably prove to be more efficient in the long run than present systems.

References

Anon. (1982). Electric Carts–Patient Simulator: Robot Slowly Moving into Hospitals. *Hospitals 56*(13), 36.

McLaren, A. (1982). High Technology in Indianapolis. *Food Mgt. 17*(10), 46–49.

Nicolaus, N. (1970). Automated Food Preparation and Service. *Hospitals 44*(6), 108–11.

Riggs, S. (1981). How Well Has Walter Reed's "Revolutionary" Food System Worked? *Restaur. Inst. 88*(11), 73–75.

U.S. Department of Agriculture. 1980. *Food Buying Guide for School Food Service,* Food and Nutrition Service, USDA, Washington, DC.

Chapter 14

Subsystem for Personnel Management

Personnel is one of the more difficult resources to manage, primarily because of the human element involved and the constant changes taking place inside and outside of the workplace. The foodservice director must have an understanding of human relations and how it relates to hiring, developing, maintaining, and utilizing an effective work force. In addition, changes in the work force, economic conditions, work environment, information technology, and outside regulatory agencies have impact on the role a manager must play in supervising employees. The manager must be flexible and able to adapt to environmental changes. A systems approach for the management of personnel, which begins with preemployment and continues through the exit interview, eliminates many of the problems confronting a manager in a dynamic milieu.

Determining Staffing Needs

Staffing is the process of determining the need for hiring employees and the level of role occupancy required to carry out the functions of the organization. In medical foodservice, staffing levels are decided by each individual facility and may be based on one or a combination of the indices used for determining staffing needs. One source recommends 1.5 full-time equivalents (FTE) for each position, based on a 7-day operation (Stokes 1979). For example, the dishroom schedule should require a minimum of two employees per shift in order to prevent cross contamination. Therefore, the minimum number of full-time equivalents for dishroom duties should not be less than three in order to provide adequate coverage ($1.5 \times 2 = 3$).

Another source (U.S. Department of Health and Human Services 1971) recommends three methods for determining dietary staffing needs.

Staffing Based on Number of Patients

Using one dietary employee for every eight patients, the following calculation is made (ratio of 1:8).

Example. Given a 100-bed facility this is explained as follows: 100-bed facility $\div$ 8 patients per employee = 12.5 employees per week, allowing for a 5-day workweek; 12.5 persons $\times$ 40-hour workweek = 500 labor hours needed per week. Since it takes 1.4 persons to cover 7 days, this is equivalent to 56 hours per person: 1.4 persons $\times$ 40 hours (1 position) = 56 hours or 7 days (1 position) $\times$ 8 hours = 56 hours.

Now divide the number of labor hours needed per week (500) by the number of hours represented by one employee (56) to get the number for the day: $500 \div 56 = 8.93$ employees. To convert this to number of labor hours, multiply by 8 hours: that is, $8.93 \times 8 = 71.4$ hours per day.

Per position, 1.6 rather than 1.4 persons are required to provide fringe benefits (i.e., sick leave, holidays, and vacations). The addition of 0.2 person at 8 hours is equivalent to 1.6 hours more per day.

These calculations were made on the basis of weekly work hours required, which remain the same. The number of persons needed varies with the actual number of work hours of each employee. If we assume there are two 15-minute relief breaks, the following adjustment must be made based on actual work hours of 7.5 hours per day: 71.4 hours per day $\div 7.5 = 9.52$ employees per day.

If we assume a 30-minute meal break and two 15-minute relief breaks, this equals 7 working hours per day, and the following adjustment must be made: 71.4 hours per day $\div 7 = 10.2$ persons per day.

The use of part-time employees alters the number of bodies needed, but does not alter the total daily hours or the FTE.

Staffing Based on Number of Positions

Count the number of positions that must be filled daily. It takes at least 1.4 persons working a 5-day week to fill each position, or seven employees for five positions. Fringe benefits, relief workers for holidays, sick leave, and vacation must be included. To allow for benefits and vacation, management may wish to budget 1.6 employees for each position, or eight employees to fill five positions.

Staffing Based on Labor Minutes per Meal

Use a figure of 14 minutes of labor required to serve one meal to one person.

Example: A 100-bed facility $\times$ 3 meals per day per bed = 300 meals per day; 300 meals $\times$ 14 minutes per meal = 4200 minutes; 4200 minutes $\div$ 60 minutes per hour = 70 hours per day; 70 hours per day $\times$ 7 days per week = 490 hours per week.

In some instances where there is a wide variety of diets and a limited use of convenience food, it has been estimated that it takes 17 minutes of employee time to prepare one meal. Using the preceding method, the result is 85 hours per day. This figure can further be reduced to number of employees required by using the procedure in Staffing Based on Number of Patients.

Professional Staffing Based on Work Activity

In addition to staffing required in the kitchen for actual food preparation, professional staffing is needed to assure quality nutritional care for the patients. A sample calculation of professional staffing requirements to achieve goals is based on the following two criteria (Brogan, Callaghan, & Mutch 1981):

1. Meet needs of 100% of patients on modified diets.
2. Conduct nutritional assessments on 25% of other patients at risk. (Assumption: 46 patients are on modified diets; 120 other patients are at risk; average hospital stay is 7 days.)

The work activity is divided into the following five categories:

1. *Service time*. Compute figures by compiling time spent on following activities.

Activities	Minutes
Reviewing chart to determine nutritional risks and problems	20
Obtaining history from patient (verbal interview or from form completed by technician)	15
Communicating with other team members (i.e., rounds, telephone, follow-up contacts)	20
Preparing and assembling materials for patient instruction	10
Developing nutritional care plan	15
Recording in chart (i.e., diet given, recommendations, progress, implementation and evaluation of instruction, and follow-up)	20
Total	100

$$A = 100 \text{ min} \times 46 \text{ patients per week} = 4600 \text{ min per week}$$

2. *Instruction time.* Compute this figure from the Client Learning Study (Callaghan, Larkin & Wright 1983), average time for each counseling session multiplied by the number of patients on each diet:

$$B = 574 \text{ min per day} \times 7 \text{ days per week} = 4019 \text{ min per week}$$

3. *Routine support service time.* Compute this figure by compiling time spent on all activities performed each day for all patients, such as checking menus:

$$C = 375 \text{ min per day} \times 7 \text{ days per week} = 2625 \text{ min per week}$$

4. *Nutritional assessment and special service time.* Compute this figure by compiling time spent on only those activities not listed in *A, B,* or *C* above, such as anthropometric measuring, or parenteral or enteral feeding formulation:

$$D = 80 \text{ min per patient} \times 20 \text{ patients per week} = 1600 \text{ min per week}$$

5. *Available staff time.* (a) Number of hours available from a dietetic practitioner per year, allowing for personal time, administrative tasks, and vacation is 6.75 hours per day × 250 days per year = 1687.5 hours per year. (The 6.75 hours per day allows for meal and break time. The 250 days per year is based on 5 days a week for 52 weeks, minus 15 days for leave time.) (b) The calculation of time needed to meet the goal in this example is as follows: $A + B + C + D =$ number of hours needed per year; that is,

$$4600 \text{ min} + 4109 \text{ min} + 2625 \text{ min} + 1600 \text{ min}$$
$$= 12{,}844 \text{ min per week}$$
$$= 30.6 \text{ hours day } 365 \text{ days per year}$$
$$= 11{,}169 \text{ hours per year}$$

$$\frac{11{,}169 \text{ staff hours needed}}{1687.5 \text{ hours available per practitioner}} = 6.6 \text{ FTE}$$

where FTE is full-time equivalent.

Although the professional staffing requirements referred only to the clinical dietitian, similar data can be collected and analyzed for all professional activities. Staffing requirements are equally important for the professional as for the nonprofessional employees. Staffing criteria should be established for both categories. It is difficult to state with any amount of specificity what the staffing requirements should be for a medical foodservice operation without consideration of the following factors:

1. Goals and objectives of the organization
2. Standards of performance
3. Efficiency of the work force
4. Type of production, distribution, and service system
5. Menu system (selective, nonselective, restaurant type)
6. Number of special activities
7. Kitchen layout and design
8. Location of kitchen from patient area
9. Number and type of diets (regular vs. modified)
10. Style of purchasing (convenience vs. scratch)
11. Sanitation and safety requirements (minimum shift requirements and amount of cleaning done by outside agencies)
12. Responsibility for distribution and service of trays to patients (dietary vs. nursing)
13. Hours of operation

Work Schedules

A work schedule is an organized procedure for ensuring staff utilization by indicating the hours of work per day, the time of work, and the number of days per week. Most workers in medical foodservice operations work a *fixed shift* of 8 hours per day, 5 days per week. However, other types of work schedules are used, such as the compressed workweek and flextime.

A *compressed workweek* is used to schedule employees for a 40-hour week in less than the normal 5 days. For example, employees may be scheduled to work 10 hours per day, 4 days per week. The schedule permits more off-time for leisure and other personal activities and is favorably regarded by some workers. Where used, employees are scheduled for 3 days off together, such as Friday through Sunday. Since medical foodservice operations must provide three meals per day, 7 days per week, the 3-day-off schedule may not be feasible.

Flextime scheduling permits flexibility in the time an employee begins and ends the work shift. For example, an employee on the early shift may report for work any time between the hours of 5:00 A.M. and 7:00 A.M. and remain on duty long enough to complete an 8-hour tour of duty. Flextime may be confined to flexible hours for lunch or break time, with the time of activity left to the discretion of the employee. Flextime may also involve working less than 8 hours on some days and more than 8 hours on other days, depending on peak periods of work. There are a number of problems that may arise in the use of flextime in a medical foodservice operation:

1. Record keeping may be increased because the manager must check to make sure that each employee's work hours comply with provisions of the *Fair Labor Standards Act.*

2. For employees requiring supervision, there may be excess time involved for supervisory personnel.
3. It may be difficult to meet prescribed mealtimes in a timely manner.
4. There may be delays in completing tasks since most work activities in a medical foodservice operation are interdependent.
5. Work activities cannot be delayed until the following day or later since meals must be served at least three times a day, 7 days a week.

Both the compressed workweek and flextime need considerable study before they can be effectively implemented in a medical foodservice operation. The procedures are more applicable to industries that operate on a Monday-through-Friday workweek.

To eliminate problems associated with making out a fixed-hour work schedule, a list of *work criteria* is recommended for use as a guide. The work criteria (see Fig. 14-1) specify the number of workers needed for each shift, the level of workers required, the number of weekends off, maximum number of workers on leave at any one time, and necessary relief coverage. By use of the criteria, the task of making out the work schedule can be a routine duty performed at the lowest supervisory level. Further, the criteria provide for uniformity, assure fair and impartial treatment for all employees, conserve supervisor's time, and make for easy construction. There should be space on the work schedule sheet (Fig. 14-2) for each assigned worker. The use of a clear, precise legend to indicate work and off-duty time eliminates confusion on the part of workers. In order to provide adequate coverage during employee vacation time, there should be a deadline for requesting vacation time. The policy will provide enough time for managerial decisions and approval. All time off, including time for vacation, personal, and other requests, should be included in the work schedule prior to posting. A sample vacation request form is shown in Figure 14-3. The work schedule should be posted in a prominent place at least 2 weeks in advance of the work period. Work schedules should remain on file for 3 years.

Volunteer Workers

The volunteer worker can be valuable asset in extending the scope of services offered by a medical foodservice department. The volunteer program should not be set up in a haphazard manner. Volunteers assigned to the department must be carefully screened either by the director of volunteer services or by the foodservice director. The volunteer worker must be in good physical condition (as evidenced by a health card) and be willing to make a commitment for regular and continuous service. The worker must be provided with a job description and given an orientation to the department's objectives, functions, and health care standards.

According to guidelines published by the American Hospital Association (1974), volunteers may be involved in patient services, departmental activities, and community outreach programs as follows:

1. *Patient services*
   a. Distributing and collecting menus.
   b. Assisting patients with menu selections.
   c. Tabulating menu selections.
   d. Helping in the preparation of materials to be used for patient instruction.

Pertinent Information:

1. Three meals are served daily to ward patients, personnel eating in the cafeteria, plus night nourishment for ward patients.
2. Hours of operation for the department: 5:30 A.M. to 7:00 P.M.
3. Meal hours are as follows:

	Cafeteria	*Ward*
Breakfast	6:30–8:00 A.M.	7:00 A.M.
Lunch	11:00 A.M.–1:00 P.M.	12:00 noon
Dinner	4:00–6:00 P.M.	5:00 P.M.
Nourishments		8:00 P.M.

4. Centralized Meals on Wheels, with eight food carts used for distribution.
5. Major clerical duties are performed by hospital secretarial staff: routine office work performed by cashiers.
6. Patient foodservice prepare approximately 150 patient trays for each meal.
7. The cafeteria serves approximately 200 persons for breakfast, 300 for lunch, and 250 for dinner.

Instructions:

1. Schedule employees for 8 hours per day, 5 days per week. *No overtime.*
2. Schedule employees for no more than 5 consecutive days together.
3. Schedule should be balanced (approximately equal number of employees daily).
4. Include all "approved" off days, such as vacation, sick leave, or personal leave.
5. Use the following legend:

    E = Early shift: 5:30 A.M.–2:00 P.M.
    L = Late shift: 10:30 A.M.–7:00 P.M.
    R = Regular shift: 8:00 A.M.–4:30 P.M.
    O = Off duty
    V = Vacation
    S = Sick leave
    P = Personal leave
    A = Administrative leave (conferences, meetings, etc.)

*Employee Categories/*Work Shift	Time Off
Director	
Regular shift, Monday—Friday	Every weekend
Administrative Dietitian	
Regular shift, Monday—Friday	Every weekend
Clinical Dietitian	
Regular shift, Monday—Friday	Every weekend
Patient Supervisor no. 1	
Early shift	Every other weekend (Rotates weekend off days with Supervisor no. 2.)
Patient Supervisor no. 2	
Late shift	Every other weekend (Rotates with no. 1.)
Production Supervisor no. 1	
Early shift	Every other weekend (Rotates with no. 2.)
Production Supervisor no. 2	
Late shift	Every other weekend (Rotates with no. 1.)
Head Cook no. 1	
Early shift	Every third weekend
Head Cook no. 2	
Late shift	Every third weekend

Figure 14-1. Criteria for work schedule.

Employee Categories/Work Shift	Time Off
Head Cook no. 3	
Swing shift as relief for no. 1 and no. 2	Every third weekend
Assistant Cooks 1, 2, 3, 4	
Early shift	Every fourth weekend
Assistant Cooks 5, 6, 7, 8	
Late shift	Every fourth weekend
Dietary Aides 1, 2, 3, 4	
Early shift	One weekend per month
Dietary Aides 5, 6, 7, 8	
Late shift	One weekend per month
Baker	
Early shift Monday—Friday	Every weekend
Cashier no. 1	
Early shift	Every third weekend
Cashier no. 2	
Late shift	Every third weekend
Cashier no. 3	
Swing shift as relief for no. 1 and no. 2	Every third weekend
Storeroom Personnel no. 1	
Early shift	Every other weekend
Storeroom Personnel no. 2	
Late shift	Every other weekend
Foodservice Workers 1, 2, 3, 4	
Early shift	One weekend per month
Foodservice Workers 5, 6, 7, 8	
Late shift	One weekend per month

Figure 14-1. *(Continued)*

      e. Making favors and decorations for patients' trays.

      f. Distributing nourishments and other in-between feedings to patients.

  2. *Department services*

      a. Serving as host or hostess in dining areas to assist patients or visitors.

      b. Acting as a guide for scheduled department tours.

      c. Arranging and preparing bulletin board displays.

      d. Assisting with clerical duties, such as supplementary typing.

      e. Hosting at special functions such as teas, parties, luncheons, and dinners for visitors, trustees, medical staff, and other groups.

  3. *Community outreach programs.* Assisting with programs and activities such as satellite clinics, diet workshops, nutrition classes, continuing education for homebound patients, and feeding programs such as Meals on Wheels. For such program activity, adequate insurance coverage for the volunteers is essential.

Volunteers should not be used to perform the work of paid employees, such as substituting for an employee who is absent from duty. The department should provide adequate training for all assigned tasks and take advantage of the special talents and attributes of the volunteers to enhance services to patients.

Work Schedule														
Date: _____ to _____ Prepared by: _____														
Employees	S	M	T	W	T	F	S		S	M	T	W	T	F	S
Director															
Administrative Dietitian															
Clinical Dietitian															
Patient Supervisor no. 1															
Patient Supervisor no. 2															
Production Supervisor no. 1															
Production Supervisor no. 2															
Head Cook no. 1															
Head Cook no. 2															
Head Cook no. 3															
Assistant Cook no. 1															
2															
3															
4															
5															
6															
7															
8															
Dietary Aide no. 1															
2															
3															
4															
5															
6															
7															
8															

Figure 14-2. Sample work schedule.

Employees	S	M	T	W	T	F	S		S	M	T	W	T	F	S
Baker															
Cashier no. 1															
Cashier no. 2															
Cashier no. 3															
Storeroom Personnel no. 1															
Storeroom Personnel no. 2															
Foodservice Worker no. 1															
2															
3															
4															
5															
6															
7															
8															
Totals															

Figure 14-2. *(Continued)*

The Hiring Process

Effective hiring procedures eliminate many of the problems related to work accomplishment. The individual should be suitable for the position for which he or she is hired. A well-planned process of ensuring that qualified persons are hired involves a series of steps, including recruitment, selection, interview, orientation, and evaluation.

Recruitment

Recruitment of personnel is most often a function of the personnel officer. Input from the foodservice director is necessary in order to seek applicants from the appropriate or most successful sources. Depending on the type of employee sought, such as professional or nonprofessional, sources of recruitment may be as follows:

1. *For professional personnel:* (a) Professional organizations, (b) professional journals, (c) private job placement agencies, (d) college and university placement services, (e) newspaper advertisements, and (f) other professional employees on the job.
2. *For nonprofessional personnel:* (a) State and city employment agencies, (b) vocational educational schools, (c) newspaper advertisements, (d) radio and television announcements, and (e) relatives, friends, and employees on the job.

Detroit-Macomb Hospital Corporation
Vacation Request

To be completed by employee

Employee name   Employee number   Job classification

Employment date: _____ Benefits (or anniversary) date: _____

Vacation preference: Note: A vacation week is Monday through Sunday.

First Choice: From _____through _____

Second Choice: From _____through _____

Third Choice: From _____through _____

Vacation Days: With pay_____Without pay_____

Remarks: _____

Date: _____ Employee signature: _____

To be completed by department head

Vacation days:

| Approved__Disapproved__With pay__Without pay__ | Vacation days available (prior to this request)_____ |
| Return to work_____
       (Month)   (Day)   (Year)
 Remarks_____ | Vacation days approved_____

 Vacation days remaining_____ |

Date:_____ Department head signature:_____

Vacation Policy

After 12 months from his date of employment and each anniversary year thereafter, each benefit status employee paid for at least 1000 hours in the 12-month period shall be entitled to vacation with pay. Full vacation benefits are as follows:

After completion of first through fourth year of employment:	10 working days
After completion of 5 or more years of employment:	15 working days
After completion of 18 or more years of employment:	20 working days

Vacation benefits will be prorated for benefit status employees receiving less than 200 paid hours in the previous year.

Vacation schedules are made biannually by the departments and posted at least 1 week in advance of the effective beginning dates, October 1 and April 1. Vacations must be scheduled with and approved by the department head at least 1 month in advance of the desired vacation time. In the event that two or more employees doing similar work request vacations for the same period, the one with the most service will be given preference if his choice is designated 1 month in advance of the posting date of the biannual vacation schedule. After the vacation schedule is established and posted, however, length of service cannot be honored in requests for revisions.

Vacations shall be scheduled within 10 months following the anniversary date. Vacation days cannot be accumulated from one year to the next. Vacations must be taken within 12 months of the benefits (or anniversary) date, or forfeited without pay. Vacations cannot be taken until they have been earned. If time off is desired prior to the time it has been earned, the employee may apply for an excused absence without pay on the proper form.

Figure 14-3. Vacation request form. *From Detroit-Macomb Hospital Corporation*

INTERNAL VS. EXTERNAL RECRUITMENT To comply with equal opportunity hiring laws, all vacancies must be advertised in some form of public media. Federal civil rights laws prohibit any recruitment that indicates discrimination based on religion, race, color, national origin, age, sex, height, weight, or marital status. Most companies also have a policy that requires a notice of all vacant positions be posted on the bulletin board, in company newsletters, and in other public places to allow for recruitment from within the organization. The main advantage to recruitment from within is a promotion to a higher position for an employee. The practice may serve to bolster morale, if employees know that they can progress from one position to another. On the other hand, hiring from within may prevent bringing in employees with new and sometimes better ideas.

Selection

After prospective employees have been recruited, a process for screening out unacceptable applicants must be in effect. A wide variety of tools are used to aid in the selection process, as described in the paragraphs that follow.

APPLICATION BLANK The application blank provides biographical data and specific information relating to the applicant's skills and abilities. All requested information should have a purpose, such as for research or for determining eligibility for the job. For example, more detailed information may be required from an applicant seeking a position as a dietitian than from an applicant seeking a position as a kitchen helper. In compliance with federal guidelines, each state government interprets and establishes basic rules and regulations. According to the Michigan Department of Civil Rights (1981), some informational items are considered unlawful preemployment inquiries, as shown in Figure 14-4. Additional information may be required for payroll and fringe benefit purposes but should not be included on the employment application. Data such as marital status, number of dependents, and other pertinent information can be lawfully secured subsequent to hiring and should have no bearings on the selection process. Sections of the Civil Rights Act provide for similar protection for the handicapped if the information is unrelated to the individual's ability to perform the duties of a particular position. For example, dietitians are employable with the following handicaps: (1) amputated limb; (2) such medical disabilities as heart trouble, tuberculosis, diabetes, and loss of hearing; (3) wheelchair bound; (4) physically dwarfed; and (5) paraplegia.

It is important for the employer to examine all job-related questions, keeping in mind that race, sex, and other stereotype information may contribute to bias in the selection process.

PREEMPLOYMENT TESTS The use of tests will vary depending on the level of the position to be filled and the required skills of the applicant. Tests are frequently administered after the initial screening and prior to the personal interview. Commonly used tests include the following:

1. *Intelligence tests* measure applicants' capacity for learning and indicate the level of their ability in problem solving. The test must be culture-free to prevent bias in the selection process.

2. *Aptitude tests* measure the probable success an applicant will achieve in a specific job classification. The test may be a combined aptitude–interest instrument designed to indicate both talent and preferences for certain jobs.

3. *Achievement tests* measure the degree of skill in specific area such as typing, spelling, cooking, and diet modification. The test may be of the norm-

SUBJECT	LAWFUL PRE-EMPLOYMENT INQUIRIES	UNLAWFUL PRE-EMPLOYMENT INQUIRIES
NAME:	Applicant's full name. Have you ever worked for this company under a different name? Is any additional information relative to a different name necessary to check work record? If yes, explain.	Original name of an applicant whose name has been changed by court order or otherwise. Applicant's maiden name.
ADDRESS OR DURATION OF RESIDENCE:	How long a resident of this state or city?	
BIRTHPLACE:		Birthplace of applicant. Birthplace of applicant's parents, spouse or other close relatives. Requirement that applicant submit birth certificate, naturalization or baptismal record.
AGE:	*Are you 18 years old or older?	How old are you? What is your date of birth?
RELIGION OR CREED:		Inquiry into an applicant's religious denomination, religious affiliations, church, parish, pastor, or religious holidays observed. An applicant may not be told "This is a Catholic, (Protestant or Jewish) organization."
RACE OR COLOR:		Complexion or color of skin.
PHOTOGRAPH:		Requirement that an applicant for employment affix a photograph to an employment application form. Request an applicant, at his or her option, to submit a photograph. Requirement for photograph after interview but before hiring.
HEIGHT:		Inquiry regarding applicant's height.
WEIGHT:		Inquiry regarding applicant's weight.
MARITAL STATUS:		Requirement that an applicant provide any information regarding marital status or children. Are you single or married? Do you have any children? Is your spouse employed? What is your spouse's name?
SEX:		Mr., Miss or Mrs. or an inquiry regarding sex. Inquiry as to the ability to reproduce or advocacy of any form of birth control.
HEALTH:	Do you have any impairments, physical, mental, or medical which would interfere with your ability to do the job for which you have applied? Inquiry into contagious or communicable diseases which may endanger others. If there are any positions for which you should not be considered or job duties you cannot perform because of a physical or mental handicap, please explain.	Requirement that women be given pelvic examinations.
CITIZENSHIP:	Are you a citizen of the United States? If not a citizen of the United States, does applicant intend to become a citizen of the United States? If you are not a United States citizen, have you the legal right to remain permanently in the United States? Do you intend to remain permanently in the United States?	Of what country are you a citizen? Whether an applicant is naturalized or a native-born citizen; the date when the applicant acquired citizenship. Requirement that an applicant produce naturalization papers or first papers. Whether applicant's parents or spouse are naturalized or native born citizens of the United States; the date when such parent or spouse acquired citizenship.

Figure 14-4. Preemployment inquiry guide. *From Michigan Department of Civil Rights (1981)*

NATIONAL ORIGIN:	Inquiry into languages applicant speaks and writes fluently.	Inquiry into applicant's (a) lineage; (b) ancestry; (c) national origin; (d) descent; (e) parentage, or nationality.
		Nationality of applicant's parents or spouse.
		What is your mother tongue?
		Inquiry into how applicant acquired ability to read, write or speak a foreign language.
EDUCATION:	Inquiry into the academic vocational or professional education of an applicant and the public and private schools attended.	
EXPERIENCE:	Inquiry into work experience.	
	Inquiry into countries applicant has visited.	
ARRESTS:	Have you ever been convicted of a crime? If so, when, where and nature of offense?	Inquiry regarding arrests.
	Are there any felony charges pending against you?	
RELATIVES:	Names of applicant's relatives, other than a spouse, already employed by this company.	Address of any relative of applicant, other than address (within the United States) of applicant's father and mother, husband or wife and minor dependent children.
NOTICE IN CASE OF EMERGENCY:	Name and address of person to be notified in case of accident or emergency.	Name and address of nearest relative to be notified in case of accident or emergency.
MILITARY EXPERIENCE:	Inquiry into an applicant's military experience in the Armed Forces of the United States or in a State Militia.	Inquiry into an applicant's general military experience.
	Inquiry into applicant's service in particular branch of United States Army, Navy, etc.	
ORGANIZA- TIONS:	Inquiry into the organizations of which an applicant is a member excluding organizations, the name or character of which indicates the race, color, religion, national origin or ancestry of its members.	List all clubs, societies and lodges to which you belong.
REFERENCES:	Who suggested that you apply for a position here?	

*This question may be asked only for the purpose of determining whether applicants are of legal age for employment.

Figure 14-4. (*Continued*)

referenced or criterion-referenced type. In the norm-referenced test, an applicant's score is compared with those of all other applicants. In the criterion-referenced test, and applicant's score is compared to an established standard, and the participant must score at a certain level in order to be considered for the position.

4. *Personality tests* are used to measure an applicant's personal traits. The test may consist of a list of personal questions requiring a *yes* or *no* answer; or it may consist of projective techniques, requiring the applicant to tell what certain images mean to him or her. Using projective type personality test, the applicant describes what he or she sees in a number of standardized inkblots. A trained psychologist analyzes the test results and can often recognize psychological tendencies that may enhance or hinder good work performance. Psychologists do not regard the results as conclusive evidence of an individual's personality.

The tests used for employee selection should be designed to predict which applicant will be the best worker for a particular job. Management must understand that test scores can provide only an estimate, rather that precise measurements, of an applicant's capabilities. If tests are used, it is recommended that more than one test be given, since several tests are considered more dependable than a single test.

According to Schmidt and Hunter (1981), the fact that many false beliefs about job aptitude test results are widely accepted by personnel psychologists may have serious consequences for productivity in the work force. The authors summarized research that contradicts the following myths.

- Employment aptitude tests' validities must be newly determined in each setting, company, or agency.
- An aptitude test may be valid for one job but invalid for another job.
- Tests that predict performance in training programs may not predict on-the-job performance, and vice versa.
- Selection procedures have very little impact on organizational productivity.
- A difference in average test scores between minority and majority groups demonstrates that the test is unfair.

The interpretation of research data can be pro or con, and from different perspectives, as indicated by the position taken by enforcement agencies responsible for ensuring equality of employment opportunity. As reported by Schmidt and Hunter (1981), the American Psychological Association's Division of Industrial and Organizational Psychology revised its standards on employment testing and selection, based of their interpretation of findings in the late 1970s. As a result of the revision, there is inconsistency in standards between the Uniform Federal Guidelines on Employment Selection Procedures and those of the professional organization for test and measurement. Since guidelines to unify federal selection procedures have only been in effect since 1978, it appears that more research is needed before federal standards are changed.

SCREENING FOR SUBSTANCE ABUSE One of the problems facing management today is the widespread use of drugs, and the resulting impact on productivity. Among the few drug addicts who are motivated to seek employment, most are discharged or dismissed within a short period of time because of absenteeism, poor performance, or theft to support their habit. Ideally, it is better to screen prospective employees for substance abuse before they are hired. One method is a new system used for screening applicants, known as Emit (Anon. 1982A). Applicants are screened for opiates, methadone, PCP ("angel dust"), cocaine, cannabis (marijuana and hashish), barbiturates, and amphetamines, as well as for tranquilizers. When such screening techniques are used, management must take care in reducing the risk of discrimination charges by requiring all applicants to undergo the same screening process and by obtaining adequate legal counsel prior to administering the test.

From a legal perspective, preemployment testing or screening may be the safest option for management because the individual is not yet an employee vested with employment rights (Henry and Parrish 1988). Testing of current employees is riskier than preemployment testing for several reasons, as follows:

1. The constitutional right to privacy (Fourth Amendment of the U.S. Constitution).
2. Equal employment laws (Federal Rehabilitation Act of 1983).
3. Wrongful discharge litigation ("good" or "just" causes or implied contract with employee).
4. Civil tort liability (invasion of privacy, defamation, and intentional infliction of emotional distress).
5. Collective bargaining agreements (National Labor Relations Act (NLRA), unemployment compensation).

In making decisions related to drug use in the workplace, organizations often implement tough policies, such as mandatory testing. According to Schreier (1988), dealing with substance abuse is more than a policy and testing issue; it involves values, motivation, stress, communication, change, and conflict management. Companies that have avoided or decreased drug use in the workplace have done so through training supervisory and management personnel, creating employee assistance programs, and emphasizing both substance abuse and management issues. In a survey to training professionals, including health care, 65 of the respondents have formed employee-assistance programs. Only 26.7% provide training, with most of the training focusing on policy and procedures and a lesser amount on confronting, counseling, and legal issues.

To assist the personnel officer in screening applications, other tools should be available, such as a job analysis, job specification, and job description.

JOB ANALYSIS Job analysis involves a detailed study of the job in terms of duties, tasks, procedures, and organizational aspects. It includes careful observation and investigation of all job essentials. The job analysis attempts to answer the following questions:

1. What is the job?
2. What kinds of tasks are involved and how do they cluster together?
3. What are the features of the job?
4. What employee behavior is required in the job?
5. What personality characteristics may be required?
6. How can the job analysis assist the selection process?

A number of techniques are used to obtain meaningful data about the job to be analyzed. The method used may or may not involve employee participation. Employees, as incumbents on the job, may provide information through a personal interview, recording in a daily diary, or completing a checklist or questionnaire about job content. A nonparticipative technique is the use of an expert job analyst to observe the incumbent as various activities are performed. When it is necessary to analyze a new position, occupational information may be obtained by means of a small survey of incumbents at other facilities, or the use of a technical conference at which experts write down activities based on recall. In addition to work activity, the method used must also provide an estimate of skills and knowledge, supervision, job and human interrelationships, and physical and mental requirements. The method used must be appropriate for the position to be analyzed. It is much easier to analyze a job composed of repetitive tasks than one that is supervisory in nature. For supervisory or managerial positions, the analysis should cover the routine day-to-day task as well as the weekly, monthly, annual, and other organizational projects involved. Figure 14-5 shows a sample job analysis for the position of assistant director of foodservice in a 400-bed hospital. The sample job analysis is a summary of activities rather than a detailed breakdown of each task. Figure 14-6 depicts a sample job analysis for a kitchen helper. The analysis is job-oriented and far less complicated than for a higher-level position. Interpersonal skills are not considered high priority for this position.

The job analysis is basic to other tools used in the management of personnel, such as the job description, job specification, job standards, and job classifications. In addition, the job analysis can serve other useful purposes:

1. Planning work activity during nonpeak periods.
2. Studying work methods as a basis for work simplification.
3. Determining work methods and procedures.
4. Preparing training needs and schedules.
5. Improving recruitment and hiring procedures.
6. Discovering job performance requirements as a basis for orientation and training.
7. Proving job content to aid in better supervision.
8. Providing facts for union negotiations and job classification.

Assistant Director—Food Service Department

Daily (A.M.)

Review mail basket for notices concerning the department, bills, meetings, etc.

Consult with Chief of Clinical Services and Production Supervisor on menu, personnel, census, etc.

Consult with Cafeteria Service Supervisor on menu, personnel, etc.

Meet with director on agenda for the day, meetings, special assignments, etc.

Review lunch menu for the day and if necessary, give special instructions to Production Supervisor.

Review menu, production worksheet, and recipes for the following day, and check with storeroom personnel on availability of food items.

Order food items as needed.

Check with storeroom personnel on deliveries for accuracy and proper storage.

Inspect kitchen and dining area for cleanliness.

Check counter setup in dining room and on tray line. Make sure lines start on time.

Sample all lunch food items.

Daily (P.M.)

Work on special project or one of weekly duties.

Check work schedule for following day. Document any and all absences and tardiness, following standard procedures.

Check dinner menu with Late Supervisor.

Check counter setup in dining room and on tray line. Make sure lines start on time.

Sample dinner meal.

Weekly

Review cycle menus and make necessary changes relative to cost, availability of food items, acceptance, and manpower.

Make meal rounds.

Monthly

Attend staff meetings, assigned committee meetings, and employee meetings.

Write report on status of department goals and objectives.

Make out work schedule for all employees.

Monitor daily record of food cost and assist with monthly inventory.

Conduct and evaluate employee in-service program, and all other external training programs assigned.

Participate in departmental quality assurance program.

Annually

Assist in the development of the department's budget.

Write performance ratings on employees.

Review and evaluate policies, procedures, job descriptions, and standards of work. Update as necessary for compliance with accrediting agencies.

Develop goals and objectives for the smooth operation of the department. Review on a timely basis.

Figure 14-5. Job analysis for assistant director.

9. Discovering related and overlapping jobs that may be combined.
10. Determining the work load when new systems, new equipment, or new work methods are introduced.
11. Providing data on safety precautions necessary to protect an employee's health.
12. Providing data on time constraints in performing various tasks.

JOB DESCRIPTION A job description is an organized list of general statements that reflects the duties and responsibilities of a job. The statements are complied from the job analysis and should include all essential duties that are

```
                              Kitchen Helper
Prepare dish machine.                   Change mop heads.
   Fill machine with water.             Fill pot and pan sink with hot water.
   Check temperatures.                  Add sanitizing solution to final rinse sink.
   Check soap dispensing levels.        Add soap to wash sink.
Operate dish machine.                   Scrape pots and pans of excess food.
Scrape, prewash, and stack soiled dishes.   Clean pots and pans.
Wash dishes, glasses, cups, and trays.  Stack and store clean pots and pans.
Wash silverware.                        Clean processing equipment.
Soak cups for removal of stains.        Clean pot and pan washing area.
Remove and store clean dishes, glasses, Assist in tray assembly.
   and cups.                            Place food items on trays.
Remove and stack clean trays.           Load food trucks.
Remove and store clean silverware.      Deliver food trucks to patient areas.
Clean dish machine inside and outside.  Dismantle tray assembly line.
Remove trash in dishroom area.          Pick up food trucks from patient areas.
Clean floors in dishroom area.          Remove trays from food carts.
Remove and dispose of old grease from   Wash and sanitize food carts.
   kitchen areas.                       Clean equipment in tray assembly area.
Empty trash in production and service   Sweep floor in tray assembly area.
   area.                                Remove all trash from tray assembly area.
Sweep floors in production and cafeteria Mop floor in tray assembly area.
   areas.                               Change mop head.
Mop floors in production and service
   areas.
```

Figure 14-6. Job analysis for kitchen helper.

routinely performed. The job description should not be cluttered with occasional tasks that may be required of a worker in the position. For those less frequently performed tasks, a statement at the end of the list of duties, such as "all related tasks," will suffice. A job description (Fig. 14-7) must be precise enough to serve as a selection tool, yet flexible enough to serve functional purposes in the organization. The job description may be written in narrative or outline form, to include identifying information, job summary, and duties and responsibilities. There should be a job description for each position shown on the organization chart. In the management of personnel, the job description can serve the following purposes:

1. Matching qualified applicants to the job.
2. Establishing orientation and training programs.
3. Establishing performance appraisal standards.
4. Establishing job classification and rate of pay.
5. Determining limits of authority and responsibility.
6. Clarifying chain of command.

JOB SPECIFICATION A job specification is a written statement of the minimum requirements that must be met by an applicant for a particular job. The specification is based on the job analysis and is used primarily by the personnel officer in screening job applicants. Typical information found in a job specification (see Fig. 14-8) include (1) experience required; (2) education required; (3) special training, knowledge, and skills needed; (4) personal requirements; (5) working conditions; (6) hours of work; (7) job classification, wage code, and grade; (8) promotional opportunities; (9) test required; and (10) professional or craft affiliation, license, and certification.

Position Title: _____ Kitchen Helper _____ Classification: _____

I. *Introduction*

Position is located in production and service areas of foodservice department, under direct supervision of production supervisor. Works in dishroom, kitchen, and patient service area as assigned.

II. *Duties and Responsibilities*

1. Operates dish machine to wash dishes, glasses, cups, trays, and silverware.
2. Stores clean serviceware.
3. Cleans dish machine and dishroom area.
4. Washes pots, pans, and processing equipment.
5. Stores clean equipment and utensils.
6. Cleans pot and pan area.
7. Assists with tray assembly.
8. Delivers food carts to patient areas.
9. Picks up food carts from patient areas.
10. Cleans and sanitizes food carts.
11. Assists in maintaining preparation and service area in sanitary condition.
12. Performs other related duties as required.

_____   _____
Signature of Foodservice Director   Date

Review Dates:

_____   _____

_____   _____

Figure 14-7. Job description for kitchen helper.

Job Specification: _____ Kitchen Helper _____ Date Reviewed: _____

Experience

None required.

Education

A minimum of eighth grade education.

Knowledge, Skills, Abilities

Able to read, write, and understand instructions.

Physical Demands

Must be able to remain standing for most of working hours.
Must be physically fit as determined by physical examination.
Must be nonallergic to a variety of soaps, detergents, and cleaning compounds.
Must be able to lift at least 35 pounds.

Working Conditions

Must be able to perform repetitive tasks.
Must be able to work flexible hours, either early or late shifts.
Must be able to work flexible days—weekdays and weekends.
May be exposed to sharp instruments, and power-driven equipment.
May be exposed to hot, humid work areas.

Figure 14-8. Job specification for kitchen helper.

Personal Interview

The personal interview is usually the final step prior to making a decision on the hiring of an employee. The interview is an important part of the selection process and should receive adequate time and attention from the foodservice director or person conducting the interview.

BEFORE INTERVIEW Some factors to consider before the interview begins are the following:

1. Determine goal of interview, such as to hire a cook in a full-time, part-time, or contingency position.
2. Prepare an outline as a guide during interview. Study all information about the prospective employee, previously obtained from the application blank, tests, and references.
3. Schedule interview at a convenient time. The time should be convenient for both the interviewer and interviewee. Provide plenty of time to obtain adequate information for effective decision making.
4. Provide privacy. The interview should be conducted in a private office, without undue interruptions by telephone calls or by other employees entering the room.

DURING INTERVIEW The following guidelines will help the person performing the interview:

1. Permit the interviewee to *settle down* before beginning the interview.
2. Make question open-ended to avoid *yes* or *no* answers. Seek information not included on application form.
3. Be a good listener. Let the interviewee finish one question before asking another, allowing time to think about the question before answering.
4. When in doubt about what the interviewee is saying, summarize the statement. Make frequent use of *why* and *how*. Do not hesitate to probe for a more complete answer.
5. Use language appropriate for the skill level of the position to be filled.
6. Do not let the interviewee know your sentiments. Avoid taking sides on issues.
7. Be in control of the interview at all times. Follow a prepared outline to make sure all pertinent questions are asked.
8. Avoid writing down answers to questions during the interview. The practice will inhibit the interviewee from talking freely.

AFTER INTERVIEW The steps to follow after the interview include the following:

1. Inform applicant when final decision will be made on selection.
2. Review and reflect on information gained through interview and record pertinent data.
3. Compare personal interview notes with references, application, and other credentials for consistency.
4. Make selection decision on the basis of objective data.
5. Inform personnel office of your decision.
6. Inform applicant of your decision.

Orientation

Orientation and training programs should be organized, consistent, and conducted by individuals knowledgeable in the job content. The practice of assigning a new employee to work with another employee until he gets the *hang of it* is one of the poorest methods of introducing a new employee to the job. The length of the orientation and training period is not as important as the thoroughness of information provided. A recommended program includes (1) general orientation and (2) specific orientation and training.

General Orientation

During this 2-day period, the trainer and employee follow a checklist (Fig. 14-9), prepared from the employee handbook, to cover all pertinent information of a general nature. The emphasis at this time is to develop an understanding of the organizational structure and the interrelationship of systems and subsystems, and to familiarize the new employee with policies, procedures, and job responsibilities. Each employee receives a copy of the handbook to keep for future reference.

Orientation and Training Guidelines

Training is for a 2-week period. During the first week, the employee has an opportunity to observe, demonstrate, and practice all functions listed in the job description (Table 14-1). Performance standards are explained during the discussion and observation periods so that the employee is aware of the quality and quantity of work expected. During the second week, the employee has an opportunity to work independently, under supervision, in all assigned work areas (Table 14-2).

At the end of the second week of training, the employee is either scheduled for a regular shift or referred for additional training, based on the performance rating (Fig. 14-10). Factors used for rating training performance are the same as those used in the performance standards.

Performance Evaluation

The terms *performance evaluation*, *performance rating*, and *performance appraisals* are often used interchangeably to indicate a process of measuring work accomplishment. The evaluation of employee performance is a serious and important part of a manager's job and should not be looked upon as a dreaded activity to be accomplished at set intervals. Employee evaluation is an ongoing process, not a once-a-year task. Each time an employee is praised for doing a good job or criticized for below-standard performance, evaluation is taking place on an informal basis. When such incidents are documented and used as a basis for evaluation, the formal evaluation process becomes less difficult.

Depending on the methods used for performance evaluation, there can be an enormous amount of fear, tension, and anxiety generated at the time of rating. After all, an employee's future may depend on, or at least may be influenced by, the rating. To alleviate the unpleasantness associated with employee evaluation, the following steps should be beneficial to both management and employees:

PART I—General Orientation

Name: _____ Date of Hire: _____

Union: _____ Nonunion: _____ Orientation Date: From _____ To _____

All new employees must be given an orientation to the Dietary Services on the first and second day of employment, by the supervisor in charge of training.

The intent of the orientation is to familiarize the new employee with various aspects of the Foodservice Department and the hospital; and to prepare him or her for a thorough on-the-job training to be followed by in-service education.

Instructions for Preparing Checklist

1. This checklist must be prepared by the supervisor in charge of training. Check √ indicates that explanation has been given.
2. Employees must sign in the appropriate section of the checklist.
3. Additional orientation must be provided for employees with a below-average rating.

	Comments	Date

___1. The functions and purposes of a hospital have been explained.

___2. The organization structure of Metropolitan Hospital has been explained.

___3. Organization of Dietary Department—Show chart.
Lines of authority
Services provided by the department
___Inpatient meal service
___Cafeteria meal service
___Therapeutic diet counseling

___4. Was given a tour of the Foodservice Department and introduced to staff members.

___5. The following policies and procedures have been explained:
___A. Wages and payroll
___Rate of pay
___Pay day
___Overtime pay
___Payroll deductions
___B. Hours of work
___Time schedule
___Mealtime, rest period
___Holidays
___Sick leave
___Vacation
___Punching of time clock
___Leave of absence with or without pay
___C. Union affiliation
___D. Personal health and appearance
___Physical examination
___Food handlers' card requirement
___Good hygiene
___Uniform regulations
___Identification nameplates
___E. Sanitation and safety
___Disaster drill
___Fire regulations and drill
___Infection control

Figure 14-9. General orientation. *From Metro Medical Group, Health Alliance Plan, Detroit, Michigan*

	Comments	Date
___F. Miscellaneous		
___Personal records		
___Correct address, telephone number requirement		
___Locker regulations		
___Personal use of telephone		
___Smoking regulations		
___G. Standards of conduct		
___Dependability		
___Absenteeism		
___Punctuality		
___Call-in		
___Emotional control		
___Patient relationship		
___Tact and courtesy		
___Staff relationship		
___Tact and courtesy		
___Use of proper name titles		
___H. Job description		
___General duties		
___Specific duties		
___Work schedule		
___I. Job performance evaluation		
___Accuracy		
___Neatness		
___Judgment		
___Initiative		
___Work standard		

I acknowledge that each topic outlined in the orientation checklist was explained to me by a supervisor prior to the on-the-job training required.

_____

Employee's signature

_____

Date

2-Day Orientation
Supervisor's recommendation and rating (Use PEP (Performance Evaluation Program) ratings)

_____ *Recommendation*

_____ Continued employment ☐

_____ Do not continue employment ☐

_____ (If recommendation is no, make comment

Evaluator's signature: _____ _____

  Date: _____ _____

Department head signature: _____ _____

  Date: _____

Figure 14-9. *(Continued)*

Table 14-1. Week 1—Orientation and Training Guidelines for Kitchen Helper[a]

Monday	Tuesday	Wednesday	Thursday	Friday
Review general orientation Function and purpose Organization structure Job description Performance standards *Discuss and observe dishwashing* Operation of dish machine Tray-veyor Prewashing and stacking soiled dishes Washing silverware Removing clean dishes Removing clean silverware Cleaning dish machine Cleaning dishroom	*Demonstrate and participate in dishwashing* Participate under supervision in operating dish machine according to procedures and standards Stripping and stacking trays Handling of clean dishes and trays, delivery to stations Washing silverware, handling and storing clean silverware Removing coffee stains from cups Cleaning dish machine Cleaning dishroom area	*Discuss and observe porter* Tour kitchen and cafeteria, pointing out areas to be swept and mopped Observe preparation of cleaning solutions and equipment used Observe time and frequency of cleaning Observe collection of trash and grease and method for disposing *Practice porter functions* Participate under supervision in: sweeping floors, mopping floors, removing trash, emptying old grease	*Discuss and observe pot and pan washing* Tour pot-washing area pointing out areas to be kept clean and sanitized Observe pot-washing procedure: filling sinks with water cleaning and sanitizing solutions disposing of food waste operation of garbage disposal cleaning pots and pans and processing equipment stacking clean pots and pans storing clean utensils cleaning work area *Practice pot and pan washing* Participate, under supervision, in washing pots, pans and utensils	*Discuss and observe tray assembly* Observe tray assembly line Placing items on patient food tray Loading food trucks according to procedures Delivering and pick-up of food trucks Cleaning tray assembly area Cleaning tray carts *Practice tray assembly functions* Participate under supervision, in assembling, loading, transporting carts to patient area and cleanup

[a]From Metro Medical Group, Health Alliance Plan, Detroit, Michigan

Table 14-2. Week 2—Orientation and Training Guidelines for Kitchen Helper[a]

Monday	Tuesday	Wednesday	Thursday	Friday
Early dishroom Employee assigned to early dishroom shift with a trained employee and, under supervision, functions independently. Evaluate and determine area for more practice.	*Late dishroom* Employee assigned to late dishroom shift with a trained employee, and under supervision functions independently. Evaluate and determine area for more practice.	*Porter* Employee assigned to porter schedule with a trained employee, and, under supervision, functions independently. Evaluate and determine area for more practice.	*Pot washer* Employee assigned to pot washer schedule with a trained employee, and, under supervision, functions independently. Evaluate and determine area for more practice.	*Tray assembly* Employee assigned to assembly with a trained employee, and under supervision, functions independently. Evaluate and determine area for additional practice. *Note:* If more training is needed in any area, retraining is scheduled. Otherwise, employee is scheduled to a shift.

[a]From Metro Medical Group, Health Alliance Plan, Detroit, Michigan

309

| Position Title: <u>Kitchen Helper</u> | | | | Department: <u>Dietary</u> |

Prepared by: _____

  Supervisor: _____ Department Head: _____

Name of Employee: _____

Training Period Date: _____ to _____

Standard Training Rates

Objective: For the new food service employee to develop a proper learning attitude, to achieve and maintain high standards of efficiency and quality.

Dishroom	Excellent	Satis-factory	Unsatis-factory	Comments

1. Properly operates dishmachine at designated temperatures using prescribed quantities of solution.
  a. Washing solution Guardian Esteem
  b. Pre-wash temperature 100°F–120°F
  c. Wash temperature 140°F–160°F
  d. Final rinse temperature 180°F–200°F				

2. Scrapes excessive food particles from patients' trays and dining room patrons' dishes.
  a. Food particles in garbage disposal.
  b. Paper waste in trash receptacle.				

3. Soiled dishes and trays stacked separately and uniformly in racks.				
4. Routinely stacks clean dishes in lowerators or appropriate containers according to description and delivers to proper kitchen areas.				

5. Soiled silverware presoaked in proper solution and cleaned according to standard procedure.
  a. Pre-soak solution (Textrox)
  b. Separate silverware place in cylinders, with handle up.				

Porter

	Excellent	Satis-factory	Unsatis-factory	Comments
1. Thoroughly cleans and sanitizes kitchen floors, dining area, offices, and rest rooms on daily basis. a. Cleaning solution: Conquest				
2. Routinely cleans and sanitizes refrigerators, freezers, and other equipment as needed.				
3. Collects trash and garbage from kitchen and dining room and disposes in dumpsters as needed.				
4. Frequently wipes up spillage on floors and work surfaces.				

Pot and Pan Washing

	Excellent	Satis-factory	Unsatis-factory	Comments

1. Prepare pot washing sinks according to standard procedure.
  a. Washes sink with hot water and solution. Solution: Textrox, 2 Tbsp to each gallon of water.
  b. Rinses sink with clear hot water only.
  c. Sanitizes sink with hot water and sanitizing solution. Solution: 3 oz. Wescodyne per $2^1/_2$ gallons of water. Note: Add Wescodyne after the water is in the sink to avoid foaming.
  d. Scrapes excessive food particles from pots, pans, and utensils.
  e. Places discarded food items in garbage disposal. Note: Do not put bones or pour grease in disposal.				

Figure 14-10. Performance rating—Orientation and Training. *From Metro Medical Group, Health Alliance Plan, Detroit, Michigan*

Pot and Pan Washing (continued)	Excellent	Satis-factory	Unsatis-factory	Comments
2. Maintains clean hot water. When the water in any sink becomes greasy or cooled, empty the sink and repeat preparation of that sink.				
3. Allows pots, pans, and utensils to air-dry. a. Stacks clean, dry pots and pans on shelves according to size and shape. b. Returns clean, dry utensils to proper storage areas.				
4. Safely cleans and sanitizes food processing equipment according to procedure. a. Food slicer b. Food chopper c. Food grinder d. Potato peeler				
5. Cleans and sanitizes work area daily. a. Sinks b. Racks c. Countertops d. Floor work area				
Tray Assembly				
1. Loads patient trays in food carts in sequential order with proper tray identification.				
2. Checks trays for neatness (no spills on trays, covers, each food item neatly arranged and properly placed on trays).				
3. Prepare and set up tray assembly work stations as assigned at each meal period (proper utensils, dishes, etc.).				
4. Accurately serves food items and/or accessories on patient trays according to prescribed diet menus regular or therapeutic ($1/2$ cup, $1/4$ cup regular, salt-free, etc.).				
Transporting Food Carts				
1. Safely and promptly transports food carts to appropriate patient areas.				
2. Safely and promptly transports food carts complete with soiled trays to dishwashing area in kitchen. a. Designated time after each meal service: Breakfast 8:45 A.M., Lunch 12:45 P.M., Dinner 5:30 P.M.				

Figure 14-10. *(Continued)*

1. *Develop job standards.* Job standards are predetermined criteria based on work samplings of duties and responsibilities as listed in the job description. For example, employees should not be told that "you are working too slow" or "your work is not of good quality," unless standards have been developed. The terms "slow" and "good" are too ambiguous and subjective to be of any value in evaluating work performance. As shown in Figure 14-11, all standards should be stated in measurable terms. Employees should know how much is to be done (quantity), how well it is to be done (quality), how fast the job is to be done (time limitations), and how the job is to be done (policies or procedures).

2. *Determine purpose of evaluation.* What is the evaluation used for? Is it routine paperwork that must be accomplished every 6 months or once a year? If the evaluation is used for a specific purpose such as promotion decisions, salary

Position: Kitchen Helper

1. *Quantity of work.* Acceptable standards are indicated when: All dishes are washed and ready for meal service.

2. *Quality of Work.* Acceptable standards are indicated when: All dishes, glasses, and silverware are free from spots.

3. *Job Knowledge.* Acceptable standards are indicated when: Instructions are followed correctly in operating equipment.

4. *Cooperation.* Acceptable standards are indicated when: Employee willingly accepts related duties.

5. *Display of Initiative.* Acceptable standards are indicated when: Employee develops a better way to perform job and reports it.

6. *Reliable.* Acceptable standards are indicated when: Employee reports for duty as scheduled.

7. *Appearance.* Acceptable standards are indicated when: Clean uniforms are worn daily.

Figure 14-11. Job standard.

increase, or employee training and development, then the employee should be so informed.

3. *Develop performance evaluation tools.* Performance evaluation is the appraisal of an employee's performance against the job standards established for the position. It represents an objective review of how well the employee has performed and the possibilities for improvement and advancement. Factors included on the performance evaluation form should be identical to those listed on the job standards. A sample form is shown in Figure 14-12. Any factor can be used to evaluate employees if it is objective and easily understood by both the rater and employee. For example, supervisory personnel may require expertise in leadership, labor relations, cost containment, resourcefulness, and interpersonal relationships.

4. *Communicate with employees.* Each employee should have a copy of the job description and job standards for the job he or she is hired to do. The manager should communicate throughout the appraisal period by letting the employee know when a job is well done or when improvements are needed. There should not be any shocking revelations during the performance appraisal conference.

5. *Encourage employee participation.* One method of involvement is to inform the employee in advance that the evaluation will take place on a specified date. Ask the employee to prepare for the conference as follows:

a. Review your job description and job standards.
b. Compare your performance against the standards. Note the areas where you have done well and areas where the improvements are needed.
c. Make suggestions on how your work performance can be more effective. Suggestions may involve your section or the entire department.
d. For the conference, scheduled on _____, bring the assessment of your performance with you so that we can fully discuss your evaluation.

METROPOLITAN HOSPITALS AND HEALTH CENTERS
EMPLOYEE PERFORMANCE EVALUATION FORM

ANNIVERSARY ☐   TERMINATION ☐   PROBATIONARY: 60-DAY ☐   80-DAY ☐   OTHER (INDICATE): _____

EMPLOYEE NAME _____POSITION_____ DEPARTMENT _____

DATE OF HIRE _____DATE OF LAST EVALUATION _____

UNION AFFILIATION: MTLA_____OPEIU_____MNA_____UPGWA_____LPNLM_____NON-UNION_____

RATING	EXCELLENT	ABOVE AVERAGE	AVERAGE	BELOW AVERAGE	UNSATIS FACTORY	NOT APPLICABLE	PERFORMANCE APPRAISAL COMMENTS (Must Be Completed for all Ratings)
FACTORS ALL ABSENCE							DAYS
PUNCTUALITY							TIMES
QUALITY							
QUANTITY							
FACTORS DEPT							

TERMINATION NOTICE: Type of Termination: Voluntary Quit ☐   Release ☐   Discharge ☐   Effective Date of Termination _____

Appropriate termination notice given: Yes ☐   No ☐   Date notified of termination: _____

Date last worked: _____ Would you recommend for rehire: Yes ☐   No ☐   (if No, explain in "General Comments")

ALL SECTIONS BELOW MUST BE COMPLETED BY EVALUATOR

GENERAL COMMENTS: _____

AREA(S) OF SUPERIOR SKILL OR PERFORMANCE: _____

AREA(S) FOR IMPROVEMENT: _____

EMPLOYEE COMMENTS: _____

EMPLOYEE SIGNATURE _____ DATE _____

TO THE EMPLOYEE	My signature means that I have read this rating and it has been discussed with me. This does not mean that I agree or disagree with the statements made.

DEPARTMENT HEAD SIGNATURE _____DATE _____EVALUATOR SIGNATURE _____DATE _____

PER-58 (1-79) REV

PERSONNEL DEPT.

Figure 14-12. Performance evaluation form. *From Metro Medical Group, Health Alliance Plan, Detroit*

During the conference, there may be some disagreement on the final evaluation. The rater should be prepared to reach mutual agreement with documents made throughout the appraisal period rather than depending on recall. The use of objective, factual documents can remove the personal element from the discussion, and the time saved can be spent on corrective action, if necessary.

Education and Training Programs

Employee training begins as soon as the individual is hired. The training may be of an informal nature such as learning from other workers how to perform certain tasks, or it can be more directed and controlled. The latter type of training is recommended for long-term operational efficiency. It is the foodservice director's responsibility to make sure that an effective education and training program is established and conducted on a continuous basis. In large- or medium-sized facilities, the education and training duties are performed by a qualified dietitian on a full-time basis. A variety of titles are used for the position, including In-Service Educator, Dietetic Educator, Director of Training and Development, among others. The individual may be responsible for all training provided by the foodservice department.

The types of education and training programs may be classified as follows.

── Required Training ──────────

These programs consist of the following:

- Orientation of new employees.
- In-service training for all employees.
- Outside education for supervisory personnel.

── Optional Training ──────────

These programs include the following:

- Outside education for all full-time employees.
- Field or work experience for high school students.
- Clinical experience for students in dietetic assistant and dietetic technician programs.
- Practicums and work experience for college students in dietetics and food systems management.
- Clinical experiences for students in Coordinated Undergraduate Programs (CUP).
- Clinical experiences for students in dietetic internships sponsored by other hospitals, public schools, and public health departments.
- Six months of practical experience for graduate students in dietetics.
- Internship program for dietetic students.

Written documentation is required for all training provided by the food-service department. For orientation, a training schedule such as the one used for the kitchen helper's position should be established and used for each position in the department. Documentation on in-service training can be accomplished each time training is conducted by using a form such as the one depicted in Figure 14-13. Space is allotted for recording names of those attending the training session, as well as space for the topic, summary, and evaluation. The form should be kept on file for future reference. All topics used for in-service training are derived from an assessment of needs and are scheduled for presentation so that employees from all work shifts can participate. Outside training for supervisory personnel may be in the form of workshops, seminars, conferences, formal classes, and other meaningful sources.

Optional education and training programs are provided by most medical foodservice operations. Contractual agreements are drawn up and signed by appropriate administrative personnel at both the requesting institution and the facility providing the training. The contract, frequently referred to as a *Master Agreement,* has provisions for continuation or termination by either party. Thereafter, a one-page document, as shown in Figure 14-14, is normally sufficient to show that the foodservice department is in accord with accepting a student for training during a specified time period. A record of affiliation (Fig. 14-15), maintained by the foodservice department, is required and should be kept on file. Training programs for students in the CUP, internship, and graduate work experience must be approved and/or accredited by the American Dietetic Association. Qualified dietitians must be available for the supervision of students when they are directly engaged in patient care activities.

Date _____

Subject: _____

Presenter–Trainer: _____

Attendance:

1. _____   9. _____

2. _____   10. _____

3. _____   11. _____

4. _____   12. _____

5. _____   13. _____

6. _____   14. _____

7. _____   15. _____

8. _____   16. _____

Summary of discussion:

Evaluation and follow-up:

Figure 14-13. Record of in-service training.

Supervised Work Experience

Student's name _____ Date _____
I.D. number _____ Telephone number _____
Major _____ Course number _____ Credit hours _____
Location of training _____
Training period: _____ to _____

Description of study

  Purpose: To gain practical experience in the operation and administration of a foodservice department.

  Scope and limitation: Student will actively participate in all phases of the foodservice operation.

Procedure–activities:

1. Review the foodservice department organizational chart, policies, and procedures.
2. Study the administration of food production in the following areas: menu planning, purchasing, receiving, storing, pre-preparation, salad units, sanitation, equipment maintenance, use, and care.
3. Work on special assignments, such as banquets and luncheons, at the discretion of the coordinator.
4. Turn in written report of each assignment.
5. Use attached assignment sheet as study guide.

Approved by:

_____
Coordinator's signature

_____
Academic advisor's signature

Figure 14-14. Agreement form for work experience.

Record of Affiliation

Trainee experience site _____

Address _____

City _____ State _____ Zip code _____

Name of trainee _____ Title _____

Area of learning experience _____

Number of weeks _____ Date: From _____ to _____

Signature of trainee _____ Date _____

College attended _____ Date: From _____ to _____

_____   _____

Signature of in-service educator   Date

_____   _____

Signature of Executive Director, Dietetics   Date

Figure 14-15. Record of affiliation form. *From Detroit-Macomb Hospital Corporation*

___ In-Service Training _____

There are four basic steps involved in establishing an in-service training program:

1. *Assessing needs.* Allow employee participation during this stage. Employees will suggest topics for which they feel a need and are of interest to them. This approach will serve to get the program off to a good start. Include areas where work improvement is needed by referring to previous evaluations or inspection reports. Topics such as safety, sanitation, infection control, proper production and service techniques, personal hygiene, and new policies and procedures are always important.

2. *Planning.* Compile all topics gathered during the assessment stage. Prioritize topics for presentation based on relevancy and degree of urgency. Be prepared to answer the following questions:

   a. Who will conduct training sessions?
   b. Who will attend training sessions?
   c. Where will training sessions take place?
   d. When will training take place?
   e. Will the training schedule include convenient time periods for employees on all shifts?
   f. How much advance time is required for posting notice of training sessions so that supervisors can plan assignments?
   g. How will employees be informed of training sessions?
   h. What methods of teaching will be used?
   i. Where are resources located?
   j. What form of evaluation will be used?

3. *Implementation.* Be prepared for each training session. Have all materials, supplies, and equipment ready before the session begins. Trial-test all equipment to make sure that it is working properly. Complete a written lesson plan for each scheduled session (Fig. 14-16). Adjust training methods to meet needs of individuals or groups; that is, it is necessary to consider factors such as length of session, learning speed, language barriers, attention span, state of

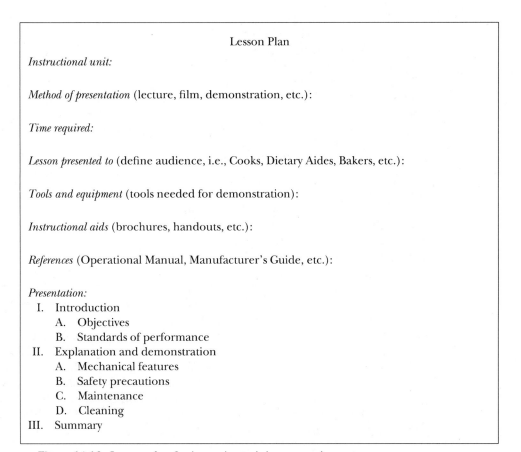

Lesson Plan

Instructional unit:

Method of presentation (lecture, film, demonstration, etc.):

Time required:

Lesson presented to (define audience, i.e., Cooks, Dietary Aides, Bakers, etc.):

Tools and equipment (tools needed for demonstration):

Instructional aids (brochures, handouts, etc.):

References (Operational Manual, Manufacturer's Guide, etc.):

Presentation:
  I. Introduction
     A. Objectives
     B. Standards of performance
 II. Explanation and demonstration
     A. Mechanical features
     B. Safety precautions
     C. Maintenance
     D. Cleaning
III. Summary

Figure 14-16. Lesson plan for in-service training on equipment.

learning readiness, motivation, nature of material or task, and the amount of guidance needed. Provide an atmosphere that is conducive to learning. Allow trainees an opportunity to ask questions and take part in discussions and demonstrations. Provide feedback throughout the training session to promote the learning concept of reinforcement.

4. *Evaluation.* This final step actually begins with the assessment stage of training. When an employee is observed to be performing a task at less than the established proficiency rate, training is indicated. For corrective action to take place, a transfer of knowledge is required to improve particular skills, knowledge, and/or attitudes. Assuming that appropriate training was used, the evaluation tool should measure any change in behavior that has taken place. Depending on training objectives, the evaluation may be in the form of (a) written test questions, (b) oral responses, or (c) demonstrations (actual or simulated). The evaluation tool should be criterion-referenced, based on performance standards. Training evaluations are confidential, and therefore precautions should be used throughout the training process to protect employee rights.

One important in-service training topic is in the area of infection control, and more specifically, of human immune deficiency virus (HIV) or acquired immune deficiency syndrome (AIDS). Medical facilities are required to have infection control committee and establish policies and procedures to protect employees and patients (JCAH 1988). Although medical facilities have always treated patients with infectious diseases, AIDS has generated a high degree of fear in that the disease is fatal with no cure. Another reason for the fear is that the general population is not convinced that transmission routes are limited to those identified at this time.

318   Foodservice Subsystems

The Center for Disease Control (CDC) expects that with 1.5 million persons now believed to be infected by HIV, the number of AIDS cases may grow to 270,000 by 1991 from the 40,000 that had been reported as of August 1987; thus, there is an increased potential for exposure to health care workers (USDL–USDHHS 1987). CDC has recommended universal precautions for all patients, eliminating the need for the isolation category of blood and body fluid precautions. The recommendations have been endorsed by the American Hospital Association and by proposed guidelines of the National Committee for Clinical Laboratory Standards. In a survey of Society of Hospital Epidemiologists (SHEA) to determine their opinion on and their hospital's actual practice of universal precautions, HIV screening, and informed consent (Miller and Farr 1988). Of the respondents, 57% opposed the CDC recommendations to eliminate the category of blood and body fluid precautions, preferring to continue use of the category for patients with documented infections. This may explain why some medical facilities have discontinued use of isolation, whereas others continue to isolate patients with infectious diseases, including those with AIDS.

Foodservice employees do not have direct patient contact, but they must be aware of the potential for exposure. Training sessions to inform employees of known transmission routes will serve to dispel misinformation, and thus fear of casual contact. The trainer needs to be aware of facility policies on isolation and other procedures for infection control, present factual information, and document training to meet standards of Occupational Safety and Health Administration (OSHA) and those of the Joint Commission on Accreditation of Hospitals (JCAH). Consultant Dietitians in Health Care Facilities (1988) have developed an excellent training tool for in-service education on infection control and other foodservice-related topics. Foodservice directors in hospitals should collaborate with human resource development personnel to develop appropriate training tools.

Union–Management Relations

Unionization can be defined as a process whereby a group of employees, sharing similar interests, voluntarily agree to form an association for the purpose of maintaining or improving wages, hours of work, and working conditions. Although unions have been legally active since the mid-thirties, it was not until passage of the 1974 Amendment to the National Labor Relations Act (Public Law 93-518, 93rd Congress, 2nd Session) that medical care facilities felt the impact of unionization.

Major Legislation

Legislation designed to ensure the rights of both labor and management, includes the following:

1. *Norris-LaGuardia Act (Anti-Injunction Act)* of 1932 (U.S. Code Service. Title 18, Section 3692) was the first major federal legislation dealing with union activity. The intent of the law was to remove some of the hostility associated with employees' attempts to organize by placing restraints on employers and courts in dealing with union efforts and labor disputes. The act guaranteed the right to strike, to pay strike benefits, to picket, to ask other employees to strike, to assist financially in labor disputes, and to meet on strike strategy.

2. *Wagner Act (National Labor Relations Act—NLRA)* of 1935 (U.S. Code Service. Title 29, Section 151+), encouraged the growth and strength of unions by promoting practices and procedures of collective bargaining and the choosing

of representation for negotiation purposes. The Act made it legal for employees to organize and illegal for employers to interfere in such efforts. Unfair labor practices by an employer were specified as (a) interference with an employee's right to join a union or with union activity, (b) discrimination in hiring or discharging of employee based on union activity, and (c) refusal to bargain in good faith.

3. *Taft-Hartley Act (Labor Management Relations Act—LMRA) of 1947* (U.S. Code Service. Title 29, Section 141+) was passed to provide a balance of labor and management rights by (a) amending the NLRA, (b) providing additional facilities for mediation of labor disputes, and (c) equalizing legal responsibilities of labor organizations and employers. The act specifically exempted health care facilities from union activity.

4. *Landrum-Griffin Act (Labor Management Reporting and Disclosure Act— LMRDA) of 1959* (U.S. Code Service. Title 29, Sections 153, 158-160, 164, 186, 187, 401+) served to redefine and state unfair management–labor practices in more specific terms.

5. *1974 Amendment to the NLRA and the LMRDA* included nonprofit medical care facilities under jurisdiction of the National Labor Relations Board (NLRB) for the first time. The amendment defined health care facilities to include any hospital, convalescent hospital, health maintenance organization, health clinic, nursing home, extended care facility, or any other institution devoted to the care of sick, infirm, or aged persons. Due to the nature of activities conducted in medical care facilities, special collective bargaining provisions were included in the amendment as follows:

a. The employer or union must adhere to a 90-day notification period versus a 60-day period for other industries.
b. For negotiation of contract renewal or modification, a 90-day notice by the employer or union is required versus a 60-day notice period for other industries.
c. Prior to the termination or expiration of a collective bargaining contract, the Federal Mediation and Conciliation Service (FMCS) must be given a 60-day notice versus 30-day notice for other industries.
d. The health care facility and the union may be required to participate in the mediation process for both renewal and initial contracts, at the discretion of the FMCS versus no such provisions for other industries.
e. The union must give the health care facility and the FMCS a 10-day notice prior to any picketing, strike, or other form of refusal to work versus no such provision for other industries.
f. When there is a threatened or actual work stoppage that would impair health care delivery, the FMCS has the authority to establish an impartial board of inquiry to investigate the labor–management dispute and to make a written report of the findings.

▬ Managerial Responsibilities ▬▬▬▬▬▬▬▬▬

In order to carry out responsibilities related to union activity, a manager needs to understand the collective bargaining process and the strategy and tactics to use during organizing campaigns. *Collective bargaining* is a method of negotiation to resolve problems of employment. Employers must negotiate in good faith on wages, hours of work, fringe benefits, and conditions of work. Other items, such as grievance procedures, disciplinary actions, vacation times, holidays, leaves of absence, and seniority rights may also be part of the bargaining package. If a settlement is not agreed upon by the ninetieth day of collective bargaining, a mediator may be brought in to assist in reaching a decision. A *mediator* is an impartial third party whose primary purpose is to restate the positions of each side, to ensure harmonious agreement, and to encourage continuation of the collective bargaining process. Interventions by a mediator are not binding; the role is to assist or influence parties. *Arbitration* is also a process of involving a third party in the negotiation process. The difference between a mediator and an arbitrator is that the decision made by the arbitration is binding for both parties. Unresolved controversies result in an impasse, culminating in a strike or lockout by the party willing to impose the most pressure.

The union is authorized to strike if a majority of its members vote in favor of withdrawing services. The strike is normally called at a time when the most pressure can be exerted on management. When a strike is called, management may use its prerogative and hire replacements for the strikers. Striking employees that have been replaced by permanent new hires have no right to their job at the end of a strike. If the employer has not replaced the striking workers during the strike, then the employer must take the strikers back at the end of the strike.

Managerial strategy and tactics used during an impending union election must be within guidelines established under fair labor practices (Azoff & Friedman 1982). Management can do the following:

1. Restrict solicitation in immediate patient areas, such as patient rooms, operating rooms, and places where patients receive treatment, including corridors adjacent to patient rooms, sitting rooms on patient floors adjacent to or used by patients, and elevator and stairs used primarily to transport patients.

2. Prohibit solicitation and distribution during an employee's working time. Meal and break times are considered nonwork time even when paid for by the health care facility.

3. Prohibit outside organizers from entering the property.

4. Include the following information in a letter to employees: (a) encouragement to vote, (b) cost of union dues, and (c) fringe benefits provided and how they compare with other health care facilities.

The laws also provide for protection against unfair employer practices as follows:

1. Employers cannot interfere with the formation or administration of labor organizations. (a) They should not make promises or threaten employees in any way that may influence voting outcome. (b) They should not spy on union activities, ask employees about union activities, advise employees in their union activities, or make charges against unions during the union drive.

2. Employers cannot discriminate against employees in hiring or tenure because of their union activity. They should not fire or threaten to fire an employee because of union activity, favor certain employees without merit consideration, discipline without sufficient warning, or transfer any employee in efforts to dilute union activity.

3. Employers cannot discharge or discriminate against employees because they have filed charges against the company. Employees should be allowed to file charges and testify to illegal employer actions without fear of reprisal from management.

4. Employers cannot interfere with employees in their right to bargain collectively with their own representatives. (a) They should avoid any appearance of interference with union activities. (b) They should assure employees that they will not be discriminated against for union activities.

5. Employers cannot refuse to bargain collectively with the employee representatives. They should become thoroughly familiar with union proposals and counterproposals from management.

It may appear that management is confronted with undue restraints in the formation of administration of labor organizations, but unions also have legal responsibilities. The laws provide for six unfair union practices as follows (Azoff & Friedman 1982).

1. Unions cannot force employees to join a union unless a legal union shop exists. A *union shop* is a security provision in which all workers must join the union within a specified period of time after hiring. (Union shops are illegal in the public employment sector.) A *closed shop* is a union security whereby the employer is required to hire union members only. Membership in the union is also a condition of continued employment. (Closed shops are also illegal in the public employment sector.) An *agency shop* is a union security provision that calls for nonunion employees in the bargaining unit either to join the union or pay the union fee, usually equal to union dues. A conscientious clause allows individuals who oppose joining organizations for religious or deeply felt philosophical beliefs to be exempted from payment of union dues or fees. However, they may be required to contribute an amount equal to union dues to a tax-exempt charitable organization.

2. Unions cannot pressure employers to force employees to join a union or discriminate against employees who have denied union membership, unless they have failed to pay dues under a union shop agreement.

3. Unions cannot refuse to bargain collectively with an employer if they are the legal representative of employees.

4. Unions cannot engage in secondary boycotts to force an employee to not do business with any other person or business. Unions cannot strike to force an employer to assign work to one union rather than another, or to force an employer to recognize a union that is not certified as the legal representative of the employees.

5. Unions cannot charge excessive or discriminatory fees.

6. Unions cannot cause an employer to pay for services that are not performed.

The negotiated contract is binding for both the employer and employees. It is a manager's responsibility to study the contract, to know the rights and power of management, to know the employees rights, to know the duties and rights of the steward, and to understand procedures for settlement of grievance and disciplinary action.

___ Grievances _____

A *grievance* is defined as any difference of opinion or any dissatisfaction arising between the health care facility and employee(s) in the interpretation or application of any provision of the contract agreement.

The grievance procedure is normally part of the negotiated contract. If no procedure exists, an employee has the right to file a grievance as outlined in Section 9 of the Taft-Hartley Act. Grievance procedure may vary from one facility to another, especially in the time involved for resolution. Depending on a grievance step, the time may vary from 2 to 30 days. A sample grievance procedure is outlined below.

Step One: The foodservice employee shall discuss the grievance with his or her immediate supervisor, with or without the steward at the option of the employee. In the event the grievance is not satisfactorily settled within five (5) working days, it shall be referred to step two.

Step Two: The foodservice employee and/or steward shall reduce the grievance to writing and submit it to the employee's department head with a copy to the personnel office. The department head shall meet with the employee, the steward and unit chairman within two (2) working days. The department head will give the steward his or her written answer, with a copy to the unit chairman within three (3) working days after the meeting. If a satisfactory settlement is not reached, the grievance shall be referred to step three within three (3) working days after receipt of the written answer.

Step Three: The grievance committee, representative(s) from the union, the steward and the foodservice employee shall take the grievance up with the executive administrator or his or her designate. A meeting with the executive administrator or designate will be held within three (3) to ten (10) working days. The executive administrator or his or her designate shall give the union representative and the unit chairman written answer within five (5) working days after the meeting. If a satisfactory settlement is not reached, the grievance shall be referred to step four within five (5) working days after receipt of the written answer.

Step Four: An impartial arbitrator shall be mutually agreed to within five (5) working days between the union and the employer. In the event that mutual agreement on an arbitrator cannot be reached within the above period, either the union or the employer will submit the grievance to the American Arbitration Association. The employer and the union agree to follow the rules of the American Arbitration Association. The arbitrator shall be empowered to rule on all grievances within the established contract and wage structure. The cost of arbitration shall be shared equally by the employer and the union. No arbitrator shall have any right to change, add to, subtract from, or modify any of the terms of any written agreement existing between the parties. The decision of the arbitrator shall be final and binding on both parties.

It is unrealistic to expect a foodservice department to operate without employee gripes, complaints, and grievances. A manager's responsibility is to resolve complaints as promptly and correctly as possible. Regardless of how minor or invalid a grievance appears to be, serious consideration must be given to all complaints. The objective is to handle gripes and complaints before they develop into formal grievances.

GUIDES TO HANDLING GRIEVANCES The following five steps will help the manager in dealing with complaints.

1. *Define nature of grievance.* Pinpoint the main issues involved so that the reply can address each point. Determine whether the grievance refers to a provision of the contract agreement or other policies and procedures in the department or facility.

2. *Gather all facts.* Answer questions of who, what, when, where, and how. Be precise in documenting day, month, year, and time of day the incident occurred. Check files for precedent. Review the employee's past record for pertinent facts that may have a bearing on the decision.

3. *Assemble and verify facts.* Do not take anything for granted. Can facts be substantiated by departmental or facility records? Can certain facts be supported by reliable witnesses? Do you have written statements from witnesses? If not, you may not be able to rely on a witness to testify since many individuals are

subjected to pressures from peers or other sources. Has the contract been violated? Has the employee been unfairly treated?

4. *Make decisions.* Be consistent with contract and facility policies. Make sure that the decision is based on facts that will be considered fair and just, should the grievance progress to the arbitration step. Check with higher administration in any areas of uncertainty.

5. *Communicate decision.* The written reply should be well organized, arranged by subject or by order of events. Make sure the words used in denying a formal grievance state precisely your reason for denial. Cite the exact provisions of the contract or policies and procedures of the facility that gives you the authority for your decision. Follow technical regulations, and comply with time limits as provided in grievance procedures.

Disciplinary Action

The term *disciplinary action* refers to the steps taken to correct undesirable behavior. All managers must take disciplinary actions at one time or another because employees do not always follow policies and standard operating procedures. Since the word "discipline" implies some form of punishment, careful attention is needed to make sure that the action taken does not result in negative attitudes toward work accomplishment. The aim of management should be to change behavior or attitude rather than just to invoke a punishment. Most union contracts include provisions for disciplinary actions similar to procedures for settling grievances.

Types of Disciplinary Actions

The type of disciplinary action taken depends upon the nature of the offense. Normally, a progressive system is used, beginning with an oral warning and continuing, if necessary, to the final step of discharge, as follows:

1. *Oral warning.* An oral warning is a privately conducted interview between the supervisor and the employee to discuss the nature, cause, and corrective actions pertaining to the violation. The employee has an opportunity to give a full explanation of circumstances under which the violation occurred. Based on facts and the employee's explanation, the supervisor can either accept the explanation or make it clear to the employee why the explanation is not acceptable and how improvements can be made. A notation is made in employee's record for follow-up action. The employee is informed of the written notation and subsequent notations on improvements. Oral warnings are considered as *temporary* in the employee record.

2. *Written warning.* A written warning is given for a repeat violation or as the first disciplinary action if the circumstance warrants. The employee is given an opportunity to explain and express his or her view of the circumstances. The employee is informed of the written warning by letter of a standardized form, as shown in Figure 14-17. The employee may reply to the written warning. The disciplinary report and the employee's reply are forwarded to the personnel department and become a permanent part of the employee's record.

3. *Suspension.* A suspension is a forced leave of absence, without pay. The length of time depends on the nature of the violation. The procedure for administration and reply by the employee are similar to that for a grievance, with time allowed for reply. The disciplinary action becomes a permanent part of an employee's record.

To: Personnel Department

From: Foodservice Department

Re: (Name of employee, position, or classification)

The following (warning or separation) was issued today, and it is to be made part of the official record.

1. ( ) Defective and improper work	9. ( ) Reporting under influence of drugs
2. ( ) Insubordination	
3. ( ) Carelessness	10. ( ) Gambling
4. ( ) Unauthorized activities	11. ( ) Firearms or other weapons
5. ( ) Tardiness	12. ( ) Confidential information
6. ( ) Disorderly conduct	13. ( ) Safety
7. ( ) Unauthorized absence	14. ( ) Destruction of property
8. ( ) Pilferage	15. ( ) Other violations

Remarks (Set forth all facts in detail including time, date, and circumstances):

_____

_____

_____

_____

_____
Signature of supervisor   Date

I have read this report
_____
Signature of employee   Date

Employee reply attached: yes ( ) no ( )

The above offense has been noted and is made a part of the above employee's record, as of this date.

_____
Offense no. 1 2 3 4   Personnel Department   Date

_____
Name of Health Care Facility

Figure 14-17. Employee disciplinary report.

4. *Dismissal.* Dismissal is the most severe type of disciplinary action. In some instances, it may be used for the first offense, but normally a progression of actions has been taken prior to terminating an employee. This disciplinary action is used less frequently than types 1, 2, and 3 because of the cost of training a new employee. Procedures to follow should be provided in the contract agreement or in organizational policies and procedures.

The use of demotion as a disciplinary action is seldom used because of the effect it will have on the work environment. Transfers are considered more appropriate. Disciplinary actions can be abusive if left to the discretion of individual supervisors. Care must be taken to make sure that penalties are appropriate for the offenses and are applied in a consistent and fair manner. The guidelines shown in Table 14-3 can be helpful to both supervisor and employees in maintaining an atmosphere of good discipline in the workplace. The violations and penalties should be posted so that employees are aware of consequences.

Table 14-3. Guidelines for Disciplinary Action

Offenses	Penalties			
	First Offense	Second Offense	Third Offense	Fourth Offense
Defective and improper work—work below standard in quality and quantity.	Oral warning	Written warning	Suspension	Dismissal
Insubordination—direct refusal or delay in carrying out instruction.	Oral warning	Written warning	Suspension	Dismissal
Carelessness—significant waste of food or supplies; attempt to cover-up waste or destroy evidence of waste.	Oral warning	Written warning	Suspension	Dismissal
Unauthorized activities—significant participation in unauthorized activities during work hours; sleeping; leaving assigned work areas; promoting non-work-related activities.	Oral warning	Written warning	Suspension	Dismissal
Tardiness—reporting late for assigned work shift; returning late from authorized breaks.	Oral warning	Written warning	Suspension	Dismissal
Disorderly conduct—use of abusive language; quarreling; boisterous acts, causing disruption in production and service.	Written warning	Suspension	Dismissal	
Unauthorized absence—leaving work without permission. Failure to report for work one day, except in case of emergency. Failure to report for work three consecutive days, except in case of emergency.	Written warning Suspension Dismissal	Suspension	Dismissal	
Pilferage—theft or attempts to steal organizational property, or the property of others.	Suspension to dismissal	Dismissal		
Reporting under influence of drugs—reporting to work under the influence of alcohol, drugs or narcotics; drinking while on duty; use of drugs or narcotics.	Written warning to suspension	Suspension to dismissal	Dismissal	
Gambling—misuse of organization time for gambling.	Suspension to dismissal	Dismissal		
Firearms or other weapons—concealing weapons, or the use of any weapon against another person on organization property.	Dismissal			
Confidential information—revealing confidential information about patients and their families.	Dismissal			
Safety—acts considered dangerous to self and others:				
Minor infraction	Written warning	Suspension	Dismissal	
Major infraction	Written warning to suspension	Suspension	Dismissal	

Table 14-3. Guidelines for Disciplinary Action (Continued)

Offenses	Penalties			
	First Offense	Second Offense	Third Offense	Fourth Offense
Destruction of property—intentional destruction of organization property or property of others:				
Minor infraction	Written warning to suspension	Suspension	Dismissal	
Major infraction	Suspension to dismissal	Dismissal		
Other violations—other administrative policies, rules, and regulations not listed; penalties based on employee's awareness of rules and regulations, and adverse affect on maintenance of discipline in the department.	Oral to written warning	Written warning to suspension	Suspension to dismissal	Dismissal

Guides to Constructive Disciplinary Action

The purpose of disciplinary action should be to correct or change an employee's action or attitude before circumstances reach the dismissal stage. The following guidelines should be helpful:

1. When it is necessary to discipline an employee, use the opportunity to train and control by making constructive criticism and following up with an explanation of how the incident should be handled.

2. Refrain from reprimanding a worker at the height of an emotional state or in the presence of other employees.

3. Practice fair and consistent treatment of all violations. A supervisor cannot afford to overlook incidents involving a certain employee simply because it will be difficult to replace the individual. Employees are constantly aware of what other employees are "getting away with."

4. Handle the interview or counseling session so that the employee will realize the seriousness of the violation and will be open to future cooperation.

5. Understand progressive discipline. Document efforts made to rehabilitate the employee prior to suspension or dismissal stages.

6. Investigate and review all facts prior to making a final decision on penalty. If necessary, check with higher administration before informing the employee of your decision. A supervisor loses credibility when decisions are rescinded at a higher level.

Employee Turnover

The rate of employee turnover in the medical care industry is high as compared with other industries. A survey of nonbusiness groups, nonmanufacturing groups, and finance was conducted by the Bureau of National Affairs (Anon. 1982B). Results indicated that the health care industry was tied with finance for the highest turnover rate. A contributing factor for high turnover may be the low salary scale associated with the nonprofessional service-type jobs in hospitals and other health care facilities. The concern of management should be to determine the cause of high turnover and take corrective action over areas of control. One method of determining the cause of turnover is the use of an exit interview.

THE EXIT INTERVIEW The exit interview is equally as important as the hiring interview, and should be a routine management practice whenever an employee leaves the organization. Management should be aware of reasons for turnover with detailed figures on causes of separation for reasons such as death, retirement, accidents and illness, dismissals, layoffs, marriage, moving to another area, obtaining a better job, and attending school. It is less expensive to maintain a stable labor force than to hire and train new personnel.

Classifying departure, regardless of the reasons given by the employee, into specific categories can provide valuable information for use in recruitment, hiring, job design, and other areas of managerial control. Categories used for why individuals leave the work force may include:

1. Performance ratings—marginal, satisfactory, outstanding.
2. Work shift—early, late.
3. Length of time on job—0–1 year, 1–3 years, 3–5 years, 5–10 years, 10 years or more.
4. Rate of pay—step I, II, III, IV.
5. Type of job—cashier, dishwasher, cook, etc.
6. Education level—K–8, 9–12, 1–2 years in college, 3–4 years in college.
7. Previous work experience—0–1 year, 2–3 years, 4–5 years, 6–10 years, 10 years or more.
8. Previous job tenure—0–1 year, 2–3 years, 4–5 years.

Personnel Record Keeping

Personnel records may be defined as records kept by an employer that may be used for employment, promotion, salary decisions, or disciplinary action. A separate record is maintained for each employee assigned to the department. The manager must be aware of what can or cannot be included in an employee's file and the rights of employees to the information therein. Federal, state, and local laws have been passed to protect the privacy and confidentiality of records maintained on employees.

Employee Right to Know Act

In Michigan, the *Bullard-Plawecki Employee Right to Know Act* (Department of Management and Budget 1978) established new restrictions on the manner in which Michigan employers may legally manage their work force. The law was based on the concept that individuals have the right to know the nature of information being kept about them. The provisions of the act include employee access, disputes over accuracy of data, record-keeping restrictions, and release of information to a third party.

EMPLOYEE ACCESS Upon written request, which describes the file in question, an employer must give an employee the opportunity to review that file. The review may be during hours or at some other convenient time and place. If an on-site review is impossible, the employer must mail to the employee a written copy of the record specifically requested. Reviews may be limited to two times in a calendar year. Upon completion of a *review*, an employee so requesting must be given an opportunity to copy all or part of the information in the file.

EXEMPTIONS TO EMPLOYEE ACCESS The following parts of the file do not have to be released to the employee:

1. Letters of references, if the identity of the source is disclosed.
2. Staff planning materials relating to compensation projections, promotions, and job assignments if materials relate to more than one person.
3. Medical reports if the employee can secure access through the medical facility or doctor involved.
4. Information that could infringe upon another individual's privacy.
5. Separate files pertaining to grievance investigations if the grievance records are not used relative to an employee's qualification for employment, promotion, transfer, compensation, or discipline.
6. Records kept by individual managers not shared with other persons. However, if employee access to such information is denied, the data may not be entered in a personnel file later than 6 months after the information was recorded.

DISPUTES OVER ACCURACY OF DATA If agreement cannot be reached over the accuracy of information in the personnel file, the employee has the right to amend the file with a statement of his or her position, not to exceed five sheets of standard size paper. Either party can invoke legal action to remove false information knowingly put into the file by either party.

RECORD-KEEPING RESTRICTIONS Employers are barred from keeping a record of an employee's political activity, associations, publications, or communications relating to nonemployment issues unless they occur on the employer's premises, or during working hours, or written authorization is given by the employee.

Records of criminal investigators may be excluded from review only if they are kept separately from all other personnel record information. Upon completion of investigation or after 2 years, whichever comes first, the employee must be notified of the investigation. If disciplinary action is not taken, the file must be destroyed.

RELEASE OF INFORMATION TO A THIRD PARTY Employers are required to notify employees by first class mail if any information relative to discipline is divulged to third party, unless:

1. The information is disseminated to the employee's labor organization.
2. The disclosure is ordered in a legal action or arbitration.
3. Dissemination is made to a government agent pursuant to claim or complaint made by an employee.
4. The employee has waived such requirements by signing a written statement to that effect on the employment application of another employer.

Managers should review record-keeping practices for assurance of complaints with applicable laws. Depending on how the *open-file* policy is approached and presented, it can serve to enhance employer-employee relations. In addition to requirements and restrictions just stated, the Bureau of Employment Standards (Michigan Department of Labor 1980) requires that an employer must keep employment records for each employee as follows:

1. An employer shall keep employment records for each employee showing all of the following: (a) name; (b) home address; (c) date of birth; (d) occupation in which employed; (e) total daily hours worked, computed to the

nearest unit of 15 minutes; (f) total hours worked in each pay period; (g) total hours worked in each work period when the work does not coincide with the pay period; (h) total hourly, daily, or weekly basic wage; (i) total wages paid each pay period; (j) itemization of all deduction made each pay period; and (k) separate itemization of all credits for meals, tips, and lodging against the minimum wage taken for each pay period, if any.

2. If a credit is taken for meals and/or lodging provided to an employee, the employment records shall contain a statement signed by the employee that acknowledges that the meals and/or lodging were received.

3. If employees of a hospital or institution agree to have their overtime computed on the basis of a 14-day work period pursuant to section 4a(3) of the act, the employment records shall contain the written agreement or written employment policy arrived at between the employer and the employee and shall be dated prior to the effective date of the agreement.

4. Records required under this rule shall be preserved by the employer for 3 years after the date thereof.

Employee Safety

An orientation on the hazards of safe practice related to specific job assignments should be incorporated into the orientation and training program recommended for each new employee. Management has a responsibility to train employees in safe work practices. Employees have a responsibility to cooperate by the application of safe work practices. Since work-related accidents and illnesses are costly for the employer, most organizations established and maintained effective safety programs before they were mandated by federal law.

Occupational Safety and Health Administration — (OSHA)

According to OSHA guidelines (U.S. Department of Labor, 1972), a safety program depends on three essentials: (1) leadership by the employer, (2) safe and healthful working conditions, and (3) safe work practices by the employees. A safety and health committee, composed of top executives, supervision, and employees should be established.

The committee should hold regular monthly meetings to discuss recommendations, accidents, records, and program plans. Policies should include:

1. Establishing procedures for handling suggestions and recommendations.
2. Inspecting an area of the establishment each month for the purpose of detecting hazards.
3. Conducting regularly scheduled meetings to discuss accident and illness prevention methods, safety and health promotions, hazards noted on inspections, injury and illness records, and other pertinent subjects.
4. Investigating accidents as a basis for recommending means to prevent recurrence.
5. Providing information on safe and healthful working practices.
6. Recommending changes or additions to improve protective clothing and equipment.
7. Developing or revising rules to comply with current safety and health standards.

8. Promoting safety and first aid training for committee members and other employees.
9. Promoting safety and health programs for all employees.
10. Keeping records of minutes of meetings.

In the event an accident does occur, the immediate supervisor on duty must assist the injured employee in obtaining medical attention. The employee may refuse medical treatment. Whether the employee receives medical treatment or not, the supervisor must complete a written report of the incident (Fig. 14-18). The report must provide detailed information including what happened and why, what could have been done to prevent the incident, and what can be done in the future. Documented in-service training records can be helpful in completing the investigation report (Fig. 14-19).

Additional standards issued by OSHA (U.S. Department of Labor 1983) known as "Hazard Communications," require chemical manufacturers and importers to assess the hazards of chemicals that they produce or import and require all employers to provide information to their employees concerning hazardous chemicals by means of hazard communication programs. OSHA defines a hazardous chemical as "any chemical which is a physical hazard or a health hazard." Employers can reply on the information provided by the chemical's manufacturer or importer on the Material Safety Data Sheet (see Appendix L) to determine whether the chemical is hazardous. Employers are not required to test independently or otherwise evaluate the hazard potential of chemicals purchased and used in the workplace.

All employees who are exposed, or may be accidently exposed to hazardous chemicals must be trained, as must employees of contractors and subcontractors who are working at the facility and are exposed to hazardous chemicals—for example, outside cleaning contractors, especially if the facility provides cleaning compounds. It is also important to know what chemicals are used by exterminators.

The foodservice director has the responsibility to:

1. Review and become familiar with the organization's written policies and procedures on its Hazard Communication Program.
2. Develop and maintain lists of each chemical used in the department. Keep list current. A list of discontinued chemicals should be on file for 30 years with information on where and why it was used.
3. Maintain file on all Material Safety Data Sheets, preferably in a loose-leaf notebook, arranged in alphabetical order. There should not be any blank spaces on the sheet. If information requested is not applicable, then the designation "NA" should be entered.
4. Develop safe use instructions from MSDAs and make them available in workplace for employee review, updated as necessary. If employees are interested in more detailed information, they must be shown the actual MSDA. If an employee requests copies of MSDA, chemical materials lists, or written programs, the request must be in writing.
5. Use label format for all containers designated as hazardous (see Appendix M).
6. Provide in-service training for all employees who are exposed or may be exposed to hazardous chemicals and for employees of contractors who are working in the department. Train all new employees before they begin work. Provide additional training when a new hazardous chemical is introduced or when new information becomes available on a chemical currently in use.

EMPLOYEE INCIDENT REPORT

This form is to be used in reporting any injuries involving employees:

DMH _____
SMH _____
JMH _____
DMHA _____

Date of Incident _____ Time _____ a.m. p.m.   Exact Location _____
                                                                            (department and room no.)

Name of Injured:

_____
          (Last)   (First)   (Middle Initial)   (Age)

Describe in Factual Terms:
    What Happened:

    Incident Site (foot of bed, etc.):

    Who Witnessed the Incident:

Name of Individual   a.m.
Reporting Incident:_____Date _____ Time _____ p.m.

Reviewed By: _____ Position:_____

Physician's Statement of Medical Findings _____

Medical Treatment _____

X-Ray Indicated: Yes _____ No _____ Results _____

Signature of Examining Physician _____

Important   Complete Form 2112, Occurrence/Incident Supplemental Information, and send to administration/DMHA, SMH or JMH with the *buff* copy of this form.

Immediately after any incident, this form is to be completed and routed as follows: The original *(white)* and *yellow* copies both go to the emergency room with the employee, or as soon as possible. The *buff* copy is to be sent to the department head, who will review and forward to administration/DMHA, SMH or JMH. The emergency room will forward the original *(white)* copy to personnel and the *yellow* copy to administration/DMHA, SMH or JMH when the bottom portion of the form is completed.

Figure 14-18. Employee incident report form. *From Detroit-Macomb Hospital Corporation*

SUPERVISOR'S INVESTIGATION REPORT

This form is to be used to supply additional information in all cases of irregular occurrences, employee incidents and incidents involving visitors, medical staff, patients and others. It is to be completed in conjunction with Irregular Occurrence Report, Form 2014, Incident Report, Form 2101, or Employee Incident Report, Form 2100.

NAME (person involved)	AGE	DATE OF OCCURRENCE
EXACT LOCATION (department and room no.)	JOB	TIME OF OCCURRENCE a.m. p.m.

WHAT HAPPENED?

_____

_____

_____

_____

Describe what took place or what caused you to make this investigation.

WHY DID IT HAPPEN?

_____

_____

_____

_____

Get all the facts by studying the job and situation involved. Question by use of WHY— WHAT—WHERE—WHEN— WHO—HOW

WHAT SHOULD BE DONE?

_____

_____

_____

_____

Determine which of the 12 items under EMP require additional attention.

Equipment	Material	People
Select	Select	Select
Arrange	Place	Place
Use	Handle	Train
Maintain	Process	Lead

WHAT HAVE YOU DONE THUS FAR?

_____

_____

_____

Take or recommend action, depending upon your authority. Follow up - was action effective?

HOW WILL THIS IMPROVE OPERATIONS?

_____

_____

OBJECTIVE
Eliminate job hindrances

Investigated by	Date	Reviewed by	Date

IMPORTANT: This form is to be sent to administration/DMHA, SMH or JMH with copy of form 2014, 2100 or 2101.

Figure 14-19. Supervisor's investigation report. *From Detroit-Macomb Hospital Corporation*

Laws Relating to Personnel

In addition to the Occupational Safety and Health Act and laws covered under the broad title of Management-Union Relations, other major laws having direct impact on personnel management are (1) Fair Labor Standards Act, (2) Worker's Compensation, and (3) Unemployment Compensation.

___ Fair Labor Standards Act ___

This law, enacted in 1938 and commonly known as the Wage-Hour Law (U.S. Code Service. Title 29, Section 210) was instrumental in establishing the 40-hour, 5-day work week and uniform minimum wage.

MINIMUM WAGE The minimum wage established by the Wage-Hour Law did not include foodservice workers until 1966. The minimum wage of $0.25 hour in 1938 has been increased over the years to a minimum of $3.35 in 1983. There are exemptions to the minimum wage law. Employers granted wage exemption certificates from the U.S. Department of Labor can pay less than the minimum wage to the following worker categories:

1. *Co-op students.* Students 16 years of age who are enrolled in a state-approved technical education program and employed in a job directly related to course of study may receive no less than 75% of the minimum wage.

2. *Full-time students.* Students at least 14 years of age, enrolled in a bona fide education institution may be employed in retail, service, or agriculture related work for no less than 85% of the minimum wage.

3. *Handicapped.* The individual must be mentally or physically handicapped. Employers may pay no less than 50% of the minimum wage without approval of the state vocational rehabilitation agency; as low as 25% with prior agency approval.

THE WORK HOURS AND DUTIES Child labor laws regulate the work hours of duties of employees. Sixteen- and 17-year-old employees may work in any occupation that is not classified as hazardous by the U.S. Department of Labor. In foodservice operations, power-driven equipment such as slicers, cutters, and mixers are declared hazardous and can be operated or cleaned by students only if they are enrolled in food-related programs. All persons under age 18 must have a work permit from school, except as follows (1) 16- or 17-year-old high school graduates; (2) 17-year-olds who have passed the General Education Development (GED) test; and (3) minors who are married or have a court order of emancipation. The employer must have proof of exemption on file.

The Act has been amended to include these additional provisions.

OVERTIME PAY Overtime pay to equal one and one-half the base pay and bonuses, must be paid for all hours worked in excess of 40 hours for a 1-week period. Salaried employees in executive, administrative, or professional classification are exempt from overtime pay if no more than 40% of their time is spent in managerial-type duties and they earn a salary of at least $150 per week.

DONATED TIME If an employee donated time to an employer, it is compensable time and must be paid accordingly. According to Stokes (1981), if a foodservice worker reports for work 30 minutes early every day because that is when the bus arrives or if an employee is willing to work *on his own time* to learn skills necessary to advance, both are interpreted as compensable time.

UNIFORMS AND UNIFORM MAINTENANCE The cost of uniforms and laundry fees cannot be charged to or deducted from salary if it will reduce wages below the minimum wage level. According to Stefanick (1981), a former wage-hour investigator with the U.S. Department Labor (DOL), the DOL will accept a payment to employees of $3.35 per week if full-time employees maintain their own uniforms; and $0.67 per day worked for part-time employees.

MEAL CREDIT An employer is allowed a meal credit, as part of the minimum wage, for the cost of providing meals for employees. The federal wage-hour law does not stipulate the amount of credit allowed. However, some state laws limit the amount of deductions for meals and housing. In Michigan, restrictions and deductions allowed from minimum wage rate for meals and lodging are as follows (Michigan Department of Labor 1980):

1. An amount not to exceed 25% of the state minimum wage rate may be credited as minimum wages paid for lodging provided to an employee if the employee is informed of the cost of the lodging, which will be deducted from the wages paid, and if the employee signs a statement that acknowledges that the lodging was received.

2. An amount not to exceed 25% of the state minimum wage rate may be credited as minimum wage paid for meals provided to an employee if the employee is informed of the cost of the meals, which will be deducted from wages paid, and if the employee signs a statement that acknowledges that the meals were received.

3. Meals shall consist of adequate portions of a variety of wholesome and nutritious foods provided by the employer to the employee at the usual mealtime or as nearly as possible thereto. A wholesome meal shall include a selection of an entree of eggs, meat, fish, or poultry, two vegetables, salad, beverage, and bread and butter.

The regulation is interpreted to mean that under no circumstance can combined total deductions for lodging and meals exceed 25% of the minimum wage. However, under the new regulation, if no other credit is taken, an employer may credit the cost of the provided meal up to 25% of the minimum wage if the employee is notified of the cost amount and acknowledges that the meals were served.

EQUAL PAY The Equal Pay Law of 1963, as part of the Wage-Hour Act, prohibits wage discrimination based on sex. All persons performing similar work and having similar qualifications must receive the same rate of pay.

Civil Rights Act

The Civil Rights Act of 1964 was amended by the Equal Employment Act of 1972. The Act prohibits discrimination in employment based on race, sex, color, religion, and national origin. The Equal Opportunity Commission is responsible for administering all federal laws relating to the Equal Employment Act, including the Uniform Guidelines on Employment Selection and Promotion, Guidelines on Sexual Harassment, and Guidelines on Discrimination Because of National Origin. The Equal Employment Act impacts on all areas of personnel management from the recruitment, selection, and hiring, to performance evaluation for the designated *protected groups*. The protected groups include blacks, Hispanics, American Indians, Pacific Islanders, women, handicapped, veterans, and older persons (40–70 years old).

___ Worker's Compensation ___

Worker's compensation insurance is paid for by the employer. The programs are designed to compensate employees for disability or death resulting from accidental injury or disease related to employment, regardless of who may be at fault. Employees are entitled to weekly compensation based on a formula established by the individual state's Department of Labor.

___ Unemployment Compensation ___

Unemployment compensation, as a part of the Social Security Act of 1935, provides for payments to an employee between jobs. Eligibility requires that an individual has worked a specified number of weeks prior to unemployment and is willing to accept a suitable position offered through a state's Employment Office. The program is funded by federal and state governments from taxes paid by the employer and calculated according to total wages paid. The employee receives approximately 50% or more of his or her wages for a period of 26 weeks. The compensation may be extended for a longer period of time by acts of Congress. When an employee voluntarily quits or is fired for theft, misconduct, or destruction of property, a penalty is imposed that disqualifies the individual for a number of weeks before payment can be made.

Laws relating to human resource management are constantly changing. An alert personnel officer will keep managers informed on changes, but the ultimate responsibility rests with the individual manager.

References

American Hospital Association. (1974). *Volunteers in the Foodservice Department of Health Care Institutions.* Chicago: AHA.

Anon. (1982A). *Personal Report for the Executive—Special Report.* New York: Research Institute of America.

Anon. (1982B). Survey of Industries Find Hospitals 1st in Turnovers, 3rd in Absenteeism. *Hospitals 56*(9), 39.

Azoff, E. S., and Friedman, P. L. (1982). Solicitation-Distribution Rules: A Developing Doctrine. *Hosp. Progr. 63*(2), 44–48, 54.

Brogan, S., Callaghan, C., and Mutch, P. (1981). *Guidelines for Clinical Dietetics Time Study: A Collection of Data on Efficiency.* Lansing: Michigan Dietetic Association, Nutritional Care Practices Committee.

Callaghan, C., Larkin, F., and Wright, D. (1983). *Guidelines for Client-Learning Time Study: A Collection of Data on Effectiveness.* Lansing: Michigan Dietetic Association, Nutritional Care Practices Committee.

Consultant Dietitians in Health Care Facilities (An ADA Practice Group). (1988). Columbus, OH: Ross Laboratories.

Henry, K. H., and Parrish, S. W. (1988). Substance Abuse in the Workplace: Drug Testing and the Health Care Industry. *Health Care Supervisor.* 7(1), 1–10.

Joint Commission on Accreditation of Hospitals (1988). Chicago: JCAH.

Michigan Department of Civil Rights. (1981). *Pre-Employment Inquiry Guide.* Detroit: Michigan Civil Rights Commission.

Michigan Department of Labor, Bureau of Employment Standards. (1980). *Michigan Administrative Code 1979.* (1981 Annual Supplement, pp. 546–549.) Lansing: Legislative Service Bureau, Department of Management and Budget.

Miller, P. J., and Farr, B. M. (1988). A Survey of SHEA Members on Universal Precautions and HIV Screening. *Infect. Control Hosp. Epidemiol. 9*(4), 163–165.

Schmidt, F. L., and Hunter, J. E. (1981). Myths Meet Realities 1980s. *Management 2*(3), 23–27.

Schreier, J. W. (1988). Combatting Drugs at Work. *Train. Develop. J. 42*(10), 56–60.

Stefanick, G. J. (1981). What You Should Know About the Wage-Hour Law. *Cornell H.R.A. Quart. 22*(1), 6–11.

Stokes, A. (1979). *Cost Effective Quality Food Service.* Germantown, MD: Aspen Systems Corp.

Stokes, A. (1981). Beware of Wage and Hour Violations. *Food Serv. Market. 43*(70), 13.

U.S. Department of Health and Human Services. (1971). *A Guide to Nutrition and Food Service* (Public Health Service, USDHHS Publication No. HSM 71-6701). Washington, DC: U.S. Government Printing Office.

U.S. Department of Labor. (1972). *Guidelines for Setting Up Job Safety and Health Programs* (Stock No. 8501-17). Washington, DC: USDL, OSHA.

U.S. Department of Labor, Occupational Safety and Health Administration. (1983). Hazard Communication. *Federal Register 48*(228), 53280–53348.

U.S. Department of Labor–U.S. Department of Health and Human Services. (1987). Joint Advisory Notice: Protection Against Occupational Exposure to Hepatitis B Virus (HBV) and Human Immunodeficiency virus (HIV). *Federal Register 52*(210), 41818–41823.

Chapter 15

Subsystem for Financial Management

Medical foodservice operations have undergone major changes during the past decade in terms of managing available resources. As a result of escalating costs of medical services, all aspects of the medical organization have become more accountable for managerial action. No longer are directors of medical foodservice operations permitted to operate with unlimited budgets. Today the emphasis is on goal setting to meet quality standards within prescribed budgetary allowances. This approach requires strict internal controls in an effort to remain solvent in view of external economic cutbacks and inflation.

Food Cost Control

Food cost is a major component of financial management, and the challenge to management is to control costs while maintaining high standards of quality. Therefore, management should strive for a balance between qualitative and quantitative controls. When food costs become excessive, the easiest form of control is to raise menu prices rather than to practice effective food cost controls. Since there is an upper limit to raising menu prices, management must seek other alternatives. Cost containment begins with effective menu planning and flows through to other subsystems.

Menu Planning

The use of cyclical menus, whether they are selective or nonselective, can serve as a reliable tool for determining budgetary allowances for food. Management can readily observe changes in food prices when the same menus are used over a set period of time. To arrive at the amount of money needed for the daily meal allowance, it is necessary to precost each item on the menu. Thus, the average daily cost of foods served will be used as the daily meal allowance. The precosting can be accomplished with the use of standardized recipes, as noted in Chapter 9.

Daily Meal Allowance

Assuming that menus have been planned in accordance with the goals and objectives of the organization and have top administrative approval, then the meal allowance will be an average cost of menu items served to patients and employees. In order to calculate the average cost of menu items, the facility must use standardized recipes and must know the daily cost of all food used. For

Table 15-1. Meal Cost Allowances

Meal	Percentage	Cost
Breakfast	20	$0.60
Lunch	37	1.11
Dinner	37	1.11
Nourishment	6	0.18
Total	100	$3.00

Table 15-2. Food Category Cost Allowances

Food Category	Percentage	Cost
Appetizer	8	$0.085
Entree	50	0.56
Potato or substitute	5	0.05
Cooked vegetable	10	0.11
Salad and dressing	7	0.08
Bread	5	0.06
Dessert	8	0.085
Beverage	5	0.06
Miscellaneous	2	0.02
Total	100	$1.11

example, if the daily meal allowance is $3.00 per person per day, then each meal and each food category should receive a certain percentage of the food dollar. A typical breakdown by meal is shown in Table 15-1.

The meal breakdown is not enough to determine whether certain food items, as listed on the menu, fall within cost allowance. To assist further in the decision-making process, food categories for each meal may be designated as a percentage of the food dollar. Table 15-2 provides a breakdown for the lunch and dinner meal.

The use of precosted standardized recipes and strict portion controls will ensure that costs will be kept within the budgetary allowance. As the price of food escalates, management is in a position to make decisions based on sound financial management practices.

Employee Meals

The price of menu items served to employees and guests in the cafeteria and the price of menu items for special activities will depend on administrative policies and procedures. In some operations the food budget is partially subsidized by the medical organization, resulting in lower menu prices for employees and guests. In such cases the food cost percentage may be as high as 70% of the total price, depending on whether the food is a convenience item or one made from scratch. In other operations the cost of employee meals is considered a fringe benefit, and therefore the cost of meals is charged to labor costs. Regardless of the system used, the foodservice department should get credit for all food served.

Food Specifications

Specifications are directly related to food cost controls and should be used for all purchases to ensure quality. Well-written specifications contribute to lower bid prices because vendors know precisely what the buyer expects and know what they are bidding on. Not only should specifications be well written, but they should also be communicated to all vendors as well as to all persons responsible for purchasing and receiving food. The most effective specifications are those that indicate different levels of quality depending on the intended use for the food item. For example, tomatoes used in soups and stews need not be perfectly shaped, and fruit used in gelatin molds need not be perfectly cut.

Forecasting

Forecasting, as related to food, can be defined as a method of using available data to project the amount of food required for a meal, day, or longer period of

	200 Portions		Cost		Portions		Cost		
Ingredients	Volume	Weight	Per pound	Total	Volume	Weight	Per pound	Total	Directions

Plain Muffins

Total Servings: 100
Serving size: 2 muffins each

Cost Data

Cost per recipe   Cost per serving

Labor
Food
Energy (Conventional)
        (Convection)
Total cost
Comments: (Type of energy used, seasonability of food
items, etc.) _____

Figure 15-1. Standardized recipe card.

time. Forecasting is used to determine the amounts to purchase, the amounts to requisition from storage, and amounts to prepare. All phases of forecasting are critical in efforts to contain food costs.

Phase 1, forecasting the amount to purchase, begins with the standardized recipe. If properly formulated, as shown on the recipe card in Figure 15-1, information pertaining to portion size can be used to project the total amount needed by multiplying each portion by the projected number of servings needed.

Another tool, useful in forecasting the amount to purchase, is the production worksheet. As shown in Figure 12-3, it provides information such as the amount of food requisitioned, amount used, projected number of meals, and actual number of meals served.

Space is provided for comments by the shift supervisor that may explain discrepancies, if any, between the projected number of meals and the actual number served. Comments may refer to weather conditions, employee payday, special activities, and so on. For example, during inclement weather conditions, more employees tend to eat in the cafeteria than on fair, sunny days when they prefer to leave the facility for meals elsewhere. Also, employees tend to go out for lunch on paydays in order to cash checks. Special activities may include scheduled conferences at the facility, patient tours or outings as practiced in many nursing homes, and holidays when guests often eat with patients. The day of the week is an important variable, because the census is usually lower on weekends than during the week.

At the end of each meal, data should be recorded on the number of meals served in various categories to provide a cumulative daily total. As shown in Figure 15-2, information helpful to management is the number of meals served to patients, employees, and others. The data are necessary for the computation of daily food costs.

The record of meals served may vary from data on patient census sheets for several reasons. First, the official patient census may include patients who did not consume a meal due to NPO (instructions to not feed by mouth), leaves of absence during mealtime, or other reasons. Second, meals are frequently delivered to wards for patients who have been discharged. Third, all patients are counted on the official census—even newborn babies who receive commercial-type formulas provided by the pharmacy. Although records maintained in the dietary department may not be totally accurate, the data provide general guidelines for cost control.

Phase 2, determining amounts to requisition, is based on the type of menu item and the state of purchase (frozen, fresh, etc.). It may be necessary to requisition certain food items from storage several days in advance. For example, frozen meats that are scheduled for service on Friday should be requisitioned on Wednesday in order to allow time for thawing. Although management is still relying on past records, a more accurate prediction can be made at this time than at the time of purchase.

Phase 3, determining the amount to prepare, is the final stage of forecasting and projections are made on the day of preparation. At this time, a more accurate projection can be made because of the current information available to management, such as the selective menu tally and daily patient census. As one progresses through the forecasting stages, the amount of food needed may be more or less than the amount originally projected. For example, based on data at the time of purchase, it was determined that 200 pounds of beef was needed for 500 servings of roast beef. At the time of requisition, the weather forecast indicated a warm, sunny day. Realizing that some employees would leave the building during the meal hour, the amount of food requisitioned was reduced by 20 pounds or 50 servings less than the amount purchased. Finally, on the day of preparation, it was determined that the beef order should be reduced further because more patients selected the alternate entree than was anticipated. Since the daily food costs reflect the amount of food actually used rather than the amount purchased, management can effect a savings by observing the step outlined above in forecasting amounts of food.

—— Receiving Food ——

Errors in delivery can be costly. Individuals authorized to accept food delivered to the facility should be designated in writing by management. A copy of the policy should be communicated to all vendors. The practice of allowing anyone in the work area to sign for deliveries is not in the best interest of management for several reasons. First, unless receiving is an assigned duty, the employee may not take the time necessary to check for quantity or quality. Second, the employee will not be familiar with amounts ordered or the quoted price. An example of the type of form that may be used to designate responsible individuals is shown in Figure 15-3.

Records of all food received should be compiled by receiving personnel to provide data for managerial control. Depending on the degree of detail, a variety of forms may be used. For example, if data are needed only on the total amount of food and other items received, a form such as the one depicted in Figure 15-4 may be used.

| Day | Patients | | | | | | Personnel | | | | | | Guests | | | Total meals served | |
| | Regular | | | Modified | | | Foodservice | | | Other | | | Guests | | | Total meals served | |
	B	L	D	B	L	D	B	L	D	B	L	D	B	L	D	Today	To-date
1																	
2																	
3																	
4																	
5																	
6																	
7																	
8																	
9																	
10																	
11																	
12																	
13																	
14																	
15																	
16																	
17																	
18																	
19																	
20																	
21																	
22																	
23																	
24																	
25																	
26																	
27																	
28																	
29																	
30																	
31																	
Total																	

_____ 19 _____
Month

Figure 15-2. Record of meals served.

Memorandum

From: Jane Doe, Foodservice Director
To: Foodservice Employees, Vendors, and Accounting Department
Re: Authorized Receiving Signatures
Date: January 1, 1989

The following foodservice personnel are authorized to sign for food and supplies delivered to the foodservice department. Nonauthorized signatures may result in nonpayment of bill.

_____

James M. Brown, Purchasing Manager

_____

Vernon Case, Storeroom Supervisor

_____

Andre Fisk, Storeroom Clerk

_____

Angela Evans, Storeroom Clerk

_____

Mark Rice, Storeroom Clerk

Figure 15-3. Authorized receiving signatures.

Daily Receiving Record

Date received _____ Received by _____

Vendor	Invoice		Description (Food, Paper, Cleaning, Office)	Cost
	Date	Number		

Figure 15-4. Receiving record.

	Invoice		Fresh meat, fish, poultry	Frozen prepared entrees	Canned entrees	Frozen fruits and vegetables	Canned fruits and vegetables	Fresh produce	Dairy	Bakery	Groceries	Other	Cost
Vendor	Date	Number											
Total													

Daily Receiving Record

Date received _____   Received by _____

Figure 15-5. Receiving record (more detailed).

The advantage of using a more detailed form such that shown in Figure 15-5 is that management can readily detect when there is an increase in food costs for a particular category. With the use of cycle menus, the increase in food cost should correspond to the inflation rate. When sharp increases occur in the food costs, management should investigate immediately.

In addition to the preceding policies, management can observe the following practices in an effort to control costs related to the receiving of food:

1. Use an invoice stamp to indicate date received, quantity check, quality check, unit price check, and signature of receiver.
2. Provide receiving personnel with copies of specifications, purchase orders, and price quotations.
3. Give receiving personnel the authority to reject unsatisfactory products.
4. Provide personnel with the tools necessary to weigh, count, and check for quality (i.e., scales and thermometers).
5. Question deliveries made to the facility either before or after scheduled hours.

Food Storage

Spoiled or deteriorated food is a waste of money. When foods are stored at the correct temperature and humidity, foods are less likely to spoil or deteriorate.

Storeroom Requisition and Issue Form							
Unit: _____			Date _____				
Requisitioned							
Amount	Unit	Description	Amount issued	Amount returned	Amount used	Unit cost	Total cost
Requisitioned by: _____				Issued by: _____			

Figure 15-6. Requisition and issue form.

To ensure freshness, date all perishables and follow the first-in-first-out (FIFO) system for storing and issuing food. Finally, to prevent contamination, store all food items at least 6 inches off the floor in a storage area that is tightly sealed to keep out insects and rodents.

___ Requisitions and Issues ___

Only authorized personnel should be allowed to requisition from storage. Depending on the size of the operation, one person may be responsible for requisitioning food for all units. An example is the supervisor in a nursing home or small hospital. In large operations, storeroom personnel may receive requisitions from each unit, such as cook, salad, bakery, tray setup, and nourishment. Control forms should provide information, as shown in Figure 15-6.

At the end of the serving period, all unopened or unused food items should be returned to storage. After returns, storeroom personnel can compile total amounts of food used, thus giving management a daily food cost record on a form such as the one shown in Figure 15-7. The amount of food used—not the amount requisitioned—is the basis for computing daily food costs.

For operations with an ingredient room, the requisitioning and issuing procedures are simplified. All foods are requisitioned by personnel assigned to the ingredient room and all issues are delivered to one unit (ingredient room), thus adding controls in the use of food items.

	Total Food Costs		Total Meals		Cost per Meal		Budgeted Food Cost
Day	Today	To-date	Today	To-date	Today	To-date	To-date
1							
2							
3							
4							
5							
6							
7							
8							
9							
10							
11							
12							
13							
14							
15							
16							
17							
18							
19							
20							
21							
22							
23							
24							
25							
26							
27							
28							
29							
30							
31							
Total							

_____ 19_____

Figure 15-7. Daily food cost record.

Inventory

All foods purchased by the department should be accounted for. The use of both perpetual and physical inventory systems can aid in the accountability process. To maintain a perpetual inventory, the use of a 5- × 7-inch cardex system is suggested. Using this procedure, each food item is listed on a separate card, as shown in Figure 11-18. When a cardex folder is used to hold the cards, the information on the bottom of each card is readily visible. The policy of returning unused and unopened foods to storage will prevent undue accumulation of food in the preparation and service areas.

A physical inventory is obtained by actually counting each item in the storeroom. It should be taken at least once a month or more often, if warranted. The monetary value of the physical inventory should equal the value of the perpetual inventory. When discrepancies occur, they should be thoroughly investigated and corrected immediately. Figure 11-19 shows information needed on a physical inventory.

In the use of physical inventory forms, the column for perpetual inventory should not be completed until after the physical inventory is taken. Any discrepancies between the two should appear in the remarks column.

The cost of food used for a month or longer is based on the physical inventory. To compute the cost of food for a given period, the following formula is used:

$$B + P - E = C$$

where   B = Beginning inventory
         P = Purchases
         E = Ending inventory
         C = Food cost

Pilferage

To secure food is to save money. The following precautions are suggested to provide adequate security:

1. Secure storage areas during nonoperating hours.
2. Permit storeroom keys to be used only by storeroom personnel.
3. Require storeroom personnel to sign for and turn in keys at the beginning and at the end of shift. (Key may be left at the front desk of the facility.)
4. Establish policies on package take-out by employees.
5. Secure preparation and service refrigerators during nonoperating hours.
6. Control trash and other pickup operations from the department.

Pre-preparation

Use of the ingredient room where pre-preparation is centralized is the best form of control. For departments without ingredient rooms, each employee must be instructed in techniques of pre-preparation in order to minimize waste. Some forms of waste are considered unavoidable, such as bones, fat, certain fruit and vegetable peelings and cores, and some outside leaves. Special attention should be given to the amount of outside leaves trimmed from vegetables, the amount of skin peeled from fruit and vegetables, and the amount of usable meat left on bones after the boning process. Even techniques that may appear minor can add up to big savings over a period of time.

___Preparation of Food _____

The most important tool to consider in the preparation of food is the use of standardized recipes that have been tested for yield. If instructions are followed from the recipes, along with information from the production worksheet on the time to begin preparation, then management need not be concerned about shrinkage, overcooking, or other wasteful practices. Use of these techniques set limits on time and temperature, which are important factors in quality control. Food of poor quality may not be consumed and therefore will constitute waste.

___Service of Food _____

Whether from a tray line or from a cafeteria counter, employees must be instructed to practice prescribed portion control in the service of food. Much of the portioning can be at the time of purchase, during pre-preparation, or prior to service in the case of prepared foods. For bulk foods that must be portioned as served, proper utensils should be provided such as ladles, scoops, and scales. Refer to portion control as presented in Chapters 12 and 13.

When patients select double portions, the menu tally should reflect two servings instead of one. Employees may request double servings from cafeteria lines, and therefore cashiers should be alerted so that charges can be made accordingly. Also tapes from computerized cash registers, as discussed in Chapter 13, will serve as a control in the handling of cash. Cost of condiments can be controlled to some extent for patient service by limiting food items only to those selected. The practice of serving dressings with salads, or routinely serving salt, pepper, and sugar should not be allowed since all items returned on trays must be discarded.

___Employee Meals _____

The cost of meals served to employees should receive careful scrutiny. Several practices are followed in terms of employee meals:

1. Employees pay full menu price for all food consumed.
2. Employees pay a reduced price for all food consumed.
3. Employees receive meals (one or more) as part of wages.
4. Employees receive meals as a fringe benefit.

If meals are served as fringe benefits, they should be charged to the cost of labor. In efforts to control costs in this area, management should review policies on the following:

1. Are employees allowed to eat as much as desired?
2. Are employees limited on the more expensive menu items?
3. How many meals are employees entitled to eat during a regular 8-hour shift?
4. Are part-time employees entitled to eat a meal?
5. Are employees entitled to eat during scheduled rest periods?
6. Is coffee or other beverages (such as soda) available to employees throughout the scheduled shift?

___Special Activities _____

All food prepared and served in the department should be charged to some account. This includes coffee breaks, special luncheons, teas, banquets, coffee

Special Activity Cost Record			
To: Accounting Office			
From: H. Faunleroy, Director of Dietetics			
Subject: Monthly Charges			
Month: _____			
Date	Group	Account No.	Amount
	Accreditation Committee	1-905-570	
	Administration	2-905-570	
	Administrator's Meeting	1-905-570	
	Admission and Utilization Committee	2-905-570	
	Applied Management Program	2-960-570	
	Board of Trustees	1-905-570	
	Case Presentation 2-1	2-617-570	
	Data Processing and Information System	1-930-570	

Figure 15-8. Special activity cost record form. *From Detroit-McComb Hospital Corporation*

served at committee meetings, and others. Forms that may be useful in controlling cost of special activities are shown in Figures 15-8 and 15-9.

The form exhibited in Figure 15-8 provides a listing of organizations and committees that frequently request food and/or services from the department. Since account numbers are assigned by accounting department, it is easier to maintain records and control.

Menus for special luncheons and other activities are precosted and updated as often as necessary. The menus and instructions for making selections are given to groups requesting service. After the selection has been made, the menu is typed on a meeting reservation form and submitted to administration for approval, as shown in Figure 15-9.

___ Leftovers ___

The optimal form of operation is to eliminate leftovers completely. Since this is not always possible, management should provide for the economic use of leftover foods. A review of the production worksheet (Figure 12-3) will show a column for disposition of foods left after the serving period. This column should be used to indicate how the food will be used. Most foods can be used again in a different form. A list of suggested ways to use leftovers can be compiled and available for cooks or personnel in the ingredient room.

Frequently overlooked in the control of leftovers is a check of unused trays delivered to patients on the wards. At one hospital, a daily check of unused trays revealed a starting number of 240 unused trays over a 1-month period. Management used a form to keep records of unused trays, as depicted in Figure 15-10.

The number of unused trays, multiplied by the average cost per meal, equals the dollar amount lost. Since all food returned to the dietary department must be discarded, control in this area alone could amount to savings in the thousands of dollars over a 1-year period.

MEETING RESERVATIONS

GROUP: _____

CHAIRMAN: _____ DEPT.: _____ PHONE: _____

DATE: _____ TIME: _____ NO. ATTENDING: _____

PLACE: **DMH: DDR** ☐ **SDR** ☐ **Cafeteria** ☐ **G 146** ☐ **ACR 109** ☐ **147** ☐ **ACR 206** ☐ **Stair Lobby** ☐ **Other** ____

       SMH: DDR ☐ **CCR-A** ☐ **CCR-B** ☐ **CCR-C** ☐ **CCR-D** ☐ **ACR-1113** ☐ **ACR-1123** ☐ **Other** ____

TYPE OF SERVICE: Cafe. Line ☐ Cafe. Table ☐ Buffet ☐ Waitress ☐ Meeting Only ☐

CHARGE TO: (ACCOUNT NO.) _____

REMARKS: _____

_____   MENU (For Dietary Use Only)

ADMINISTRATION
APPROVAL.: _____

Form 3107 — Rev. 10/75   Submit Original and Two Copies To Administration

Figure 15-9. Special activity approval form. *From Detroit-Macomb Hospital Corporation*

Record of Tray Return

Date	ICU	1-1	2-1	2-2	2-3	2-4	3-1	3-2	3-3	4-1	4-2	4-3	Total
													Breakfast _____ Lunch _____ Dinner _____ Total _____
													Breakfast _____ Lunch _____ Dinner _____ Total _____
													Breakfast _____ Lunch _____ Dinner _____ Total _____

Ward

Figure 15-10. Records of trays returned. This sample form is used for recording the number of unused trays returned from wards. Abbreviations are used to denote reasons such as: NPO—nothing by mouth, D—discharged, DC—diet change, and T—transferred. Collected data are used to improve cost savings through employee in-service, better communication with nursing staff, and close monitoring of patient census. *From Detroit-Macomb Hospital Corporation*

— Nourishments ——————————————————

Standard operating procedures should indicate what foods are stocked on the wards routinely and what foods should be delivered by request only. Since nourishments make up part of the cost per meal served to patients, management must make sure that nourishments are being consumed by patients and not by personnel on the wards. All requests in excessive amounts and all unusual requests should be investigated. A form such as the one shown in Figure 15-11 can serve as a control tool.

It is important that all requisitions are approved by supervisory staff, rather than the dietary clerk responsible for nourishment preparation. Special attention should be given to the amount left over from the previous day and whether ward personnel are using the FIFO system in distributing to patients. Cost records should be maintained for both bulk nourishments and individual between-meal feeding for patients.

			Nourishment Order Sheet			
Ward _____				Date _____		
Unit	Food Item	Quantity on Hand	Quantity Ordered	Quantity Delivered	Unit Cost ($)	Total Cost ($)
Ordered by:		Approved by:		Filled by:		
_____		_____		_____		

Figure 15-11. Nourishment ordering form.

Labor Cost Control

Labor costs are directly related to the number of full-time equivalents (FTE) employed by the facility and the amount of salary paid, including wages and benefits. When the labor cost percentage is higher than established limits for staffing, management must either increase the number of meals served, reduce the number of employees, or develop and maintain effective labor cost controls. The last alternative is suggested.

Direct and Indirect Labor Costs

Labor costs can be classified as direct or indirect. *Direct costs* are those related to wages paid for productive work hours or actual hours on the job. *Indirect costs* refer to activities and benefits such as vacation, sick leave, holidays, personal leave, employee meals, insurance (life, health, and accident), FICA, workers' compensation, unemployment compensation, pension, retirement, and other benefits that may be part of the labor agreement. Indirect labor costs, frequently referred to as nonproductive labor costs, can equal as much as 50% of the total labor costs (Rose 1980).

Labor costs can be broken down further into *noncontrollable* and *controllable* costs. Wages and benefits that have been negotiated and agreed upon, as well as costs established by external agencies (i.e., FICA, Workers' Compensation) may be classified as noncontrollable costs. The following discussion will concentrate on labor costs that can be controlled, in varying degrees, by the foodservice department. There are some areas in which management can exert some control in reducing labor costs.

Menu Planning

Consider changing labor-intensive menu items, such as complex, gourmet-type foods that require highly skilled chefs to prepare. Since highly skilled chefs expect and get higher wages, the labor cost per FTE will be higher.

The coordination of menu items served to patients on regular and modified diets and employees in the cafeteria is another factor to consider. A menu policy that requires the use of the same food item for all areas of service whenever feasible reduces the handling, preparation, and service required of employees.

Equipment

Purchasing mechanical equipment and requiring employees to use such equipment can possibly save a fraction of a FTE. When FTE savings are used to justify the investment of funds for equipment, the total FTE should be reduced and not absorbed within the department.

Purchasing and Issuing of Food

The form in which food is purchased affects labor costs. The use of convenience foods will decrease labor cost but will increase food cost. Investigate the degree of convenience in relation to labor cost savings.

The use of an ingredient room for centralized issuing, measuring, portioning, and manipulating food saves time in the production area. An excessive amount of time can be wasted by highly paid employees in the aforementioned activities.

Production

Full utilization of scheduled employees will reduce the amount of money paid for idle time. Higher labor cost is associated with the conventional food production system due to uneven work distribution. The peak periods of operation are at mealtimes, which take up 4 to 6 hours of an 8-hour shift. Decreased activity, which occurs between meals, accounts for 2 to 4 hours of the regular shift. Management needs to monitor this period to determine exactly what employees are doing. For managers involved in planning a new facility or renovation, consideration should be given to other types of production systems that have proved to be more labor efficient.

Service

Decentralized service is more costly in terms of labor than centralized service because of the amount of supervision required. Each ward pantry requires adequate supervision for assurance of quality and quantity standards. Although there is a decrease in labor costs when the task of patient foodservice is performed by nursing personnel, the foodservice department loses control of the finished product. Depending on the location of the dietary department in relation to the patient area, ambulatory patients may be permitted to consume meals in the cafeteria. This practice is particularly applicable to small hospitals and nursing homes.

Consider the use of disposable serviceware. The use of disposables will reduce labor costs (dishwashing), but may increase costs in other areas such as trash removal, storage, and the cost of disposable serviceware.

Investigate alternative production and service patterns. The traditional three-meals-a-day plan may be substituted with a four- or five-meal plan. The major advantage of alternate patterns is that peaks and valleys are practically eliminated.

For cafeteria service, consider the use of more self-service. Quantities can be controlled in self-service food items with the size of the serving dish, scales, and selected serving utensils. Also, the self-bussing of trays, the removal of disposables such as paper napkins, and the sorting of silverware by those eating in the cafeteria will reduce labor costs.

Personnel

It is in the area of personnel utilization that the most dramatic labor cost savings can be realized without increasing other costs. Reference is made to the following factors as contributors to labor costs. (See Chapter 14 for full discussion of each entity.)

JOB ANALYSIS, DESCRIPTION, AND SPECIFICATION Has each position undergone analysis for job content, been well defined in the job description, and been specified in writing for use by personnel responsible for hiring? The hiring practice has a direct bearing on tardiness, absenteeism, productivity, and turnover.

JOB STANDARDS Decreased employee activity can be measured by using standards of performance. For labor cost savings, standards refer to the quantity of work performed. For each position, employees need to know what and how much is required for full productivity. Accumulated data based on job standards can serve as counseling tools to rehabilitate the nonproductive employee or can provide objective measures for termination.

WORK METHODS All supervisory personnel should be trained in the fundamentals of work simplification. With this knowledge, supervisors can use concepts of motion economy to analyze how tasks are performed, develop improved methods, and train employees in new procedures.

WORK SCHEDULES Establish criteria for employee work schedules based on service required and not on the convenience of the employee. The traditional method of scheduling employees with overlapping early and late shifts over a 7-day period is costly. The practice is primarily associated with the conventional production system. It is easier to change the method of scheduling than the type of production system. For cost savings, consider alternate scheduling systems such as flextime, compressed or 4-day workweek, or permanent part-time. It is reported at one facility that a schedule change to 4 days on and 3 days off for cooks resulted in lower labor costs and some favorable side effects as well (Longrigg 1981).

ABSENTEEISM AND TURNOVER The factors of absenteeism and turnover are grouped together since chronic absenteeism frequently results in employee turnover, and also since both are classified as nonproductive labor costs (paid days off and Workers' Compensation). The traditional use of strong disciplinary measures to curb absenteeism is not effective (Taylor 1981). For any meaningful cost reduction in this area, management will need to determine the underlying factors contributing to high absenteeism and turnover. Maintaining records, as described in Chapter 14, and careful scrutiny of managerial practices will supply adequate data for corrective action.

EMPLOYEE TRAINING Effective training can serve to correct undesirable employee practices that contribute to labor costs. Tools available in a well-organized department that can be used for training are policies, procedures, job analysis, job descriptions, job specifications, job standards, performance evaluation, accumulated work records, and safety and sanitation reports. The overall objective of training is to produce an efficient, cost-effective work force.

Energy Cost Control

Medical foodservice operations must become actively involved in energy conservation, not only because energy is a scarce resource but also because of the steady increase in energy costs. Foodservice directors in medical facilities encounter problems dealing with energy control that are not found in single or independent foodservice operations. The facility is complex, composed of many departments that are all energy intensive in their effort to provide required services. In most medical facilities, energy used for heat, light, ventilation, refrigeration, and hot water are not measured and charged to individual departments. Therefore, it is difficult for the foodservice director to determine whether the department is energy efficient. In spite of these problems, there is much that can be done to conserve energy and thus reduce cost in this area.

Establishing an Energy Program

The control of energy, like the control of food and labor costs, begins with the menu system and continues as an integral part of all basic resources that must be controlled. Specific techniques for energy cost controls, as discussed in Chapters 9 through 15, should become part of a long-range plan for energy conservation.

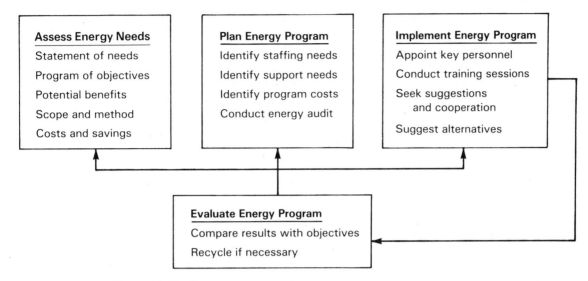

Figure 15-12. Energy management system.

The major stages to consider in establishing a long-range energy program are the same as those required in other systematic processes. As shown in Figure 15-12, management must assess, plan, implement, and evaluate.

— Assessment

Begin the assessment by stating why an energy program is needed. As part of the statement of need, include documentation on existing energy costs. The accounting department in the facility should be of help in supplying information on the amount of energy used for a given period. The data can be compared with future increases or decreases. Another concern during this state is to determine whether major changes have occurred in the operation that may have contributed to increased use of energy, such as expansion of the facility, a change in the production system, or purchase of additional equipment. It is important that the complete energy program is in writing for two reasons. First, when ideas are on paper, efforts are more effectively directed toward improved energy control. Second, the written version can serve as a guide for all employees involved in the program.

Program objectives should include broad statements, which then can be defined further in measurable terms. This procedure will prove to be an important step during the evaluation when one must determine whether objectives have been met. Make objectives and goals both realistic and attainable.

In addition to cost savings, which is the primary interest of top administrators, list other potential benefits that may occur as a result of an energy control program. For example, how will the program affect the management of other resources such as personnel? Will employee morale improve as the result of active participation? Since this is a group project, will the program foster cohesiveness among employees?

To indicate the scope and method to be used, consideration should be given to the following:

1. Will the plan cover the whole department or will it be limited to specific areas such as production and service?
2. What are the tasks to be accomplished?
3. Will all employees become involved?

4. Will written reports be required by key personnel on a daily, weekly, or monthly basis?
5. Who will run the program?
6. How much support is needed from higher administration?
7. Will outside consultants be necessary?
8. Will technical assistance from other departments within the medical facility be needed?

Finally, during the assessment stage an estimate of the annual costs and savings should be made. Estimates should include what it will cost to implement the program, as well as savings-to-cost ratio or payback period. It should be remembered that the plan will be more acceptable to higher management if both energy and money can be saved.

Planning

During the planning stage, decisions should be made in reference to questions raised during the assessment period. For example, will staffing permit use of a manager, a first-line supervisor, or head cook to run the program, or will the department head take on this task? As part of the plan, one should consider the use of an energy audit as follows:

1. Document energy usage and operating procedures for major pieces of equipment, using Forms 1 and 2, as shown in Figures 15-13 and 15-14. The findings can be used for reference during the implementation and evaluation stages.
2. Formulate a checklist to identify opportunities for cost savings. Group energy usage according to sections within the department and list on the left side of the checklist. Opposite each section, list suggested cost savings obtained from remarks section of Forms 1 and 2. In addition to techniques for energy control, as discussed in Chapters 9–14, employees should be encouraged to make additional suggestions.

Implementation

The key to effective implementation is to seek and gain the full cooperation of all employees. It may be necessary to provide some kind of incentive for employee participation based on the degree of goal fulfillment. Employees should be involved as early as possible and to the greatest extent possible. Training sessions should be initiated for one section at a time with emphasis on temperature, time, and proper use and care of equipment in order to accurately document energy usage.

To determine the amount of energy used in the preparation of a food item, management may use meters which can be attached to individual pieces of equipment or conduct studies of time and temperature. The use of meters to measure the cubic feet of gas or the kilowatt-hours of electricity is the most reliable method, but may partially defeat the purpose of cost savings since an outlay of funds is required for purchasing and installing the instruments. A less costly method, and the one recommended, is the use of time and temperature multiplied by the energy ratings for individual pieces of equipment. Using this method of estimating energy consumption, a study was conducted to determine which of four types of electric equipment was least energy intensive and produced the most acceptable product (Romanelli 1979). The technique, which requires only the use of a stopwatch and a record of dates, involves the following steps:

Form 1—Use and Cost of Electricity					
Equipment (type and location) _____ Date _____ to _____					
Electrical use per device (kW)	Number of devices	Total electrical use (kW) [(1)×(2)]	Operating hours per week	Operating weeks per year	Estimated kWh per year [(3)×(4)×(5)]
(1)	(2)	(3)	(4)	(5)	(6)

Prepared by: _____

Comments/remarks (operating procedures, temperature, time, etc.) _____

_____

_____

_____

Figure 15-13. Form detailing usage and cost of electricity.

1. Measure the on-time of the thermostat signal light immediately after placing the food item into the equipment.
2. Record the total on-time of signal light immediately after removing food product from equipment.
3. Conduct five duplications, using identical equipment, cooking temperatures, and food products. Food products should have the same size, weight, initial temperature, and final internal temperature for each replication.
4. Determine average on-time for the five replications.
5. Divide average on-time of thermostat signal light by 60 to determine percentage of 1 hour.
6. Multiply percentage by the electrical rating of the equipment to obtain estimated kilowatt-hour (kWh) consumption. (Example: 30 minutes average on-time ÷ 60 = 50%, and 50% × an equipment kWh rating of 12 = 6 kWh consumed.)
7. Record kWh consumption on standardized recipe card.

When this type of information is recorded on each standardized recipe in a cycle menu system, management can make accurate decisions in efforts to reduce energy costs. The recording of the data also provides tangible evidence

Form 2—Use and Cost of Natural Gas					
Equipment (type and location) _____ Date _____ to _____					
Fuel use per device	Number of devices	Total gas use (ft³/hr) [(1)×(2)]	Operating hours per week	Operating weeks per year	Estimated cubic feet per year [(3)×(4)×(5)]
(1)	(2)	(3)	(4)	(5)	(6)

Prepared by: _____

Comments/remarks (operating procedures, temperature, time, etc.) _____

_____

_____

_____

Figure 15-14. Form detailing usage and cost of natural gas.

that an energy control program is in effect. The cost of energy, as well as labor and food costs, should become a permanent part of each standardized recipe as a basis for establishing the selling price of a food item.

___ Evaluation ___

Results should be measured against the stated objectives. It is possible that expectations have been exceeded. Should results fail to measure up to objectives, it will be necessary to reexamine the various states to determine where difficulties exist.

Budget Systems

A budget is defined as a written financial statement, expressed in numerical terms, for a specified period of time. A budgeting system is more comprehensive and is defined as a process of planning, coordinating, and controlling financial resources in order to meet the objectives and goals of the organization. In medical operations the objective has been one of mission or service, with minimal attention to the budgetary process as practiced by profit-oriented businesses.

Recently, due to escalating costs of medical care, medical operations are faced with the challenge of seeking congruence between service and fiscal responsibility.

Traditional Budgeting System

The most widely used method of allocating funds is the use of the traditional budgeting system. In this system, use of funds are not always questioned unless there is an excessive overrun. Each year, based on last year's budgetary allowance, additional funds are added to the operating budget. The amount of increased funding is usually associated with the inflation rate. This type of budgeting may well perpetuate inefficiency because objectives are not redefined to reflect changes that may have occurred. In addition, when funds are limited, cuts in the operating budget are made across the board, regardless of departmental objectives and goals.

Although medical organizations may be reluctant to do so, they must look beyond the traditional budgeting system. The reluctance to use what has been described as more *complex systems* for financial control in medical organizations may stem from the nonfinancial background of most professionals who head various departments. According to Deters (1980), employees in nonfinancial areas are sometimes intimidated by financial jargon and should be taught basic concepts through well-developed educational programs.

Some of the more widely used systems for planning, coordinating, and controlling financial resources today are (1) management by objectives (MBO) (see Chapter 2 for a full discussion); (2) planning, programming and budgeting systems (PPBS); and (3) zero-base budgeting (ZBB). Zero-base budgeting is the latest to receive widespread managerial practice and therefore will receive a more detailed description.

Planning, Programming, and Budgeting System (PPBS)

PPBS is an integrated, analytical approach used to allocate resources in the most effective manner to meet goals of the operation. Emphasis is on planning to achieve stated goals, and then consideration is given to resources necessary to obtain desired results. In this system, budgeting plays a secondary role to setting goals and establishing plans.

Concepts of PPBS were first used in private industry by companies such as the Rand Corporation, General Motors, and DuPont (Novick 1969). As early as 1940, principles of PPBS were used for World War II production controls. The system received national attention in 1961 when it was introduced by Secretary of Defense Robert McNamara. As used in the Defense Department, it served to improve management decision making in the federal government and was mandated for use by all federal agencies in 1965 by President Johnson. The system provided a uniform language to be used by all agencies requesting funding over a multiyear period.

Pyhrr (1973) cites the major components of PPBS, as used in the Defense Department:

1. *Program structures* are the grouping of activities (intra- and interagency-wide) that have the same common goal. The basic unit of the program structure is the program element. The charting or breaking down of elements within a program structure is analogous to an organization chart, with elements defined at different organizational levels. The purpose of this phase is to analyze all

relevant activities by different agencies relating to a given objective—to eliminate overlap and to identify gaps in the services provided.

2. *Issue letters,* formulated through consensus of agencies involved, concentrate on major issues that need in-depth analysis. Issue letters are used early in the cycle so that agreement can be reached on the nature of the problem and alternatives formulated for evaluation.

3. *Special analytical studies* relate to issues identified in issue letters. Support documents used to analyze issues may include statistical models, surveys, and other data needed to support issues.

4. *Program memoranda* relate to analysis of issues as identified in and among agencies and the alternatives considered. Program memoranda are used to summarize agency decisions.

5. *Program and financial plans* include the actual data for the 2 preceding years, plus the projected funds for the next 5 years. Since the time plan for spending was increased to 5 years or more, the plans attempted to bridge the gap between long-range objectives and the current year's budget allocation; to identify future commitment based on past decisions; and to identify consequences of current decisions.

Since PPBS is more complex than this simplistic description portrays, some federal and private organizations fail to utilize all components of the system fully.

⎯ Zero-Base Budgeting (ZBB) ⎯⎯⎯⎯⎯⎯⎯⎯⎯⎯

ZBB is a relatively new managerial technique developed by Peter A. Pyhrr. The budgeting system was first applied at the Texas Instruments Company in Dallas for its staff and research budget for 1970 (Pyhrr 1970). It is a well-known concept today in the business world, with over 300 businesses and a dozen state governments using the technique (Carter 1977).

The budgeting process received its widest application when Governor Carter of Georgia decided to use it for the 1973 state budget. He was convinced at that time that ZBB was a most effective method for analyzing and evaluating all activities, both current and new, before allocating funds. As president, Carter was equally convinced that the same general principles of budgeting could be successfully applied to most federal funding.

To clarify and provide mutual understanding, it may be necessary to define briefly certain terms related to the discussion of ZBB.

> *Activity* is the basic work or action of an individual or group in the accomplishment of objectives established for a program.
> *Alternative* is the comparison of two or more methods of accomplishing or performing the operation or activity and choosing the one that is considered best.
> *Cost-benefit* is an analytical approach to solving problems of choice. It involves alternative ways of achieving objectives that yield the greatest benefit for the least cost.
> *Decision package* is a document that identifies and describes a specific activity so that management can evaluate and rank it against other activities competing for funds in terms of approval or disapproval.
> *Incremental packages* reflect different levels of effort that may be expended on a specific function.
> *Issue identification* results in the review of decision packages and the ranking process in which additional issues, alternatives, and policy questions may

arise as analysts evaluate the impact of the operations on program objectives.

Mutually exclusive packages identify alternative means for performing the same function. The best alternative is chosen, and the other packages are discarded.

Program structure is a clear identification of the interaction of operations in the program.

Special analysis is a method of offering a ready-made data source as a result of the mass of information and analysis provided.

Zero-base budgeting is a technique for starting from scratch in identifying, analyzing, and evaluating all activities (current and new) before funds are allocated. Each manager evaluates and considers the need for each function, different levels of effort, and alternative ways of performing different functions.

Implementation of ZBB involves two major or basic steps: (1) Describing each decision unit as a *decision package*. (2) Evaluating and ranking all decision packages by cost-benefit analysis to develop the budget request and the profit-and-loss statements.

In defining decision units, ZBB attempts to focus management's attention on evaluating activities and making decisions related to their continuation. Each organization must determine for itself what is meaningful in terms of the decision units. In practice, the organization or program level at which decision units are defined is usually determined by top management.

After the decision units have been identified, top management must then explain the decision package concept to all levels of management and present guidelines for individual managers to use in breaking down their areas into workable packages. The decision package is the building block of the ZBB process and is designed to identify activity, function, or operation in a definitive manner for management evaluation and comparison with other activities. The decision package should include the purpose, consequences of not performing the activity, measures of performance, alternative course of action, and cost-benefit.

The ranking process is accomplished by managers in the various departments as they identify all packages in order of decreasing benefit to the organization. The process then pinpoints the benefits to be gained at each level of expenditure and considers the consequences of not approving additional decision packages ranked below a certain expenditure level. This process allows upper management an opportunity to trade off expenditures among cost centers and other larger divisions of the organization (Pyhrr 1976).

The initial implementation of ZBB is often done by a task force of operating and financial managers who are responsible for the design and administration of the process throughout the organization. Each organization must decide whether to install ZBB throughout the organization or only within special departments first. Duties of the task force in managing the process are as follows:

1. Designing the process to fit the needs of the organization.
2. Preparing a simplified budget manual that illustrates examples of analysis required and explains the decision package and ranking concepts.
3. Presenting the process to management and training operating managers in the application of the technique.
4. Working with division unit managers to improve and expedite the analysis.

5. Working with middle management to review and rank decision packages.

6. Evaluating the process and revising it accordingly.

There are distinct problems associated with ZBB. The major causes of problems in implementation stem from the lack of support from top management, ineffective design of the system to meet the needs of the user organization, and ineffective management of the system. Administrative problems may arise (1) if operating managers are apprehensive of the process because their functions are being scrutinized, (2) if there is a lack of communication of goals, objectives, and purpose, (3) if there is a lack of planning assumptions, and (4) because extra time is required during the first year.

The benefits of ZBB far outweigh the possible problems that may be encountered. One of the unique features of ZBB is that it requires the participation of all managers at all levels of the organization, whereas in many organizations the planning and budgeting process is done by financial and fiscal people with participation of only top management. The benefits that each organization can derive from ZBB can be divided into three general categories:

1. Improved plans and budgets
2. Residual benefits, realized during the operating years
3. A skilled management team

The improved plans and budgets offer the most immediate benefits because of the identification, evaluation, and justification of all activities proposed rather than just the increase or decrease from current operating levels. Great flexibility is also provided to top management in reallocating resources. Zero-base budgeting combines planning, goal setting, budgeting and operational decision making and results in an integrated approach. Duplication of efforts among organizational units will be identified and can be eliminated with this system.

A major follow-up benefit is that managers' effectiveness can be measured against the goals, performance, and benefits to which they commit themselves, as indicated in the decision packages and in their budgets. In addition, ZBB trains managers to continue to think along the analytical lines that the process requires.

In developing the managerial team, ZBB can be considered an educational process. The identification and evaluation required in ranking decision packages can become an ingrained thought process, where managers evaluate their planning, operations, efficiency, and cost effectiveness on a continuous basis.

In the sample *decision package* format (Fig. 15-15), the problem relates to deleting an unfilled position in storeroom section in order to effect a cost-benefit. It is clearly up to the manager of that section to identify and evaluate alternatives. This process need not be accomplished by the manager alone, all employees in the section may assist in reaching a decision. Note that the sample format is the first of three decision packages and concentrates on the minimum level of performance required to deliver services. It reflects the loss of one technical assistant and the savings of $13,000 while at the same time letting management know the consequences as a result of this change.

The alternatives suggested in section 10 of Figure 15-15 offer two levels of effort with recommendations for adoption of package 2 of 3 packages. In section 11, different ways of performing the same activity are suggested with resulting consequences. Management may require a detailed explanation relating to the poor logistic set-up alluded to in that section. In section 12, management can readily review and analyze the resources required, which will be important in the ranking process. Formulating alternatives in terms of effort and identifying

(1) *Package Name*	(2) *Division*	(3) *Department*	(4) *Cost Center*	(5) *Rank*
Basic Plan (1 of 3)	Storeroom	Foodservice	56	3

(6) *Statement of Purpose*

To provide minimum level of storeroom operation in terms of receiving, storing, and issuing of food, and maintenance of records.

(7) *Description of Actions (Operations)*

Receive food and check for quantity according to purchase order.
Verify all items listed for quality as stated in food specifications.
Store foods according to safety and sanitation codes, using FIFO.
Issue foods as requisitioned by production and service units.
Maintain perpetual and physical inventory records.
                    1 Professional, 1 Technical Assistant

(8) *Benefits*

This is a minimum level of planning required to deliver services.
                    Personnel: 2   Cost: $29,640

(9) *Consequences of Not Approving Package*

Elimination of technical assistant position results in zero incremental costs, but a breakdown in control standards plus excessive delays in receiving and issuing would develop.

(10) *Alternatives (Different Levels of Effort) and Cost*

Package 2 of 3 (cost $37,960): provides the storeroom section with more manpower during its heaviest work period (early A.M.) by hiring two part-time assistants at lower rates (20 hours per week @ $4.00 per hour). *Recommended Package.*
Package 3 of 3 (cost $42,640): retain technical assistant position @ $13,000.

(11) *Alternatives (Different Ways of Performing the Same Activity)*

Combine storeroom and production sections (rotate assistant cooks to storeroom duties).
Shift other production and service personnel to storeroom duties on a short term basis.
NOTE: Both alternatives would result in poor logistic setup—in addition to possible lowering of control standards.

(12) *Resources Required*

1989	$42,640	Personnel: 3	(1 Professional + 2 Technical Assistants)
1990	$37,960	Personnel: 4	(1 Professional + 1 Technical Assistant and 2 Part-time Assistants)
	−4,680	+1	

Manager	J.P. Doe	Prepared by	J.P. Doe	Date 10-10-89	Page 1

Figure 15-15. Zero-base budgeting decision package. *Adapted from Decision Package developed by Peter A. Pyhrr*

different ways of performing the same task are the most important aspects of the decision package.

Implications for medical foodservice management are apparent. Since ZBB is becoming more and more popular in business, industry and government, the foodservice director should be aware of its implications for foodservice management. Also, since most medical organizations receive some type of state or federal funding, it is advantageous for the foodservice director to understand how these funds are allocated.

The foodservice director has the major responsibility for exerting leadership in developing financial plans; therefore it is imperative that the managerial staff remain alert to new and innovative techniques. Current economic conditions dictate that one means of accountability will surely be in the form of finance. Funds are no longer handed out based on status quo but require detailed scrutiny at all levels.

Uniform System of Accounting

There are similarities among various types of foodservice operations, yet each is uniquely different. One difference is in the accounting procedures. Because of this difference, each major segment of the foodservice industry (hotels, restaurants, school lunch program, hospitals) has developed a uniform system for reporting costs. For hospitals, the uniform system of accounting (American Hospital Association 1973) is performed by the Hospital Administrative Services (HAS).

Hospital Administrative Services

The primary function of HAS is to provide comparative cost data to hospital administrators. Statistical indicators are used to compare hospitals according to size, type, and geographical location. To obtain cost data, based on group mediums, hospitals must pay a fee and submit data on income and expenses, using uniform accounting procedures. Hospital Administrative Services has developed specific guidelines for determining the number of patient meals served; equivalent number of cafeteria meals served; where and how to report personnel salaries and labor hours; food and other direct expenses; and procedures for reporting all revenue (cafeteria, vending, coffee shop, etc.).

A confidential monthly report is sent to each participating hospital so that the administrator can compare his or her operation to a group medium in eight categories. The HAS indicators and possible reasons for deviation from the group medium are shown in Table 15-3. It should be pointed out that although resolution of problem areas is not the responsibility of HAS, it does suggest possible causes for extreme deviations. Hospitals may use the information in a number of ways to evaluate the effectiveness of the department. Should it become necessary to investigate significant differences, management can begin with a check on accuracy of data as reported by the department head. If data are reported accurately, then management might refer to factors of food and labor cost controls as discussed earlier in this chapter.

Budget Preparation

The degree to which department heads are involved in budget preparation varies from one institution to another, based on (1) administrative policies and procedures, (2) the degree of accountability for cost controls, (3) the amount of budget information communicated from top management, and (4) the level of budgeting knowledge possessed by the foodservice director.

The following questions help discern the administrative policies that may affect department head involvement: Are the policies of the organization one of participatory budget preparation or are all budget estimates made by the

Table 15-3. Hospital Administrative Service Indicators[a]

HAS Monthly Indicators	Possible Reasons for Significant Differences
1. Total Dietary Expense Percent Total dietary direct expense ÷ total hospital expense	The percentage indicates the proportion of hospital funds expended by the dietary department. Significant deviations above medium may suggest overstaffing, waste of food or other materials, or that too high a price is paid for food and supplies. A percentage that is far below the medium may indicate insufficient resources allotted to dietary or that quality of service is far below standard.
2. Total Meals per Patient Day Total no. of meals ÷ patient days	This indicator is designed to verify the accuracy of the meal count statistics. A large variation from previous periods suggests that the meal count should be investigated so that other dietary indicators will not be distorted.
3. Total Dietary Direct Expense per Meal Total dietary direct expense ÷ total no. of meals served	Total dietary expense per meal indicates the cost effectiveness of the dietary department. A very high per-meal cost may point to overstaffing, inadequate scheduling, waste, poor purchasing practice, or unusual policies. This indicator should be examined along with the indicator for salary expense per meal in order to distinguish area of excessive cost.
4. Total Dietary Salary Expense per Meal Total dietary salaries ÷ total no. of meals served	This indicator reflects the labor expense component of dietary department total expense. A high indicator may suggest unusually high wage rates, low productivity, or a combination of the two. This indicator should be examined along with the indicator for meals served per labor hour.
5. Total Meals Served per Labor Hour Total no. of meals served ÷ total dietary labor hours	This is a productivity indicator that reflects on labor utilization. A low indicator will result in high salary expense per meal.
6. Inpatient Meals Served per Day Inpatient meals served obstetrical and medical and surgical patients	This is another indicator for verifying the meal count statistics. The indicator will generally be close to 2.8 meals per patient day. Extreme variations should result in an examination of the meal count in order to ensure reliability.
7. Cafeteria Meals Percentage of Total Meals Cafeteria meals ÷ total all meals	This indicator provides a check on the accuracy of the cafeteria meal count. Extreme variations from month to month may indicate inconsistency in calculating the equivalent meal count. A decrease may be attributed to inaccurate meal counting or reduced patronage.
8. Cafeteria Meals per Labor Hours Cafeteria meals ÷ cafeteria labor hours	This is a productivity indicator for the cafeteria. Cafeteria productivity is always greater than total productivity because it does not include food preparation, dishwashing, etc. A low indicator may be the result of overstaffing, inadequate use of part-time personnel during peak serving periods, and inefficient cafeteria layout.

[a]From the American Hospital Association.

365

accounting department? On what basis are budget estimates approved or dis-approved before they become effective or a part of the general budget? What is the procedure for making changes in the budget?

The amount of information communicated to the foodservice director has the most direct bearing on his or her involvement. In addition to accurate records of prior costs, the foodservice director needs information on both short- and long-range goals of the organization. For example, major policy changes, significant increases in patient census, major renovations, or plans for a new facility could have direct effects on the foodservice budget.

One method of communication is through the use of a budget question-naire. This procedure requires more than just a listing of items and dollar amounts. It also requires the individual to state departmental objectives and justifications for expenditures. Sample questions asked by one organization are shown in Figure 15-16.

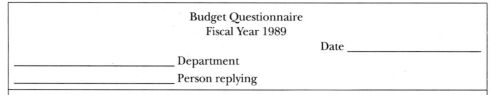

Budget Questionnaire
Fiscal Year 1989

Date _____

_____ Department

_____ Person replying

1. (A) During the present fiscal year, what changes in departmental responsibilities, func-tions, or other factors have increased or decreased your department's volume of work?
   (B) What 1989 budgetary changes are you making to reflect revised needs for (1) FTE personnel? (2) Space? (3) Equipment? (4) Other expense?
2. What functions are you and your department performing that are unrelated to your basic purpose and should be eliminated, transferred, or curtailed? What cost savings will result?
3. What routines or procedures can be simplified or obsoleted from your department during this next year? How and why?
4. What "paperwork" does your department perform or receive that is no longer of value or use, is overly time-consuming, or for other reasons should be simplified, eliminated, or computerized?
5. What nonrecurring service did you perform this year that will not be an expense factor next year?
6. What deficiencies of other departments, or lack of coordination, made work for your department?
7. What overlap by other departments can be eliminated, and why?
8. In what ways do you plan to maintain or modify your department's function and reduce payroll and other costs, where the census or service demand has declined?
9. If you plan an increase in full-time personnel equivalents, what justification do you offer? What income will be available to offset the expense?
10. What items are you presently storing in your department that can be more effectively kept in central storage?
11. What significant changes in supply items (recent or planned) will have an appreciable effect on your operation expense for fiscal year 1989?
12. What other ideas do you have for reducing work and expense in your department? In other departments?
13. In the event that new Blue Cross economic controls reduce our income significantly below current levels, what reductions in the scope and cost of your departmental services could you effect and still maintain service for patients at an acceptable level? (List in order of your preferred priority).
14. How does the ratio of personnel (FTE) to departmental activity compare for 1987, 1988, and the proposed 1989 budget? How do you explain changes?

Figure 15-16. Budget questionnaire form. *From Detroit-Macomb Hospital Corporation*

In addition to the questionnaire, department heads are required to complete another form, which lists departmental objectives, how objectives will be accomplished, and the time frame for completion. This method of budget preparation is not as complex as the budget systems discussed earlier, but it does require more than the superficial planning associated with the traditional method.

The foodservice director is probably more prepared to participate in budget preparation than most department heads in a medical operation, since accounting and cost control courses are included in the curriculum for foodservice management. Department heads in other areas are professionally competent in their specialty areas but may have little interest or knowledge in financial management. Therefore, participative financial management practices are not fully utilized in some medical organizations.

The foodservice budget, in numerical terms, should include the following costs (Fig. 15-17): (1) raw food, (2) labor, (3) supply, (4) equipment, and (5) other.

Food Costs

The budget amount for food will depend on the projected number of meals multiplied by the projected cost per meal. Unless there has been a change in menu offerings, a good estimate can be made from current food costs. A review of current food costs compared with costs during the previous year will give the rate of increase in cost. The projection is only as accurate as the records that have been maintained.

Labor Costs

Labor costs include wages, FICA, and fringe benefits. To arrive at a projected cost figure for nonmanagement employees, multiply the number of labor hours required by the hourly wage for each worker classification. The amount to add for fringe benefits can be obtained from the accounting office. In some cases an estimate can be made by adding a certain percentage to the base salary. Fringe benefits and other employee costs may include holiday pay, vacation pay, sick leave, funeral leave, personal days, group hospital insurance, group life, pension, workman's and unemployment compensation. In addition to FICA and fringe benefits, consider wage increases that have been negotiated, promotions, minimum wage increases as a result of federal regulations, projected overtime, and differential pay. Labor costs for management level employees is not subject to overtime or differential pay, but consideration must be given to annual increases and promotions. It is estimated that managerial costs can run from 6% to 20% of total labor cost and still result in an efficient operation (Kotschevar 1973).

Supply Costs

In this category, funds should be allocated for cleaning materials, disposables, china, glassware, flatware, office supplies, and small equipment. Here again, usage records can be used to project funds needed for optimal operation. The amount needed for cleaning supplies (detergent, soap, sanitizers, dishwashing compounds, mop heads, etc.) will depend on who is responsible for cleaning. If housekeeping or outside contractors are used, then the supply costs will be less, but the contractual fee will be higher. Cleaning supplies should be securely stored and issued in the same manner as food supplies. Employees responsible for cleaning duty should be fully informed on the use of all cleaning compounds, including amounts for different types such as "full strength" or "diluted." The

		Total Amount Spent		
Monthly Expense Report Department _____ Date _____				

Monthly Expense Report

Department _____ Date _____

Expense Item	Account No.	Total Amount Spent		Total Amount Budgeted ($)
		Month ($)	YTD (Year to Date)	
Food (Costs based on amounts pur-chased minus inventory.)				
Meat, fish, poultry				
Groceries				
Fruits and vegetables				
Dairy products				
Bakery				
Total		$	$	$
Labor				
Wages				
FICA				
Overtime premium				
Differential pay				
Vacation pay				
Holiday pay				
Sick leave				
Funeral				
Personal time				
Group hospital insurance				
Group life				
Workman's compensation				
Unemployment compensation				
Pension				
Total		$	$	$
Supply				
Cleaning materials				
Disposables				
China				
Glassware				
Silverware				
Office supplies				
Small equipment				
Total		$	$	$
Equipment				
Total		$	$	$
Other costs				
Laundry				
Uniforms				
Utilities				
Education				
Administrative over-head				
Printing				
Contractural services				
Contingency				
Total		$	$	$

Figure 15-17. Monthly expense report form.

use of automatic dispensers in areas such as dish machines, kitchen hand sinks, and employee facilities can result in savings.

Disposables include all paper and plastic supplies needed, such as napkins, plates, cups, trays for isolated patients, straws, sandwich wrap, and aluminum foil. To reduce costs of paper supplies, consider group purchasing or purchasing in bulk, if storage space is available. The use of dispensers for paper supplies such as napkins, straws, and cups tend to discourage taking more than one at a time. The amount of office supplies needed will depend on the form, type, and amount of paperwork generated in the foodservice department.

Small equipment costs refer to pots and pans, trays, serving utensils, knives, and so on. Pilferage and improper handling by employees are major causes of cost escalation in this category; therefore replacement is warranted on an annual basis. Make employees aware of the cost of each piece of small equipment, china, and silverware. Take pre- and postinventories for a period of time and share information on shortages with employees. Post the price of each item on the bulletin boards in the work areas so that employees will know the monetary loss to the department as the result of improper handling and breakage. Check trash for silverware thrown away as dishes and trays are scraped. Savings from the above practices can outweigh the cost of time involved.

Equipment Costs

Funding for large equipment (new, replacement, repair, and maintenance) is included in the capital budget. The need for effective capital budgeting is emphasized, not only because of the increasing costs of capital items but also because the failure to make timely replacement of inefficient equipment can impair the quantity and quality of food production and service. Capital budgeting practices require long-range planning, consistent with the needs of the organization. Since the medical organization may not have enough funds to meet all budgeted requests, careful consideration is given to approval. In most instances, a separate request form is used for each piece of equipment or project, such as the example shown in Figure 15-18.

Justifications are required for each request and should be submitted with the budget. Records of repair and maintenance, as shown in Figure 15-19, can serve as part of the justification. If your records show that the amount of *down time* for a piece of equipment or the cost of repairs results in inefficiency, you are more likely to get the budget request approved. Keep in mind that the foodservice budget is in competition with other departments of the facility, which may (in the eyes of the equipment committee) have a higher priority for funds.

Other Costs

In addition to food, labor, supply, and equipment costs, consideration should be given to the following: laundry, uniforms, utilities, continuing education, administrative overhead, printing, contractual services, and contingency. In most organizations, laundry is a contractual service. Whether this service is contracted or accomplished in-house, the cost will be minimal since most uniforms are of the noncotton permanent press type. Dish towels are not permitted for drying dishes or utensils, but clean sanitized cloths are needed for cleaning tabletops and other areas of food preparation and service. If disposable cleaning cloths are used, the cost should be included in the supply category. The costs associated with uniform purchase, if paid for by the organization, should be part of the fringe benefits. Some organizations prefer to provide both the uniform and the upkeep in order to ensure that employees are neat and clean for duty.

Capital Equipment Budget Request
Fiscal Year 19___

Department: _____ Date Submitted: _____

Capital Expenditure No. _____ Date Approved: _____

Directions: Complete *one* form for each item requested.

1. Item (equipment) _____

2. Description (manufacturer, model, serial no., etc.) _____
   _____

3. *Classification*   4. *Priority*
   ____Initial   ____Absolutely Essential
   ____Replacement   ____Necessary
   ____Expansion   ____Desirable

5. What is the anticipated cost (include expenses below) $_____
   Basic Equipment $_____   Auxiliary Cost $_____
   Freight $_____   Installation $_____
   Other Expenses (explain) $_____

6. Warranty Period _____ months/years   7. Estimated useful life _____

8. If maintenance contract is required, what is monthly cost? $_____

9. If replacement item, state plans for disposition of replaced item?
   _____
   _____

10. Briefly justify the expenditure (cost savings, quality control, revenue generated, new
    service, etc.) _____
    _____
    _____
    _____

                                    Requested by _____

Administrative Action:

Approved _____   Disapproved _____   Date _____

Comments: _____
_____

Figure 15-18. Capital equipment budget request form.

Equipment Record

Equipment _____ Purchase date _____

Cost _____ Full depreciation date _____

Location _____

Motor serial no. _____ Model _____

Motor specifications: (W) _____ (V) _____ (amp) _____ (hp) _____

Description: (type) _____ (size) _____

  (capacity) _____ (design) _____

Repair Maintenance and Replacement

Date	Nature	By Whom	Cost	Remarks

Figure 15-19. Equipment record form.

Utility costs are those such as heat, electricity, and water. Since the foodservice department is unlikely to have separate meters for the above costs, they are usually prorated. Check with the accounting department to determine the percentage of utility costs charged to foodservice.

Continuing education is an ongoing cost and should receive adequate attention to provide for in-service training of employees; attendance at conventions, workshops, and seminars; formal courses taken by employees; and books and other reference materials. To make sure that an adequate amount of funds is allotted for travel to out-of-town educational meetings, determine the number of employees attending, the mode of travel, and the cost of lodging and meals. For most annual meetings, the location is determined at least 1 year in advance. If formal courses taken by employees are counted as fringe benefits, cost should be reflected in the labor category.

Administrative overhead may include occupancy space, interest, mortgage depreciation, and salaries for staff and functional employees. All of these costs are prorated. Most organizations have calculations for operational cost based on square footage and may charge a percentage of that cost to foodservice or make the charges to the general fund.

Printing costs refer to expenses incurred for the printing of standardized forms. Color-coded "front-of-the-house" menus are a major part of this cost, in addition to other forms used on a regular basis.

Contractual services may include garbage and trash removal, housekeeping duties, exterminating services, and cleaning of vents, hoods, and windows. Consider reducing the amount of garbage and trash by using heavy-duty disposals and compactors. Investigate the sale of discarded fat, as well as compacted or compressed paper waste, especially corrugated boxes. Compare the cost and quality of outside versus in-house housekeeping. Exterminating services are essential for high standards of sanitation and safety, but cost and effectiveness of these services should be scrutinized. For all contractual services, know what you are being charged for by keeping records of services rendered. Compare services with bills submitted by contractors, especially on the number of hours spent in the department.

Contingency funds may be allowed, depending on the policies of the organization. Some organizations permit the inclusion of a certain percentage of the total budget for unexpected financial outlay.

Operating Reports and Analysis

Operating reports are provided at designated intervals as feedback for the department head. The most useful report is a comparison of costs on a monthly basis. As shown in Figure 15-17, the foodservice director can readily determine whether costs are out of line by comparing cost to date with budgeted amount. The analysis of costs on a monthly basis will provide enough time to investigate significant deviations from the budgeted amount and thus take corrective action.

References

American Hospital Association. Hospital Administrative Services. (1973). *Uniform System of Accounts*. Chicago: American Hospital Association.

Carter, J. E. (1977). Jimmy Carter Tells Why He Will Use Zero-Base Budgeting. *Nation's Bus. 65*(1), 24–26.

Deters, J. R. (1980). Teaching Finance to the Non-Financial Manager. *Financ. Exec. 48*(1), 28–34.

Hospital Administrative Services. (1973). *Uniform System of Accounts.* Chicago: American Hospital Association.

Kotschevar, L. H. (1973). *Foodservice for the Extended Care Facility.* Boston: Cahners Books.

Longrigg, J. (1981). Casebook No. 165: How to Reduce Staff Turnover. *Hosp. Nurs. Homes 16*(10), 98.

Novick, D. (1969). The Origin and History of Program Budgeting. *Calif Mgt Rev 11*(1), 7–12.

Pyhrr, P. (1970). Zero-Base Budgeting. *Harvard Bus. Rev. 48,* 111–121.

Pyhrr, P. (1973). *Zero-Base Budgeting.* New York: Wiley.

Pyhrr, P. (1976). Zero-Base Budgeting: Where to Use It and Where to Begin. *SAM Adv. Mgt. J. 41*(3), 4–14.

Romanelli, F. (1979). Study Shows How to Measure Energy Use, Costs, in Food Service. *Hospitals 53*(3), 77–78, 91.

Rose, J. C. (1980). Containing the Labor Cost of Foodservice. *Hospitals, 54*(6), 93–98.

Taylor, W. C. (1981). Absenteeism in Health Care Food Service. *J. Am. Diet. Assoc. 79*(6), 699–701.

APPENDIXES

APPENDIXES

Appendix A. Dietary Information

Table A-1. Food and Nutrition Board, National Academy of Sciences–National Research Council Recommended Daily Dietary Allowances, Revised 1980[a]

	Age (years)	Weight (kg)	Weight (lb)	Height (cm)	Height (in)	Energy Needs (kcal)	Energy Needs (with range)	(MJ)	Protein (g)	Vitamin A (μg RE)[b]	Vitamin D (μg)[c]	Vitamin E (mg α-TE)[d]	Vitamin C (mg)	Thiamin (mg)	Riboflavin (mg)	Niacin (mg NE)[e]	Vitamin B$_6$ (mg)	Folacin (μg)[f]	Vitamin B$_{12}$ (μg)	Calcium (mg)	Phosphorus (mg)	Magnesium (mg)	Iron (mg)	Zinc (mg)	Iodine (μg)
Infants	0.0–0.5	6	13	60	24	kg × 115	(95–145)	kg × 0.48	kg × 2.2	420	10	3	35	0.3	0.4	6	0.3	30	0.5	360	240	50	10	3	40
	0.5–1.0	9	20	71	28	kg × 105	(80–135)	kg × 0.44	kg × 2.0	400	10	4	35	0.5	0.6	8	0.6	45	1.5	540	360	70	15	5	50
Children	1–3	13	29	90	35	1300	(900–1800)	5.5	23	400	10	5	45	0.7	0.8	9	0.9	100	2.0	800	800	150	15	10	70
	4–6	20	44	112	44	1700	(1300–2300)	7.1	30	500	10	6	45	0.9	1.0	11	1.3	200	2.5	800	800	200	10	10	90
	7–10	28	62	132	52	2400	(1650–3300)	10.1	34	700	10	7	45	1.2	1.4	16	1.6	300	3.0	800	800	250	10	10	120
Males	11–14	45	99	157	62	2700	(2000–3700)	11.3	45	1000	10	8	50	1.4	1.6	18	1.8	400	3.0	1200	1200	350	18	15	150
	15–18	66	145	176	69	2800	(2100–3900)	11.8	56	1000	10	10	60	1.4	1.7	18	2.0	400	3.0	1200	1200	400	18	15	150
	19–22	70	154	177	70	2900	(2500–3300)	12.2	56	1000	7.5	10	60	1.5	1.7	19	2.2	400	3.0	800	800	350	10	15	150
	23–50	70	154	178	70	2700	(2300–3100)	11.3	56	1000	5	10	60	1.4	1.6	18	2.2	400	3.0	800	800	350	10	15	150
	51–75	70	154	178	70	2400	(2000–2800)	10.1	56	1000	5	10	60	1.2	1.4	16	2.2	400	3.0	800	800	350	10	15	150
Females	11–14	46	101	157	62	2200	(1500–3000)	9.2	46	800	10	8	50	1.1	1.3	15	1.8	400	3.0	1200	1200	300	18	15	150
	15–18	55	120	163	64	2100	(1200–3000)	8.8	46	800	10	8	60	1.1	1.3	14	2.0	400	3.0	1200	1200	300	18	15	150
	19–22	55	120	163	64	2100	(1700–2500)	8.8	44	800	7.5	8	60	1.1	1.3	14	2.0	400	3.0	800	800	300	18	15	150
	23–50	55	120	163	64	2000	(1600–2400)	8.4	44	800	5	8	60	1.0	1.2	13	2.0	400	3.0	800	800	300	18	15	150
	51–75	55	120	163	64	1800	(1400–2200)	7.6	44	800	5	8	60	1.0	1.2	13	2.0	400	3.0	800	800	300	10	15	150
Pregnant						+300			+30	+200	+5	+2	+20	+0.4	+0.3	+2	+0.6	+400	+1.0	+400	+400	+150	h	+5	+25
Lactating						+500			+20	+400	+5	+3	+40	+0.5	+0.5	+5	+0.5	+100	+1.0	+400	+400	+150	h	+10	+50

[a] The allowances are intended to provide for individual variations among most normal persons as they live in the United States under usual environmental stresses. Diets should be based on a variety of common foods in order to provide other nutrients for which human requirements have been less well defined.

[b] Retinol equivalents. 1 retinol equivalent = 1 μg retinol or 6 μg β-carotene.

[c] As cholecalciferol. 10 μg cholecalciferol = 400 IU of vitamin D.

[d] α-Tocopherol equivalents. 1 mg d-α-tocopherol = 1 α-TE.

[e] 1 NE (niacin equivalent) is equal to 1 mg of niacin or 60 mg of dietary tryptophan.

[f] The folacin allowances refer to dietary sources as determined by *Lactobacillus casei* assay after treatment with enzymes (conjugases) to make polyglutamyl forms of the vitamin available to the test organism.

[g] The recommended dietary allowance for vitamin B$_{12}$ in infants is based on average concentration of the vitamin in human milk. The allowances after weaning are based on energy intake (as recommended by the American Academy of Pediatrics) and consideration of other factors, such as intestinal absorption.

[h] The increased requirement during pregnancy cannot be met by the iron content of habitual American diets nor by the existing iron stores of many women; therefore, the use of 30–60 mg of supplemental iron is recommended. Iron needs during lactation are not substantially different from those of nonpregnant women, but continued supplementation of the mother for 2–3 months after parturition is advisable in order to replenish stores depleted by pregnancy.

Table A-2. Estimated Safe and Adequate Daily Dietary Intakes of Additional Selected Vitamins and Minerals[a]

Age group (years)	Vitamins			Trace elements[b] (mg)						Electrolytes (mg)		
	Vitamin K (μg)	Biotin (μg)	Pantothenic acid (mg)	Copper	Manganese	Fluoride	Chromium	Selenium	Molybdenum	Sodium	Potassium	Chloride
Infants												
0.0–0.5	12	35	2	0.5–0.7	0.5–0.7	0.1–0.5	0.01–0.04	0.01–0.04	0.03–0.06	115–350	350–925	275–700
0.5–1.0	10–20	50	3	0.7–1.0	0.7–1.0	0.2–1.0	0.02–0.06	0.02–0.06	0.04–0.08	250–750	425–1275	400–1200
Children and adolescents												
1–3	15–30	65	3	1.0–1.5	1.0–1.5	0.5–1.5	0.02–0.08	0.02–0.08	0.05–0.1	325–975	550–1650	500–1500
4–6	20–40	85	3–4	1.5–2.0	1.5–2.0	1.0–2.5	0.03–0.12	0.03–0.12	0.06–0.15	450–1350	775–2325	700–2100
7–10	30–60	120	4–5	2.0–2.5	2.0–3.0	1.5–2.5	0.05–0.2	0.05–0.2	0.1–0.3	600–1800	1000–3000	925–2775
11+	50–100	100–200	4–7	2.0–3.0	2.5–5.0	1.5–2.5	0.05–0.2	0.5–0.2	0.15–0.5	900–2700	1525–4575	1400–4200
Adults	70–140	100–200	4–7	2.0–3.0	2.5–5.0	1.5–4.0	0.05–0.2	0.05–0.2	0.15–0.5	1100–3300	1875–5625	1700–5100

[a] From Food and Nutrition Board, National Research Council, 1980. Recommended Dietary Allowances, Ninth Edition. National Academy of Science, Washington, D.C. Because there is less information on which to base allowances, these figures are not given in the main table of the RDAs and are provided here in the form of ranges of recommended intakes.

[b] Since the toxic levels for many trace elements may be only several times usual intakes, the upper levels for the trace elements given in this table should not be habitually exceeded.

Table A-3. Mean Heights and Weights and Recommended Energy Intake [a]

Age (years) and Sex Group	Weight kg	Weight lb	Height cm	Height in.	Energy Needs MJ [b]	Energy Needs kcal	Range (kcal)
Infants							
0.0–0.5	6	13	60	24	kg × 0.48	kg × 115	95–145
0.5–1.0	9	20	71	28	kg × 0.44	kg × 105	80–135
Children							
1–3	13	29	90	35	5.5	1300	900–1800
4–6	20	44	112	44	7.1	1700	1300–2300
7–10	28	62	132	52	10.1	2400	1650–3300
Males							
11–14	45	99	157	62	11.3	2700	2000–3700
15–18	66	145	176	69	11.8	2800	2100–3900
19–22	70	154	177	70	12.2	2900	2500–3300
23–50	70	154	178	70	11.3	2700	2300–3100
51–75	70	154	178	70	10.1	2400	2000–2800
76+	70	154	178	70	8.6	2050	1650–2450
Females							
11–14	46	101	157	62	9.2	2200	1500–3000
15–18	55	120	163	64	8.8	2100	1200–3000
19–22	55	120	163	64	8.8	2100	1700–2500
23–50	55	120	163	64	8.4	2000	1600–2400
51–75	55	120	163	64	7.6	1800	1400–2200
76+	55	120	163	64	6.7	1600	1200–2000
Pregnancy						+300	
Lactation						+500	

[a]From Food and Nutrition Board, National Research Council. 1980. Recommended Dietary Allowances, Ninth Edition. National Academy of Science, Washington, DC. The data in this table have been assembled from the observed median heights and weights of children, together with desirable weights for adults for mean heights of men (70 in.) and women (64 in.) between the ages of 18 and 34 years as surveyed in the U.S. population (DHHS data).

Energy allowances for the young adults are for men and women doing light work. The allowances for the two older age groups represent mean energy needs over these age spans, allowing for a 2% decrease in basal (resting) metabolic rate per decade and a reduction in activity of 200 kcal per day for men and women between 51 and 75 years; 500 kcal for men over 75 years; and 400 kcal for women over 75. The customary range of daily energy output is shown for adults in the range column and is based on a variation in energy needs of ±400 kcal at any one age, emphasizing the wide range of energy intakes appropriate for any group of people.

[b]MJ is megajoule. One joule equals 0.24 kcal.

Appendix B. Equivalent Measures and Weights

Table B-1. Equivalent Measures and Weights of Commonly Used Foods[a]

Food Item and Form	Approximate Weight per Cup	
	(g)	(oz)
Dairy products		
Butter	224	7.9
whipped	152	5.4
Cheese		
cheddar (natural or processed), grated or chopped	113	4.0
cottage	236	8.3
cream	230	8.1
spread		
Parmesan	92	3.3
Cream		
light (table)	240	8.5
heavy (whipping), whipped	236	8.3
sour	241	8.5
half and half (cream, milk), sweet	242	8.5
half and half, sour	242	8.5
Milk		
whole or skim	242	8.5
buttermilk	242	8.5
sweetened condensed	306	10.8
evaporated, whole or skim, reconstituted	252	8.9
dry, whole, reconstituted	121	4.3
dry, nonfat		
instant, reconstituted	75	2.6
noninstant, reconstituted	131	4.6
Milk desserts		
ice cream	142	5.0
ice milk	187	6.6
sherbet	193	6.8
Yogurt	246	8.7
Eggs		
whole	248	8.8
frozen	248	8.8
dried, sifted	86	3.0
whites		
fresh	246	8.7
frozen	246	8.7
dried, sifted	89	3.1
yolks		
fresh	233	8.2
frozen	233	8.2
dried, sifted	80	2.8
Fats and oils		
oils: corn, cottonseed, olive, peanut, and safflower	210	7.4
margarine	224	7.9
whipped	149	5.3
hydrogenated fat	188	6.6
lard and rendered fat	220	7.8
Fruits		
Apples		
pared and sliced	122	4.3
sauce, sweetened (not canned)	252	8.9
frozen, sliced, sweetened	205	7.2
canned, sliced	204	7.5
juice	249	8.8
sauce	259	9.1
dried	104	3.7
cooked	244	8.6

(continued)

Table B-1. Equivalent Measures and Weights of Commonly Used Foods (Continued)

Food Item and Form	Approximate Weight per Cup	
	(g)	(oz)
Apricots		
fresh, whole	115	4.1
sliced or halved	156	5.5
canned whole (medium)	225	7.9
halved (medium)	217	7.7
dried	150	5.3
cooked	249	8.8
Avocado		
sliced, diced, wedges	142	5.0
Banana		
fresh, sliced	142	5.0
mashed	232	8.2
dried	100	3.5
Blueberries		
fresh	146	5.2
frozen	161	5.7
canned	170	6.0
Cherries		
fresh, red, pitted	154	5.4
frozen	210	7.4
canned	177	6.2
Cranberries		
fresh	114	4.0
sauce	215	7.6
canned		
sauce	278	9.8
juice	250	8.8
Currants, dried	140	4.9
Dates, pitted, cut	178	6.3
Figs		
canned	230	4.9
dried, cut fine	168	5.9
Fruit juice		
canned	247	8.7
Fruits		
canned, cocktail or salad	229	8.1
Grapefruit		
fresh sections	194	6.8
frozen sections	219	7.7
canned, sections	241	8.5
Grapes, fresh		
seeded	184	6.5
seedless	169	6.0
Lemons		
fresh, juice	247	8.7
frozen, juice	283	10.0
canned, juice	245	8.6
Melon		
frozen	231	8.2
Oranges		
fresh, diced or sectioned	214	7.5
juice	247	8.7
frozen, juice, concentrated	268	9.5
canned, juice	247	8.7
Peaches		
fresh, sliced	177	6.2

Table B-1. **(Continued)**

Food Item and Form	Approximate Weight per Cup	
	(g)	(oz)
Peaches		
frozen, halves	220	7.8
canned		
halves	224	7.9
slices	218	7.7
dried	160	5.6
cooked	224	8.6
Pears		
fresh, sliced	158	5.6
canned, halves	227	8.0
Pineapples		
fresh, cubed	146	5.2
frozen, chunks	204	7.2
canned, chunks, tidbits	198	7.0
crushed	260	9.2
sliced	208	7.3
Plums		
fresh, halved	185	6.5
canned, whole	223	7.9
Prunes		
canned	196	6.9
dried, whole	176	6.2
cooked	229	8.1
pitted	162	5.7
cooked	210	7.4
Raisins		
seeded		
whole	142	5.0
chopped	182	6.4
seedless		
whole	146	5.2
cooked	183	6.5
chopped	189	6.7
Rhubarb		
fresh		
cut	122	4.3
cooked	242	8.5
frozen, sliced	168	5.9
Strawberries		
fresh		
whole	144	5.1
sliced	148	5.2
frozen		
whole	204	7.2
sliced or halved	235	8.3
Cereals		
Bulgur		
uncooked	162	5.7
cooked	230	8.1
Cornmeal		
white, uncooked	129	4.6
yellow		
uncooked	152	5.4
cooked	238	8.4
Farina		
cooked	238	8.4

(continued)

Table B-1. Equivalent Measures and Weights of Commonly Used Foods (Continued)

Food Item and Form	Approximate Weight per Cup (g)	(oz)
Hominy, whole		
cooked	182	6.4
Grits		
uncooked	154	5.4
cooked	236	8.3
Oats, rolled		
uncooked	72	2.5
cooked	240	8.5
Ready-to-eat		
flaked	32	1.1
granulated	87	3.1
puffed	23	0.8
shredded	37	1.3
Flours		
corn	116	4.1
gluten, sifted	142	5.0
rice		
sifted	126	4.4
stirred, spooned	158	5.6
rye		
light, sifted	88	3.1
dark, sifted	127	4.5
soy		
full-fat, sifted	60	2.1
lowfat	83	2.9
wheat, all-purpose		
sifted	115	4.1
unsifted, spooned	125	4.4
instant	129	4.6
bread, sifted	112	4.0
cake		
sifted	96	3.4
spooned	111	3.9
pastry, sifted	100	3.5
self-rising, sifted	106	3.7
whole-wheat, stirred	132	4.7
Starch		
corn, stirred	128	4.5
potato, stirred	142	5.0
Sweetening Agents		
Sugar		
brown, light	200	7.1
dark, packed	212	7.5
cane or beet granulated	200	7.1
superfine	196	6.9
confectioner's unsifted	123	4.3
confectioner's sifted	95	3.4
Corn syrup, light and dark	328	11.6
Honey	332	11.7
Maple syrup	312	11.0
Molasses, cane	309	10.9
Sorghum	330	11.6
Vegetables		
Asparagus, spears		
fresh, cooked	181	6.4
canned	195	6.9
frozen spears, cuts, and tips	181	6.4

Table B-1. (Continued)

Food Item and Form	Approximate Weight per Cup	
	(g)	(oz)
Beans, green		
fresh	114	4.0
cooked	125	4.4
frozen	161	5.7
canned	135	4.8
Beans, kidney, canned	187	6.6
dried		
uncooked	184	6.5
cooked	185	6.5
Beans, lima, shelled		
fresh		
raw	155	5.5
cooked	166	5.9
frozen	173	6.1
canned	170	6.0
dried		
uncooked	180	6.3
cooked	186	6.6
Beans, navy		
dried	190	6.7
cooked	191	6.7
Beans, soybeans, dried	210	7.4
Beets, without tops		
fresh		
uncooked	145	5.1
cooked	180	6.3
canned	167	5.9
Broccoli		
fresh, cooked	164	5.8
spears, chopped, frozen	188	6.6
Brussels sprouts		
fresh		
uncooked	102	3.6
cooked	180	6.4
Cabbage		
fresh, shredded	80	2.8
cooked	146	5.2
Carrots, without tops		
fresh	112	4.0
shredded	137	4.8
diced	160	5.6
cooked		
frozen, cooked	165	5.8
canned	159	5.6
Cauliflower, fresh		
raw	104	3.7
cooked	125	4.4
frozen		
uncooked	152	5.4
cooked	179	6.3
Celery, fresh		
raw	121	4.3
cooked	153	5.4
Corn, fresh ears		
cooked	165	5.8
frozen		
uncooked	135	4.8
cooked	182	6.4

(continued)

Table B-1. Equivalent Measures and Weights of Commonly Used Foods (Continued)

Food Item and Form	Approximate Weight per Cup	
	(g)	(oz)
Corn		
canned, cream style	249	8.8
whole kernel	169	6.0
Eggplant, fresh		
diced		
uncooked	99	3.5
cooked	213	7.5
Greens, fresh		
raw	77	2.7
cooked	190	6.7
frozen	187	6.6
Lentils		
dried	191	6.7
cooked	202	7.1
Mixed vegetables		
frozen	182	6.4
canned	179	6.3
Mushrooms, fresh, sliced		
raw	68	2.4
canned	161	7.4
Okra, fresh		
cooked	177	6.2
frozen	209	7.4
canned	171	6.0
Onions, fresh		
chopped, uncooked	135	4.8
cooked	197	6.9
dried	64	2.3
Parsnips, fresh		
cooked	211	7.4
Peas, green, fresh, in pod		
shelled		
raw	138	4.9
cooked	163	5.7
frozen		
raw	156	5.5
cooked	167	5.9
canned	168	5.9
dried, split		
uncooked	200	7.1
cooked	194	6.8
Peas, black-eyed, fresh		
raw	144	5.1
cooked	162	5.7
frozen, cooked	171	6.0
canned	205	7.2
dried, split		
uncooked	200	7.1
cooked	248	8.7
Potatoes, white, fresh		
raw	164	5.8
cooked	163	5.7
mashed	207	7.3
canned, whole	179	6.3
dried flakes	36	1.3
reconstituted	212	7.5
dried granules	201	7.1
reconstituted	212	7.5

Table B-1. (Continued)

Food Item and Form	Approximate Weight per Cup	
	(g)	(oz)
Pumpkin, fresh		
cooked, mashed	247	8.7
canned	244	8.6
Rutabaga, fresh, cubed		
raw	139	4.9
cooked	163	5.7
Sauerkraut, canned	188	6.6
Spinach, fresh		
raw	54	1.9
cooked	200	7.1
frozen	190	6.7
canned	221	7.8
Squash, winter, fresh		
cooked, mashed	244	8.6
frozen	242	8.5
Squash, summer, fresh		
raw	136	4.8
cooked, mashed	238	8.4
frozen, sliced	221	7.4
Sweet potatoes, fresh		
cooked, sliced	232	8.2
frozen	200	7.1
canned	220	7.8
dried, flakes	115	4.1
reconstituted	255	9.0
Tomatoes		
fresh	162	5.7
canned, whole	238	8.4
sauce	258	9.1
Turnips, fresh		
raw	134	4.7
cooked	196	6.9
Miscellaneous		
Bread, sliced		
crumbs, soft	46	1.6
dry	113	3.6
Catsup, tomato	273	9.6
Chocolate, bitter or semisweet	225	7.9
Cocoa		
prepared drink	112	4.0
instant, prepared drink	139	4.9
Coconut, long thread	80	2.8
canned	85	3.0
Coffee		
brewed	85	3.0
instant	38	1.4
Crackers		
graham, crumbs	86	3.0
soda, crumbs		
soda, crumbs, fine	70	2.5
Gelatin		
unflavored, granulated, unprepared	150	5.3
flavored, unprepared	179	6.3
prepared	557	19.5
Mayonnaise	243	8.6

(continued)

Table B-1. Equivalent Measures and Weights of Commonly Used Foods (Continued)

Food Item and Form	Approximate Weight per Cup	
	(g)	(oz)
Nuts, shelled		
almonds, blanched	152	5.4
filberts, whole	134	4.7
peanuts	144	5.1
pecans		
halved	108	3.8
chopped	118	4.2
pistachio	125	4.4
walnuts, Persian, English		
halved	100	3.5
chopped	119	4.2
Pasta		
macaroni, 1-in. pieces		
raw	123	4.3
cooked	140	4.9
macaroni, shell, raw	115	4.1
noodles, 1-in. pieces	73	2.6
spaghetti, 2-in. pieces		
raw	94	3.3
cooked	160	5.6
Peanut butter	251	8.9
Salad dressing, french	248	8.8
Salt, free-running	288	10.2
Soups		
canned, ready-to-serve	227	8.0
dried, reconstituted	231	8.2
Tapioca, quick-cooking	152	5.4
Tea, leaves		
brewed	72	2.5
instant	34	1.2
Water	237	8.4

	Approximate Weight (g)	
	(per tsp)	(per Tbsp)
Leavening agents		
Baking powder		
phosphate	4.1	12.7
SAS–phosphate	3.2	10.2
tartrate	2.9	9.2
Baking soda	4.0	12.2
Cream of tartar	3.1	9.4
Yeast		
active dry	2.5	7.5
compressed	4.2	12.8

[a]American Home Economics Association. 1975. Handbook of Food Preparation. AHEA, Washington, DC.

Appendix C. Adjusting Yield of Weight Amounts

The following instructions explain the use of Table C-1.

1. Locate the column which corresponds to the original yield of the recipe you wish to adjust. For example, assume your original recipe for meat loaf yields 100 portions. Locate the 100 column.

2. Run your finger down this column until you come to the amount of the ingredient required (or closest to this figure) in the recipe you wish to adjust. Say that your original recipe for 100 portions of meat loaf requires 21 lb of ground beef. Run your finger down the column headed 100 until you come to 21 lb.

3. Next, run your finger across the page, in line with that amount, until you come to the column which is headed to correspond with the yield you desire. Suppose you want to make 75 portions of meat loaf. Starting with your finger under the 21 lb (in the 100 column), slide it across to the column headed 75 and read the figure. You see you need 15 lb 12 oz ground beef to make 75 portions with your recipe.

4. Record this figure as the amount of the ingredient required for the new yield of your recipe. Repeat steps 1, 2, 3 for each ingredient in your original recipe to obtain the adjusted ingredient weight needed of each for your new yield. You can increase or decrease yield in this manner.

5. If you need to combine two columns to obtain your desired yield, follow the above procedure and add together the amounts given in the two columns to get the amount required for your adjusted yield. For example, to find the amount of ground beef for 225 portions of meat loaf (using the same recipe for 100 used above) locate the figures in columns headed 200 and 25 and add them. In this case they would be: 42 lb + 5 lb 4 oz, and the required total would be 47 lb 4 oz.

6. The figures in Table C-1 are given in exact weights including fractional ounces. After you have made yield adjustments for every ingredient, refer to Appendix F for "rounding-off" fractional amounts which are not of sufficient proportion to change product quality. No rounding-off is required for amounts needed for adjusted ingredients in the examples we have used here.

Table C-1. Direct-Reading Table for Adjusting Yield of Recipes with Ingredient Amounts Given in Weights [a,b]

25 portions		50 portions		75 portions		100 portions		200 portions		300 portions		400 portions		500 portions	
lb	oz	lb	oz	lb	oz	lb	oz	lb	oz	lb	oz	lb	oz	lb	oz
	2		4		6		8	1		1	8	2		2	8
	2¼		4¼		6½		8½	1	1	1	9½	2	2	2	10½
	2¼		4½		6¾		9	1	2	1	11	2	4	2	13
	2½		4¾		7¼		9½	1	3	1	12½	2	6	2	15½
	2½		5		7½		10	1	4	1	14	2	8	3	2
	2¾		5½		8½		11	1	6	2	1	2	12	3	7
	3		6		9		12	1	8	2	4	3		3	12
	3¼		6½		9¾		13	1	10	2	7	3	4	4	1
	3½		7		10½		14	1	12	2	10	3	8	4	6
	3¾		7½		11¼		15	1	14	2	13	3	12	4	11
	4		8		12	1		2		3		4		5	
	4½		9		13½	1	2	2	4	3	6		8	5	10

(continued)

385

Table C-1. (Continued)

25 portions		50 portions		75 portions		100 portions		200 portions		300 portions		400 portions		500 portions	
lb	oz	lb	oz	lb	oz	lb	oz	lb	oz	lb	oz	lb	oz	lb	oz
	5		10		15	1	4	2	8	3	12	5		6	4
	5½		11	1	½	1	6	2	12	4	2	5	8	6	14
	6		12	1	2	1	8	3		4	8	6		7	8
	6½		13	1	3½	1	10	3	4	4	14	6	8	8	2
	7		14	1	5	1	12	3	8	5	4	7		8	12
	7½		15	1	6½	1	14	3	12	5	10	7	8	9	6
	8	1		1	8	2		4		6		8		10	
	8½	1	1	1	9½	2	2	4	4	6	6	8	8	10	10
	9	1	2	1	11	2	4	4	8	6	12	9		11	4
	9½	1	3	1	12½	2	6	4	12	7	2	9	8	11	14
	10	1	4	1	14	2	8	5		7	8	10		12	8
	11	1	6	2	1	2	12	5	8	8	4	11		13	12
	12	1	8	2	4	3		6		9		12		15	
	13	1	10	2	7	3	4	6	8	9	12	13		16	4
	14	1	12	2	10	3	8	7		10	8	14		17	8
	15	1	14	2	13	3	12	7	8	11	4	15		18	12
1		2		3		4		8		12		16		20	
1	1	2	2	3	3	4	4	8	8	12	12	17		21	4
1	2	2	4	3	6	4	8	9		13	8	18		22	8
1	3	2	6	3	9	4	12	9	8	14	4	19		23	12
1	4	2	8	3	12	5		10		15		20		25	
1	5	2	10	3	15	5	4	10	8	15	12	21		26	4
1	6	2	12	3	2	5	8	11		16	8	22		27	8
1	7	2	14	3	5	5	12	11	8	17	4	23		28	12
1	8	3		4	8	6		12		18		24		30	
1	10	3	4	4	14	6	8	13		19	8	26		32	8
1	12	3	8	5	4	7		14		21		28		35	
1	14	3	12	5	10	7	8	15		22	8	30		37	8
2		4		6		8		16		24		32		40	
2	2	4	4	6	6	8	8	17		25	8	34		42	8
2	4	4	8	6	12	9		18		27		36		45	
2	6	5	12	7	2	9	8	19		28	8	38		47	8
2	8	5		7	8	10		20		30		40		50	
2	12	5	8	8	4	11		22		33		44		55	
3		6		9		12		24		36		48		60	
3	4	6	8	9	12	13		26		39		52		65	
3	8	7		10	8	14		28		42		56		70	
3	12	7	8	11	4	15		30		45		60		75	
4		8		12		16		32		48		64		80	
4	4	8	8	12	12	17		34		51		68		85	
4	8	9		13	8	18		36		54		72		90	
4	12	9	8	14	2	19		38		57		76		95	
5		10		15		20		40		60		80		100	
5	4	10	8	15	12	21		42		63		84		105	
5	8	11		16	8	22		44		66		88		110	
5	12	11	8	17	4	23		46		69		92		115	
6		12		18		24		48		72		96		120	
6	4	12	8	18	12	25		50		75		100		125	
7	8	15		22	8	30		60		90		120		150	
8	12	17	8	26	4	35		70		105		140		175	
10		20		30		40		80		120		160		200	
11	4	22	8	33	12	45		90		135		180		225	
12	8	25		37	8	50		100		150		200		250	

[a]From American Dietetic Association. 1967. Standardizing Recipes for Institutional Use. ADA, Chicago, IL. This table was adapted from conversion charts developed by the Nutrition Services Division of the New York State Department of Mental Hygiene, Albany, NY.

[b]This table is primarily for adjusting recipes with original and desired portion yields which can be divided by 25.

Appendix D. Adjusting Yield of Measurement Amounts

The following instructions explain the use of Table D-1.

1. Locate column which corresponds to the original yield of the recipe you wish to adjust. For example, let us assume your original sour cream cookie recipe yields 300 cookies. Locate the 300 column.

2. Run your finger down this column until you come to the amount of the ingredient required (or closest to this figure) in the recipe you wish to adjust. Say that your original recipe for 300 cookies required 2¼ cup fat. Run your finger down the column headed 300 until you come to 2¼ cup.

3. Next, run your finger across the page, in line with that amount, until you come to the column which is headed to correspond with the yield you desire. Suppose you want to make 75 cookies. Starting with your finger under the 2¼ cup (in the 300 column), slide it across to the column headed 75 and read the figure. You see you need ½ cup + 1 Tbsp fat to make 75 cookies from your recipe.

4. Record this figure as the amount of the ingredient required for the new yield of your recipe. Repeat steps 1, 2, 3 for each ingredient in your original recipe to obtain the adjusted measure needed of each for your new yield. You can increase or decrease yield in this manner.

5. If you need to combine two columns to obtain your desired yield, follow the above procedure and add together the amounts given in the two columns to get the amount required for your adjusted yield. For example, to find the amount of fat needed to make 550 cookies (using the same basic recipe as above) locate the figures in column headed 500 and 50 and add them. In this case they would be 3¾ cup + 6 Tbsp and the required total would be 1 qt + 2 Tbsp fat.

6. The figures in Table D-1 are given in measurements which provide absolute accuracy. After you have made yield adjustments for each ingredient, refer to Appendix F for *rounding-off* odd fractions and complicated measurements. You can safely *round-off* to 1 qt as shown in Appendix F, for the amount of fat needed in the recipe for 550 cookies.

Table D-1. Direct-Reading Table for Adjusting Yield of Recipes with Ingredient Amounts Given in Measurement[a,b]

25 portions	50 portions	75 portions	100 portions	200 portions	300 portions	400 portions	500 portions
1 Tbsp	2 Tbsp	3 Tbsp	¼ cup	½ cup	¾ cup	1 cup	1¼ cup
1 Tbsp + 1 tsp	2 Tbsp + 2 tsp	¼ cup	⅓ cup	⅔ cup	1 cup	1⅓ cup	1⅔ cup
2 Tbsp	¼ cup	¼ cup + 2 Tbsp	½ cup	1 cup	1½ cup	2 cups	2½ cup
2 Tbsp + 2 tsp	⅓ cup	½ cup	⅔ cup	1⅓ cup	2 cup	2⅔ cup	3⅓ cup
3 Tbsp	6 Tbsp	½ cup + 1 Tbsp	¾ cup	1½ cup	2¼ cup	3 cup	3¾ cup
¼ cup	½ cup	¾ cup	1 cup	2 cup	3 cup	1 qt	1¼ qt
¼ cup + 1 Tbsp	½ cup + 2 Tbsp	¾ cup + 3 Tbsp	1¼ cup	2½ cup	3¾ cup	1¼ qt	1½ qt + ¼ cup
⅓ cup	⅔ cup	1 cup	1⅓ cup	2⅔ cup	1 qt	1¼ qt + ⅓ cup	1½ qt + ⅔ cup
⅓ cup + 2 Tbsp	¾ cup	1 cup + 2 Tbsp	1½ cup	3 cup	1 qt + ½ cup	1½ qt	1¾ qt + ½ cup
6 Tbsp + 2 tsp	¼ cup + 4 Tbsp	1¼ cup	1⅔ cup	3⅓ cup	1¼ qt	1½ qt + ⅔ cup	2 qt + ⅓ cup
¼ cup + 3 Tbsp	¾ cup + 2 Tbsp	1¼ cup + 1 Tbsp	1¾ cup	3½ cup	1¼ qt + ¼ cup	1¾ qt	2 qt + ¾ cup

(continued)

Table D-1. Direct-Reading Table for Adjusting Yield of Recipes with Ingredient Amounts Given in Measurement (Continued)

25 portions	50 portions	75 portions	100 portions	200 portions	300 portions	400 portions	500 portions
½ cup	1 cup	1½ cup	2 cup	1 qt	1½ qt	2 qt	2½ qt
½ cup + 1 Tbsp	1 cup + 2 Tbsp	1½ cup + 3 Tbsp	2¼ cup	1 qt + ½ cup	1½ qt + ¾ cup	2¼ qt	2¾ qt + ¼ cup
½ cup + 4 tsp	1 cup + 2 Tbsp + 2 tsp	1¾ cup	2⅓ cup	1 qt + ⅔ cup	1¾ qt	2¼ qt + ⅓ cup	2¾ qt + ⅔ cup
½ cup + 2 Tbsp	1¼ cup	1¾ cup + 2 Tbsp	2½ cup	1¼ qt	1¾ qt + ½ cup	2½ qt	3 qt + ½ cup
⅔ cup	1⅓ cup	2 cup	2⅔ cup	1¼ qt + ⅓ cup	2 qt	2½ qt + ⅔ cup	3 qt + ⅓ cup
½ cup + 3 Tbsp	1¼ cup + 2 Tbsp	2 cup + 1 Tbsp	2¾ cup	1¼ qt + ½ cup	2 qt + ¼ cup	2¾ cup	3¼ qt + ¾ cup
¾ cup	1½ cup	2¼ cup	3 cup	1½ qt	2¼ qt	3 qt	3¾ qt
¾ cup + 1 Tbsp	1½ cup + 2 Tbsp	2¼ cup + 3 Tbsp	3¼ cup	1½ qt + ½ cup	2¼ qt + ¾ cup	3¼ qt	1 gal. + ¼ cup
¾ cup + 4 Tbsp	1⅔ cup	2½ cup	3⅓ cup	1½ qt + ⅔ cup	2½ qt	3¼ qt + ⅓ cup	1 gal. + ⅔ cup
¾ cup + 2 Tbsp	1¾ cup	2½ cup + 2 Tbsp	3½ cup	1¾ qt	2½ qt + ½ cup	3½ qt	1 gal. + 1½ cup
¾ cup + 2 Tbsp + 2½ tsp	1¾ cup + 4 Tbsp	2¾ cup + ½ tsp	3⅔ cup	1¾ qt + ⅓ cup	2¾ qt	3½ qt + ⅔ cup	1 gal. + 1⅔ cup
¾ cup + 3 Tbsp	1¾ cup + 2 Tbsp	2¾ cup + 1 Tbsp	3¾ cup	1¾ qt + ½ cup	3 qt + ¼ cup	1 gal.	1 gal. + 3¾ cup
1 cup	2 cup	3 cup	1 qt	2 qt	3 qt	1 gal.	1¼ gal.
1½ cup	3 cup	1 qt	1½ qt	3 qt	1 gal. + 2 cup	1½ gal.	1¾ gal. + 2 cup
1¾ cup	3½ cup	1¼ qt + ¼ cup	1¾ qt	3½ qt	1¼ gal. + 1 cup	1¾ gal.	2 gal. + 3 cup
2 cup	1 qt	1½ qt	2 qt	1 gal.	1½ gal.	2 gal.	2½ gal.
2¼ cup	1 qt + ½ cup	1½ qt + ¾ cup	2¼ qt	1 gal. + 2 cup	1½ gal. + 3 cup	2¼ gal.	2¾ gal. + 1 cup
2½ cup	1¼ qt	1¾ qt + ½ cup	2½ qt	1¼ gal.	1¾ gal. + 2 cup	2½ gal.	3 gal. + 2 cup
2¾ cup	1¼ qt + ½ cup	2 qt + ¼ cup	2¾ qt	1¼ gal. + 2 cup	2 gal. + 1 cup	2¾ gal.	3¼ gal. + 3 cup
3 cup	1½ qt	2¼ qt	3 qt	1½ gal.	2¼ gal.	3 gal.	3¾ gal.
3¼ cup	1½ qt + ½ cup	2¼ qt + ¾ cup	3¼ qt	1½ gal. + 2 cup	2¼ gal. + 3 cup	3¼ gal.	4 gal. + 1 cup
3½ cup	1¾ qt	2½ qt + ½ cup	3½ qt	1¾ gal.	2½ gal. + 2 cup	3½ gal.	4¼ gal. + 2 cup
3¾ cup	1¾ qt + ½ cup	2¾ qt + ¼ cup	3¾ qt	1¾ gal. + 2 cup	2¾ gal. + 1 cup	3¾ gal.	4½ gal. + 3 cup
1 qt	2 qt	3 qt	1 gal.	2 gal.	3 gal.	4 gal.	5 gal.
1¼ qt	2½ qt	3¾ qt	1¼ gal.	2½ gal.	3¾ gal.	5 gal.	6¼ gal.
1½ qt	3 qt	1 gal. + 2 cup	1½ gal.	3 gal.	4½ gal.	6 gal.	7½ gal.
1¾ qt	3½ qt	1¼ gal. + 1 cup	1¾ gal.	3½ gal.	5¼ gal.	7 gal.	8¼ gal.
2 qt	1 gal.	1½ gal.	2 gal.	4 gal.	6 gal.	8 gal.	10 gal.
2¼ qt	1 gal. + 2 cup	1½ gal. + 3 cup	2¼ gal.	4½ gal.	6¾ gal.	9 gal.	11¼ gal.
2½ qt	1¼ gal.	1¾ gal. + 2 cup	2½ gal.	5 gal.	7½ gal.	10 gal.	12½ gal.
2¾ qt	1¼ gal. + 2 cup	2 gal. + 1 cup	2¾ gal.	5½ gal.	8¼ gal.	11 gal.	13¾ gal.
3 qt	1½ gal.	2¼ gal.	3 gal.	6 gal.	9 gal.	12 gal.	15 gal.
3 qt + 1 cup	1½ gal. + 2 cup	2¼ gal. + 3 cup	3¼ gal.	6½ gal.	9¾ gal.	13 gal.	16¼ gal.
3½ qt	1¾ gal.	2½ gal. + 2 cup	3½ gal.	7 gal.	10½ gal.	14 gal.	17½ gal.
3½ qt + 1 cup	1¾ gal. + 2 cup	2¾ gal. + 1 cup	3¾ gal.	7½ gal.	11¼ gal.	15 gal.	18¾ gal.
1 gal.	2 gal.	3 gal.	4 gal.	8 gal.	12 gal.	16 gal.	20 gal.

[a]From American Dietetic Association. 1967. Standardizing Recipes for Institutional Use. ADA, Chicago, IL.

[b]This table is primarily for adjusting recipes with original and desired portion yields which can be divided by 25. *Abbreviations in table:* tsp is teaspoon; Tbsp, tablespoon; qt, quart; and gal., gallon. *Basic information:* For ¾ tsp, combine ½ tsp + ¼ tsp; for ⅛ tsp use half of the ¼ tsp. Equivalents are: 3 tsp, 1 Tbsp; 4 Tbsp, ¼ cup; 5 Tbsp + 1 tsp, ⅓ cup; 8 Tbsp, ½ cup; 10 Tbsp + 2 tsp, ⅔ cup; 12 Tbsp, ¾ cup; 16 Tbsp, 1 cup; 4 cups, 1 qt; and 4 qt, 1 gal.

Appendix E. Purchase Units for Commonly Used Foods[1]

Table E-1. Meats

Meat as Purchased; Unit of Purchase, lb	Yield, Cooked As Served (%)	Yield, Cooked Lean Only (%)	Description of Portion as Served	Size of Portion As Served (oz)	Size of Portion Lean Only (oz)	Portions per Purchase Unit (no.)	Approximate Purchase Units for— 25 Portions (no.)	Approximate Purchase Units for— 100 Portions (no.)
Beef, fresh or frozen								
Brisket:								
corned, bone out	60	41	Simmered	4	2.8	2.40	10½	41¾
				3	2.1	3.20	8	31¼
fresh:								
bone in	52	36	Simmered, bone out	4	2.8	2.08	12¼	48¼
				3	2.1	2.77	9¼	36¼
bone out	67	46	Simmered	4	2.8	2.68	9½	37½
				3	2.1	3.57	7¼	28¼
Ground beef:								
lean	75	75	Broiled	3	3.0	4.00	6¼	25
				2	2.0	6.00	4¼	16¾
regular	72	72	Pan-fried	3	3.0	3.84	6¾	26¼
				2	2.0	5.76	4½	17½
Heart	39	39		2	2.0	3.12	8¼	32¼
Kidney	39	39		2	2.0	3.12	8¼	32¼
Liver	69	69	Braised	3	3.0	3.68	7	27¼
				2	2.0	5.52	4¾	18¼
Oxtails	29	29		a	a	a	a	a
Roasts:								
chuck:								
bone in	52	42	Roasted, moist heat, bone out	4	3.2	2.08	12¼	48¼
				3	2.4	2.77	9¼	36¼
bone out	67	54	Roasted, moist heat	4	3.2	2.68	9½	37½
				3	2.4	3.57	7¼	28¼
7-rib (shortribs removed):								
bone in	65	42	Roasted, dry heat, bone out	4	2.6	2.60	9¾	38½
				3	1.9	3.47	7¼	29
bone out	73	47	Roasted, dry heat	4	2.6	2.92	8¾	34¼
				3	1.9	3.89	6½	25¾
round:								
bone in	69	56	Roasted, dry heat, medium, bone out	4	3.3	2.76	9¼	36¼
				3	2.5	3.68	7	27¼
bone out	73	60	Roasted, dry heat, medium	4	3.3	2.92	8¾	34¼
				3	2.5	3.89	6½	25¼
rump:								
bone in	58	43	Roasted, dry heat, bone out	4	3.0	2.32	11	43¼
				3	2.2	3.09	8¼	32½
bone out	73	55	Roasted, dry heat	4	3.0	2.92	8¾	34¼
				3	2.2	3.89	6½	25¾
shortribs	67	32	Braised, bone in	6	2.9	1.79	14	56
				4	1.9	2.68	9½	37½
Steaks								
club								
bone in	73	33	Broiled, bone in	6	2.7	1.95	13	51½
				4	1.8	2.92	8¾	34¼
bone out	73	42	Broiled	4	2.3	2.92	8¾	34¼
				3	1.7	3.89	6½	25¾

(continued)

[1] All Appendix E tables are from U.S. Department of Agriculture, 1976. Food Purchasing Guide for Group Feeding, Agriculture Handbook No. 284. Superintendent of Documents, U.S. Government Printing Office, Washington, DC.

Table E-1. Meats (Continued)

Meat as Purchased; Unit of Purchase, lb	Yield, Cooked As Served (%)	Yield, Cooked Lean Only (%)	Description of Portion as Served	Size of Portion As Served (oz)	Size of Portion Lean Only (oz)	Portions per Purchase Unit (no.)	Approximate Purchase Units for— 25 Portions (no.)	Approximate Purchase Units for— 100 Portions (no.)
Steaks								
flank	67	67	Braised	3	3.0	3.57	7¼	28¼
				2	2.0	5.36	4¾	18¾
hip								
bone in	73	32	Broiled, bone in	6	2.6	1.95	13	51½
				4	1.8	2.92	8¾	34¼
bone out	73	40	Broiled	4	2.2	2.92	8¾	34¼
				3	1.6	3.89	6½	25¾
minute, cubed	75	75	Pan-fried	3	3.0	4.00	6¼	25
				2	2.0	6.00	4¼	16¾
porterhouse:								
bone in	73	36	Broiled, bone in	8	4.0	1.46	17¼	68½
				6	3.0	1.95	13	51½
				4	2.0	2.92	8¾	34¼
bone out	73	42	Broiled	4	2.3	2.92	8¾	34½
				3	1.7	3.89	6½	25¾
round								
bone in	73	56	Broiled, bone in	4	3.1	2.92	8¾	34¼
				3	2.3	3.89	6½	25¾
bone out	73	60	Broiled	4	3.3	2.92	8¾	34½
				3	2.5	3.89	6½	25¾
sirloin (wedge and round):								
bone in	73	44	Broiled, bone in	6	3.6	1.95	13	51½
				4	2.4	2.92	8¾	31¼
bone out	73	48	Broiled	4	2.6	2.92	8¾	31¼
				3	2.0	3.89	6½	25¾
T-bone:								
bone in	73	34	Broiled, bone in	8	3.8	1.46	17¼	68½
				6	2.8	1.95	13	51½
				4	1.9	2.92	8¾	34¼
bone out	73	41	Broiled	4	2.2	2.92	8¾	34¼
				3	1.7	3.89	6½	25¾
Stew meat (chuck), bone out	67	54	Cooked, moist heat	3	2.4	3.57	7¼	28¼
				2	1.6	5.36	4¾	18¾
Tongue:								
fresh	59	59	Cooked, moist heat	3	3.0	3.15	8	31¾
				2	2.0	4.72	5½	21¼
smoked	51	51	Cooked, moist heat	3	3.0	2.72	9¼	37
				2	2.0	4.08	6¼	24¾
Beef, canned								
Beef, corned	100	100	Heated	3	3.0	5.33	4¾	19
6-lb can	100	100	Heated	2	2.0	8.00	3¼	12½
				3	3.0	32.00	1	3¼
Beef, dried								
Beef, chipped	125	125	Cooked, moist heat	3	3.0	6.67	3¾	15
				2	2.0	10.00	2⅓	10
Lamb, fresh or frozen								
Chops								
loin	76	41	Broiled, bone in	5.0	2.7	2.43	10½	41¼
rib	76	34	Broiled, bone in	5.0	2.2	2.43	10½	41¼
shoulder	70	41	Broiled, bone in	5.0	2.9	2.24	11¼	44¾
Ground lamb	68	68	Broiled patties	3.0	3.0	3.63	7	27¾
				2.0	2.0	5.44	4¾	18½

Table E-1. (Continued)

Meat as Purchased; Unit of Purchase, lb	Yield, Cooked		Description of Portion as Served	Size of Portion		Portions per Purchase Unit (no.)	Approximate Purchase Units for—	
	As Served (%)	Lean Only (%)		As Served (oz)	Lean Only (oz)		25 Portions (no.)	100 Portions (no.)
Roasts								
leg								
bone in	54	45	Roasted, bone out	4.0	3.3	2.16	11¾	46½
				3.0	2.5	2.88	8¾	34¾
bone out	70	58	Roasted	4.0	3.3	2.80	9	35¾
				3.0	2.5	3.73	6¾	27
Shoulder								
bone in	55	41	Roasted, bone out	4.0	3.0	2.20	11½	45½
				3.0	2.2	2.93	8¾	34¼
bone out	70	52	Roasted	4.0	3.0	2.80	9	35¾
				3.0	2.2	3.73	6¾	27
Stew meat,[b] bone out	66	—	Simmered	3.0	—	3.52	7¼	28½
				2.0	—	5.28	4¾	19
Pork, cured (mild)								
Bacon (2–4 slices per pound)	32	—	Fried or broiled	2 slices	—	12.00	2¼	8½
Canadian bacon	63	63	Broiled, sliced	2	2.0	5.04	5	20
				1	1.0	10.08	2½	10
Ham								
bone in	67	54	Roasted, slices and pieces	4	2.9	2.68	9½	37½
				3	2.2	3.57	7¼	28¼
	56	44	Roasted, slices	4	2.4	2.24	11¼	44¾
				3	1.8	2.99	8½	33½
bone out	77	72	Roasted, slices and pieces	4	2.9	3.08	8¼	32½
				3	2.2	4.11	6¼	24½
	64	60	Roasted, slices	4	2.4	2.56	10	39¼
				3	1.8	3.41	7½	29½
ground	77	77	Patties	3	3.0	4.11	6¼	24½
				2	2.0	6.16	4¼	16¼
Shoulder, Boston butt								
bone in	67	52	Roasted, bone out	4	3.1	2.68	9½	37½
				3	2.3	3.57	7¼	28¼
bone out	74	58	Roasted	4	3.1	2.96	8½	34
				3	2.3	3.95	6½	25½
Shoulder, picnic								
bone in	56	41	Roasted, bone out	4	3.9	2.24	11¼	44¾
				3	2.2	2.99	8½	33½
bone out	74	53	Roasted	4	3.9	2.96	8½	34
				3	2.2	3.95	6½	25½
Pork, fresh								
Chops:								
loin	69	42	Broiled, bone in	5	3.0	2.21	11½	45¼
				3	1.8	3.68	7	27¼
rib	70	37	Broiled, bone in	5	2.6	2.24	11¼	44¼
				3	1.6	3.73	6¾	27
Cutlet, tenderloin	75	75	Broiled	3	3.0	4.00	6¼	25
				2	2.0	6.00	4¼	16¾
Ground pork	57	57	Broiled, bone in	3	3.0	3.04	8¼	33
				2	2.0	4.56	5½	22
Liver	60	60	Pan- or oven-fried	3	3.0	3.20	8	31¼
				2	2.0	4.80	5¼	21

(continued)

Table E-1. Meats (Continued)

Meat as Purchased; Unit of Purchase, lb	Yield, Cooked		Description of Portion as Served	Size of Portion		Portions per Purchase Unit (no.)	Approximate Purchase Units for—	
	As Served (%)	Lean Only (%)		As Served (oz)	Lean Only (oz)		25 Portions (no.)	100 Portions (no.)
Roasts								
ham								
bone in	54	40	Roasted, bone out	4	3.0	2.16	11¾	46⅓
				3	2.2	2.88	8¾	34¾
bone out	68	50	Roasted	4	3.0	2.72	9¼	37
				3	2.2	3.63	7	27¾
loin:								
bone in	68	37	Roasted, bone in	5	2.8	2.18	11⅓	46
				4	2.2	2.72	9¼	37
	47	37	Roasted, bone out	4	3.2	1.88	13½	53¼
				3	2.4	2.51	10	40
bone out	68	54	Roasted	4	3.2	2.72	9¼	37
				3	2.4	3.63	7	27¾
shoulder, Boston butt:								
bone in	62	49	Roasted, bone out	4	3.2	2.48	10¼	40½
				3	2.4	3.31	7¾	30¼
bone out	68	54	Roasted	4	3.2	2.72	9¼	37
				3	2.4	3.63	7	27¾
Shoulder, picnic:								
bone in	47	35	Simmered, bone out	4	3.0	1.88	13½	53¾
				3	2.2	2.51	10	40
bone out	64	47	Simmered	4	3.0	2.56	10	39¼
				3	2.2	3.41	7½	29½
Sausage:								
brown and serve	81	81	Heated	3	3.0	4.32	6	23¼
				2	2.0	6.48	4	15½
bulk or link	48	48	Oven-fried	3	3.0	2.56	10	39¼
				2	2.0	3.84	6¾	26¼
Spareribs	66	26	Braised, bone in	6	2.3[c]	1.76	14¼	57
				4	1.6[c]	2.64	9½	38
Pork, canned								
Ham, chopped	100	100	Sliced	3	3.0	5.33	4¾	19
				2	2.0	8.00	3¼	12½
Ham, smoked	77	75	Slices and pieces	3	2.9	4.11	6¼	24½
				2	1.9	6.16	4¼	16¼
	73	71	Slices	3	2.9	3.89	6½	25¾
				2	1.9	5.84	4½	17¼
Pork luncheon meat (with natural juices)	89	89	Unheated	3	3.0	4.75	5½	21¼
				2	2.0	7.12	3¾	14¼
Sausages								
Frankfurters:								
8/lb	98	—	2 frankfurters	—	—	4.00	6¼	25
			1 frankfurter	—	—	8.00	3¼	12½
10/lb	98	—	2 frankfurters	—	—	5.00	5	20
			1 frankfurter	—	—	10.00	2½	10

Table E-1. (Continued)

Meat as Purchased; Unit of Purchase, lb	Yield, Cooked As Served (%)	Yield, Cooked Lean Only (%)	Description of Portion as Served	Size of Portion As Served (oz)	Size of Portion Lean Only (oz)	Portions per Purchase Unit (no.)	Approximate Purchase Units for 25 Portions (no.)	Approximate Purchase Units for 100 Portions (no.)
Luncheon meats (all meat varieties)	100	100	—	3	3.0	5.33	4¾	19
				2	2.0	8.00	3¼	12½
Vienna sausage (all meat) (drained weight)	100	100	About 4 sausages	2	2.0	8.00	3¼	12½
			About 2 sausages	1	1.0	16.00	1¾	6¼
Veal, fresh or frozen								
Chops:								
loin	78	47	Broiled, bone in	5	3.0	2.50	10	40
				3	1.8	4.16	6	24¼
rib	69	38	Broiled, bone in	5	2.8	2.21	11½	45¼
				3	1.6	3.68	7	27¼
shoulder	66	40	Broiled, bone in	5	3.0	2.11	12	47½
				3	1.8	3.52	7¼	28½
Cutlet, bone out	75	75	Broiled	4	3.0	3.00	8½	33½
				3	2.2	4.00	6¼	25
Ground	64	64	Oven- or pan-fried	3	3.0	3.41	7½	29½
				2	2.0	5.12	5	19¾
Heart	35	35	Braised	2	2.0	2.80	9	35¾
Liver, calf	58	58	Fried or braised	3	3.0	3.09	8¼	32½
				2	2.0	4.64	5½	21¾
Roasts:								
chuck (shoulder):								
bone in	46	40	Braised, bone out	4	3.4	1.84	13¾	54½
				3	2.6	2.45	10¼	41
bone out	66	56	Braised	4	3.4	2.64	9½	38
				3	2.6	3.52	7¼	28½
leg:								
bone in	44	36	Roasted, bone out	4	3.3	1.76	14¼	57
				3	2.5	2.35	10¾	42¼
bone out	66	54	Roasted	4	3.3	2.64	9½	38
				3	2.5	3.2	7¼	28½
plate (breast):								
bone in	45	33	Stewed, bone out	4	2.9	1.80	14	55¾
				3	2.2	2.40	10½	41¾
bone out	66	48	Stewed	4	2.9	2.64	9½	38
				3	2.2	3.52	7¼	28½
Stew meat	66	48	Stewed	4	2.9	2.64	9½	38
				3	2.2	3.52	7¼	28½

[a]Size of portion and number of portions per purchase unit are determined by use.
[b]Breast, flank.
[c]Fat and lean.

Table E-2. Combination Foods Containing Meat

Meat Combinations, Canned or Frozen, as Purchased	Unit of Purchase	Weight per Unit[a] (lb)	Cooked Meat (%)	Size of Portion (oz)	Meat in Portion (oz)	Portions per Purchase Unit (no.)	Approximate Purchase Units for—	
							25 Portions (no.)	100 Portions (no.)
Beans with frankfurt-	Pound	1.00	20	8	1.6	2.00	12½	50
ers in sauce	No. 3 cylinder	3.12	20	8	1.6	6.24	4¼	16¼
	No. 10 can	6.75	20	8	1.6	13.50	2	7½
Beans with ham in	Pound	1.00	12	8	1.0	2.00	12¼	50
sauce	No. 3 cylinder	3.19	12	8	1.0	6.38	4	15¾
Beans with meat in	Pound	1.00	8	8	0.6	2.00	12½	50
chili sauce	No. 10 can	6.50	8	8	0.6	13.00	2	7¼
Beef goulash								
Canned	Pound	1.00	18	8	1.4	2.00	12½	50
	No. 3 cylinder	3.12	18	8	1.4	6.24	4¼	16¼
frozen	Carton	5.00	18	8	1.4	10.00	2½	10
	Carton	6.75	18	9	1.6	12.00	2¼	8½
	Carton	8.25	18	11	2.0	12.00	2¼	8½
Beef stew	Pound	1.00	18	8	1.4	2.00	12½	50
	No. 3 cylinder	3.12	18	8	1.4	6.24	4¼	16¼
	No. 10 can	6.62	18	8	1.4	13.24	2	7¾
Beef with barbecue	Pound	1.00	50	6	3.0	2.67	9½	37½
sauce	No. 3 cylinder	3.25	50	6	3.0	8.67	3	11¾
	No. 10 can	6.50	50	6	3.0	17.33	1½	6
Beef with gravy	Pound	1.00	50	6	3.0	2.67	9½	37½
	No. 3 cylinder	3.00	50	6	3.0	8.00	3¼	12¾
	No. 10 can	6.50	50	6	3.0	17.33	1½	6
Brunswick stew	Pound	1.00	18	8	1.4	2.00	12½	50
	No. 10 can	6.62	18	8	1.4	13.24	2	7¾
Chili con carne	Pound	1.00	28	8	2.2	2.00	12½	50
	No. 3 cylinder	3.19	28	8	2.2	6.38	4	15¾
	No. 10 can	6.75	28	8	2.2	13.50	2	7½
Chili con carne with	Pound	1.00	18	8	1.4	2.00	12½	50
beans	No. 3 cylinder	3.19	18	8	1.4	6.38	4	15¾
	No. 10 can	6.75	18	8	1.4	13.50	2	7½
Chili mac	Pound	1.00	18	8	1.4	2.00	12½	50
	No. 3 cylinder	3.19	18	8	1.4	6.38	4	15¼
	No. 10 can	6.50	18	8	1.4	13.00	2	7¾
Chop suey or chow mein vegetables with meat								
Canned	Pound	1.00	8	8	0.6	2.00	12½	50
	No. 3 cylinder	3.06	8	8	0.6	6.12	4¼	16½
Frozen	Carton	5.00	8	8	0.6	10.00	2½	10
Hash, corn beef, roast	Pound	1.00	35	7	2.4	2.29	11¼	44¼
beef, beef	No. 3 cylinder	3.19	35	7	2.4	7.29	3½	14
	No. 10 can	6.50	35	7	2.4	14.86	1¾	7

Table E-2. (Continued)

Meat Combinations, Canned or Frozen, as Purchased	Unit of Purchase	Weight per Unit[a] (lb)	Cooked Meat (%)	Size of Portion (oz)	Meat in Portion (oz)	Portions per Purchase Unit (no.)	Approximate Purchase Units for—	
							25 Portions (no.)	100 Portions (no.)
Lamb stew	Pound	1.00	18	8	1.4	2.00	12½	50
	No. 3 cylinder	3.19	18	8	1.4	6.38	4	15¾
	No. 10 can	6.62	18	8	1.4	13.24	2	7¾
Macaroni and beef in	Pound	1.00	8	8	0.6	2.00	12½	50
tomato sauce	No. 10 can	6.50	8	8	0.6	13.00	2	7¾
Meatballs with gravy								
canned	Pound	1.00 (10 count)	38	6	2.3 (4 count)	2.67	9½	37½
	No. 10 can	6.50 (70 count)	38	6	2.3 (4 count)	17.33	1½	6
frozen	Carton	8.00 (160 count)	38	6	2.3 (7½ count)	21.33	1¼	5
	Carton	10.00 (100 count)	38	6	2.3 (4 count)	26.67	1	4
Pork with barbecue sauce:								
canned	Pound	1.00	50	6	3.0	2.67	9½	37½
	No. 3 cylinder	3.19	50	6	3.0	8.51	3	12
	No. 10 can	6.62	50	6	3.0	17.65	1½	5¾
in waxed tub (perishable)	4-pound tub	4.00	50	6	3.0	10.67	2½	9½
	5-pound tub	5.00	50	6	3.0	13.33	2	7¾
Pork with gravy	Pound	1.00	50	6	3.0	2.67	9½	37½
	No. 3 cylinder	3.12	50	6	3.0	8.32	3¼	12¼
	No. 10 can	6.50	50	6	3.0	17.33	1½	6
Ravioli with meat in	Pound	1.00	7	8	.6	2.00	12½	50
sauce	No. 3 cylinder	3.19	7	8	.6	6.38	4	15¾
		3.62	7	8	.6	7.24	3½	14
Spaghetti with meat-balls and sauce	Pound	1.00	8	8	.6	2.00	12½	50
	No. 3 cylinder	3.19	8	8	.6	6.38	4	15¾
	No. 10 can	6.62	8	8	.6	13.24	2	7¾
Tamales, frozen	Pound	1.00 (4 tamales)	18	8 (2 tamales)	1.4	2.00	12½	50
	Carton	6.00 (24 tamales)	18	8 (2 tamales)	1.4	12.00	2¼	8½
	Carton	18.00	18	8	1.4	36.00	[b]	3
Tamales with gravy or	Pound	1.00	14	8	1.1	2.00	12½	50
sauce (Packed in sizes from 1½–6 oz. per tamale)	No. 10 can	6.50	14	8	1.1	13.00	2	7¾

[a]Net weights of containers are not standardized and may vary depending on establishment preparing the product.
[b]Number of purchase units needed is less than one.

Table E-3. Poultry

Poultry as Purchased; Unit of Purchase, lb	Yield, as Served (%)	Description of Portion as Served	Size of Portion		Portions per Purchase Unit (no.)	Approximate Purchase Units for—	
			As Served (oz)	Edible Portion[a] (oz)		25 Portions (no.)	100 Portions (no.)
Chicken, fresh or frozen							
Live							
roasters	30	Boned, excludes neck and giblets	3.0	3.0	1.60	15¾	62½
			2.0	2.0	2.40	10½	41¾
stewers	34	Boned, includes neck and giblets	3.0	3.0	1.81	14	55¼
			2.0	2.0	2.72	9¼	37
Ready-to-cook							
Broilers, ½-lb bird	70	½ bird	8.3	5.4	2.00	12½	50
fryers, 2½-lb bird	43	Boned	3.0	3.0	2.29	11	43¾
			2.0	2.0	3.44	7½	29¼
		¼ bird ·	5.8	3.9	4.00	6¼	25
	65	⅙ bird	3.9	2.6	6.00	4¼	16¾
		⅛ bird	2.9	1.9	8.00	3¼	12½
parts (from 2½-lb bird):							
breast half	67	With bone	3.2	2.6	3.35	7½	30
drumstick	72	With bone	2.1	1.4	5.49	4¾	18¼
thigh	68	With bone	2.2	1.6	4.95	5¼	20¼
drumstick and thigh	70	With bone	4.3	3.1	2.60	9¾	38½
wing	64	With bone	1.6	0.8	6.40	4	15¾
back	49	With bone	2.5	1.3	3.14	8	32
rib	65	With bone	2.5	1.3	4.16	6¼	24¼
giblets							
gizzards	26	—	2	2	2.08	12¼	48¼
hearts	38	—	2	2	3.04	8¼	33
livers	65	—	2	2	5.20	5	19¼
roasters	42	Boned, excludes neck and giblets	3	3	2.24	11¼	44¾
			2	2	3.36	7½	30
stewers	47	Boned, includes neck and giblets	3	3	2.51	10	40
			2	2	3.76	6¾	26¾
Chicken, canned							
boned	90	Meat	3	3	4.80	5¼	21
			2	2	7.20	3½	14
can (35 oz)	90	Meat	3	3	10.50	2½	9¾
			2	2	15.75	1¾	6½
boned, solid pack	95	Meat	3	3	5.07	5	19¼
			2	2	7.60	3½	13¼
Boned, with broth	80	Meat	3	3	4.27	6	23½
			2	2	6.40	4	15¾
Whole	32	Meat	3	3	1.71	14¾	58½
			2	2	2.56	10	39¼

Table E-3. (Continued)

Poultry as Purchased; Unit of Purchase, lb	Yield, as Served (%)	Description of Portion as Served	Size of Portion		Portions per Purchase Unit (no.)	Approximate Purchase Units for—	
			As Served (oz)	Edible Portion[a] (oz)		25 Portions (no.)	100 Portions (no.)
Turkey, fresh or frozen							
Live	36	Excludes neck and giblets	3	3	1.92	13¼	52¼
			2	2	2.88	8¾	34¾
Ready-to-cook							
roasters	47	Excludes neck and giblets	3	3	2.51	10	40
			2	2	3.76	6¾	26¾
parts:							
breasts, whole	60	—	3	3	3.20	8	31¼
			2	2	4.80	5¼	21
legs (thigh and drumstick)	48	—	3	3	2.56	10	39¼
			2	2	3.84	6¾	26¼
giblets							
gizzards	34	—	2	2	2.72	9¼	37
hearts	38	—	2	2	3.04	8¼	33
livers	67	—	2	2	5.36	4¾	18¾
Turkey, frozen only							
Stuffed, whole	33	Boned meat	3	3	1.76	14¼	57
			2	2	2.64	9½	38
Rolls, precooked	92	Meat	3	3	4.91	5¼	20½
			2	2	7.36	3½	13¾
Rolls, ready-to-cook	61	Meat	3	3	3.25	7¼	31
			2	2	4.88	5¼	20½
Turkey, canned							
Boned	90	Meat	3	3	4.80	5¼	21
			2	2	7.20	3½	14
can (35 oz)	90	Meat	3	3	10.50	2½	9¼
			2	2	15.75	1¾	6½
Boned, solid pack	95	Meat	3	3	5.07	5	19¾
			2	2	7.60	3½	13¼
Boned, with broth	80	Meat	3	3	4.27	6	23⅓
			2	2	6.40	4	15¾
Other poultry, fresh or frozen							
Duck, ready-to-cook	38	Boned, excludes neck and giblets	3	3	2.03	12½	49½
			2	2	3.04	8¼	33
Goose, ready-to-cook	39	Boned, excludes neck and giblets	3	3	2.08	12¼	48¼
			2	2	3.12	8¼	32¼

[a]Includes edible skin.
[b]Based on 2½-lb bird as purchased; neck and giblets not served.

Table E-4. Combination Foods Containing Poultry

Poultry Combinations, Canned or Frozen, as Purchased, Unit of Purchase,[a] lb; Weight per Unit, 1 lb	Cooked Meat (%)	Size of Portion (oz)	Meat in Portion (oz)	Portions per Purchase Unit (no.)	Approximate Purchase Units for—	
					25 Portions (no.)	100 Portions (no.)
Chicken a la king	20	8	1.60	2.00	12½	50
Chickenburgers	100	3	3.00	5.33	4¾	19
Chicken cacciatore	20	8	1.60	2.00	12½	50
Chicken chop suey	4	8	.32	2.00	12½	50
Chicken chow mein	4	8	.32	2.00	12½	50
Chicken fricassee	20	8	1.60	2.00	12½	50
Chicken noodles or dumplings	15	8	1.20	2.00	12½	50
Chicken potpie	14	8	1.12	2.00	12½	50
Chicken stew	12	8	.96	2.00	12½	50
Chicken tamales	6	8	.48	2.00	12½	50
Creamed chicken	20	8	1.60	2.00	12½	50
Creamed turkey	20	8	1.60	2.00	12½	50
Minced chicken barbecue	40	3	1.20	5.33	4¾	19
Noodles or dumplings with chicken	6	8	.48	2.00	12½	50
Sliced chicken with gravy	35	6	2.10	2.67	9½	37½
Sliced turkey with gravy	35	6	2.10	2.67	9½	37½
Turkey a la king	20	8	1.60	2.00	12½	50
Turkey fricassee	20	8	1.60	2.00	12½	50
Turkey potpie	14	8	1.12	2.00	12½	50

[a]There is no standardization of can or carton sizes for canned and frozen poultry products. Information given for a pound may be related to the weight of the contents of the can or carton.

Table E-5. Fish and Shellfish

Fish and Shellfish as Purchased	Unit of Purchase	Weight per Unit (lb)	Yield, as Served (%)	Portion as Served	Portions per Purchase Unit (no.)	Approximate Purchase Units for—	
						25 Portions (no.)	100 Portions (no.)
Fish, canned							
Gefiltefish	16-oz can (9¼ oz drained)	1.00	58	3 oz drained	3.08	8¼	32½
				2 oz drained	4.62	5½	21¾
	32-oz can (20½ oz drained)	2.00	64	3 oz drained	6.83	3¾	14¾
				2 oz drained	10.25	2½	10
	51-oz can (39 oz drained)	3.19	76	3 oz drained	13.00	2	7¾
				2 oz drained	19.50	1½	5¼
Mackerel	15-oz can (12½ oz drained)	0.94	83	3 oz drained	4.17	6	24
				2 oz drained	6.25	4	16
Salmon	3¾-oz can (2¼ oz drained)	0.23	60	2¼ oz drained	1.00	25	100
	16-oz can (13 oz drained)	1.00	81	3 oz drained	4.33	6	23¼
				2 oz drained	6.50	4	15½
	64-oz can (50 oz drained)	4.00	78	3 oz drained	16.67	1½	6
				2 oz drained	25.00	1	4
Sardines:							
Maine	3¾- to 4-oz can (3¾ oz drained)	0.23–0.25	100	3 oz drained	1.25	20	80
				2 oz drained	1.87	13½	53½
	12-oz can (10¾ oz drained)	0.75	90	3 oz drained	3.58	7	28
				2 oz drained	5.38	4¾	18¾
Pacific:							
in brine	15-oz can (11½ oz drained)	0.94	77	3 oz drained	3.83	6¾	26¼
				2 oz drained	5.75	4½	17½
in mustard or tomato sauce	15-oz can	0.94	100	3 oz drained	5.00	5	20
				2 oz drained	7.50	3½	13½
Tuna	3½- to 4-oz can (3¼ oz drained)	0.22–0.25	93	3¼ oz drained	1.00	25	100
	6- to 7-oz can (6 oz drained)	0.38–0.44	100	3 oz drained	2.00	12½	50
				2 oz drained	3.00	8½	33½
	60- to 66½-oz can (58 oz drained)	3.75–4.16	97	3 oz drained	19.33	1½	5½
				2 oz drained	29.00	[a]	3½
Fish, dried							
Salt cod	Pound	1.00	72	3 oz	3.84	6¾	26¼
				2 oz	5.76	4½	17½
Fish, fresh or frozen							
Fillets	Pound	1.00	64	3 oz	3.41	7½	29½
				2 oz	5.12	5	19¾
Steaks (backbone in)	Pound	1.00	58[b]	3 oz	3.09	8¼	32¼
				2 oz	4.64	5½	21¾
Dressed (scaled and eviscerated, usually head, tail, and fins removed)	Pound	1.00	45[b]	3 oz	2.40	10½	41¾
				2 oz	3.60	7	28

(continued)

Table E-5. Fish and Shellfish (Continued)

Fish and Shellfish as Purchased	Unit of Purchase	Weight per Unit (lb)	Yield, as Served (%)	Portion as Served	Portions per Purchase Unit (no.)	Approximate Purchase Units for—	
						25 Portions (no.)	100 Portions (no.)
Drawn (entrails removed)	Pound	1.00	32[b]	3 oz	1.71	14¾	58½
				2 oz	2.56	10	39¼
Whole, or round (as caught)	Pound	1.00	27[b]	3 oz	1.44	17½	69½
				2 oz	2.16	11¾	46½
Fish, frozen							
Portions							
breaded, fried or raw:							
5½-oz	Pound	1.00	95	1 portion	3.00	8½	33½
4-oz	Pound	1.00	95	1 portion	4.00	6¼	25
3-oz	Pound	1.00	95	1 portion	5.33	4¾	18¾
2-oz	Pound	1.00	95	1 portion	8.00	3¼	12½
unbreaded:							
4-oz	Pound	1.00	69	1 portion	4.00	6¼	25
3-oz	Pound	1.00	69	1 portion	5.33	4¾	18¾
2-oz	Pound	1.00	68	1 portion	8.00	3¼	12½
Sticks, breaded, fried or raw, 1-oz	Pound	1.00	85	4 sticks	4.00	6¼	25
				3 sticks	5.33	4¾	18¾
				2 sticks	8.00	3¼	12½
Shellfish, canned							
Clam chowder	8-oz can, ready-to-serve	0.50	100	8 oz	1.00	25	100
	10½-oz can, condensed	0.66	200	8 oz	2.62	9¾	38¼
	15-oz can, condensed	0.94	200	8 oz	3.75	6¾	26¾
	50- to 51-oz can, condensed	3.12–3.19	200	8 oz	12.50	2	8
Clam juice	8-fluid-oz can	—	100	3 fl oz	2.67	9½	37½
	12-fluid-oz can	—	100	3 fl oz	4.00	6¼	25
Clams, minced	7½-oz can	0.47	100	3 oz	2.50	10	40
				2 oz	3.75	6¾	26¾
	51-oz can	3.19	100	3 oz	17.00	1½	6
				2 oz	25.50	1	4
Crabmeat	6½-oz can (5½ oz drained)	0.41	85	3 oz drained	1.83	13¾	54¾
				2 oz drained	2.75	9¼	36½
Oysters, whole	5-oz can (5 oz drained)	0.31	100	3 oz drained	1.67	15	60
				2 oz drained	2.50	10	40
Oyster stew	10½-oz can, ready-to-serve	0.66	100	8 oz	1.31	19¼	76½
Shrimp	4½-oz can (4½ oz drained)	0.28	100	3 oz drained	1.50	16¾	66¾
				2 oz drained	2.25	11¼	44½
Shellfish, fresh, live in shell							
Clams:							
hard	Dozen	—	14[b]	6 clams on half shell	2.00	12½	50
soft	Dozen	—	29[b]	12 clams in the shell	1.00	25	100
Crabs							
blue	Pound	1.00	14	3 oz cooked	.75	33½	133½
				2 oz cooked	1.12	22½	89½
Dungeness	Pound	1.00	24	3 oz cooked	1.28	19¾	78¼
				2 oz cooked	1.92	13¼	52¼

Table E-5. (Continued)

Fish and Shellfish as Purchased	Unit of Purchase	Weight per Unit (lb)	Yield, as Served (%)	Portion as Served	Portions per Purchase Unit (no.)	Approximate Purchase Units for—	
						25 Portions (no.)	100 Portions (no.)
Oysters	Dozen	—	12[b]	6 oysters on half shell	2.00	12½	50
Shellfish, fresh or frozen							
Clams, shucked	Pound	1.00	48	3 oz meat	2.56	10	39¼
				2 oz meat	3.82	6¾	26
Crabs, cooked in shell							
blue	Pound	1.00	14	3 oz meat	.75	33½	133½
				2 oz meat	1.12	22½	89½
Dungeness	Pound	1.00	24	3 oz meat	1.28	19¾	78¼
				2 oz meat	1.92	13¼	52¼
Crabmeat	Pound	1.00	97	3 oz	5.17	5	19½
				2 oz	7.76	3¼	13
Lobster, cooked in shell	Pound	1.00	25[b]	1 lobster	1.00	25	100
				1½ lobster	2.00	12½	50
Lobster meat	Pound	1.00	91	3 oz	4.85	5¼	20¼
				2 oz	7.28	3½	13¾
Oysters, shucked	Pound	1.00	40	3 oz	2.13	11¾	47
				2 oz	3.20	8	31¼
Scallops, shucked	Pound	1.00	63	3 oz	3.36	7½	30
				2 oz	5.04	5	20
Shrimp							
cooked, peeled, cleaned	Pound	1.00	100	3 oz	5.33	4¾	19
				2 oz	8.00	3¼	12½
raw, in shell	Pound	1.00	50	3 oz meat	2.67	9½	37½
				2 oz meat	4.00	6¼	25
raw, peeled	Pound	1.00	62	3 oz meat	3.30	7¾	30½
				2 oz meat	4.96	5¼	20¼
Shellfish, frozen							
Clams, breaded:							
fried	Pound	1.00	85	3 oz	4.53	5¾	22½
				2 oz	6.80	3¾	14¼
raw	Pound	1.00	83	3 oz	4.43	5¾	22¾
				2 oz	6.64	4	15¼
Crabcakes, fried	Pound	1.00	95	3 oz	5.07	5	19¼
				2 oz	7.60	3½	13¾
Lobster, spiny tails							
8 oz	Pound	1.00	51[b]	1 tail	2.00	12½	50
6 oz	Pound	1.00	51[b]	1 tail	2.67	9½	37½
4 oz	Pound	1.00	51[b]	1 tail	4.00	6¼	25
Oysters, breaded, raw	Pound	1.00	88	3 oz	4.69	5½	21½
				2 oz	7.04	3¾	14¼
Scallops, breaded							
fried	Pound	1.00	93	3 oz	4.96	5¼	20¼
				2 oz	7.44	3½	13½
raw	Pound	1.00	81	3 oz	4.32	6	23¼
				2 oz	6.48	4	15½
Shrimp, breaded							
fried	Pound	1.00	88	3 oz	4.69	5½	21½
				2 oz	7.04	3¾	14¼
raw	Pound	1.00	85	3 oz	4.53	5¾	22¼
				2 oz	6.80	3¾	14¾

[a]Number of purchase units needed is less than one.
[b]Yield, edible portion.

Table E-6. Eggs

Eggs, In Shell, Frozen, and Dried, as Purchased	Unit of Purchase	Weight per Unit (lb)	Portions as Served or Used	Portions per Purchase Unit (no.)	Approximate Purchase Units for	
					25 Portions (no.)	100 Portions (no.)
In Shell						
large	Dozen	1.50	1 egg	12.00	2¼	8½
	Case	45.00	1 egg	360.00	a	a
medium	Dozen	1.31	1 egg	12.00	2¼	8½
	Case	39.50	1 egg	360.00	a	a
small	Dozen	1.12	1 egg	12.00	2¼	8½
	Case	34.00	1 egg	360.00	a	a
Frozen						
whole eggs	Pound	1.00	1 egg (3 Tbsp thawed)	10.00	b	b
			12 eggs (2¼ cup thawed)	0.83	b	b
	Can	10.00	1 egg	100.00	b	b
	Can	30.00	1 egg	300.00	b	b
egg yolks	Pound	1.00	1 yolk (1⅓ Tbsp thawed)	26.00	b	b
			12 yolks (1 cup thawed)	2.16	b	b
egg whites	Pound	1.00	1 white (2 Tbsp thawed)	16.00	b	b
			12 whites (1½ cup thawed)	1.33	b	b
Dried						
whole eggs	Pound	1.00	1 large egg (½ oz or 2½ Tbsp dried + 2½ Tbsp water)	32.00	b	b
			12 large eggs (6 oz or 2 cups dried + 2 cups water)	2.67	b	b
	13-oz package	0.81	1 large egg	26.00	b	b
	No. 10 can	3.00	1 large egg	96.00	b	b
	Package	25.00	1 large egg	800.00	b	b
	Package	50.00	1 large egg	1600.00	b	b
egg yolks	Pound	1.00	1 large yolk (2 Tbsp dried + 2 tsp water)	51.00	b	b
			12 large yolks (1½ cups dried 1½ cup water)	4.50	b	b
	Package	3.00	1 large yolk	162.00	b	b
egg white, spray-dried	Pound	1.00	1 large white (2 tsp dried + 2 Tbsp water)	100.00	b	b
			12 large whites (½ cup dried + 1½ cups water)	8.33	b	b
	Package	3.00	1 large white	300.00	b	b

aNumber of purchase units needed is less than one.
bNumber of purchase units needed is determined by use.

Table E-7. Nuts

Nuts in Shell and Peanut Butter as Purchased; Unit of Purchase, lb	Weight per Unit (lb)	Yield, as Served (%)	Portion as Used	Portions per Purchase Unit (no.)	Approximate Purchase Units for 25 Portions (no.)	100 Portions (no.)
Almonds						
nonpareil (softshell)	1.00	60	1 cup (0.31 lb)	1.94	a	a
peerless (hardshell)	1.00	35	1 cup (0.31 lb)	1.13	a	a
Brazil nuts	1.00	48	1 cup (0.31 lb)	1.55	a	a
Cashew nuts	1.00	22	1 cup (0.30 lb)	0.73	a	a
Chestnuts	1.00	84	8 large nuts (0.11 lb)	7.64	a	a
Coconut						
dried	1.00	100	1 cup (0.14 lb)	7.14	a	a
fresh, in shell	1.00	52	1 cup (0.21 lb)	2.48	a	a
Filberts	1.00	39	1 cup (0.30 lb)	1.50	a	a
Peanuts, roasted	1.00	68	1 cup (0.32 lb)	2.12	a	a
Peanut butter	1.00	100	2 Tbsp (0.07 lb)	14.29	1¾	7
no. 10 can	6.75	100	2 Tbsp (0.07 lb)	96.43	b	1¼
Pecans	1.00	52	1 cup halves (0.24 lb)	2.17	a	a
Walnuts						
black	1.00	22	1 cup (0.28 lb)	0.79	a	a
English	1.00	45	1 cup (0.22 lb)	2.05	a	a

a Number of purchase units needed is determined by use.
b Number of purchase units needed is less than one.

Table E-8. Dairy Products

Dairy Products as Purchased	Unit of Purchase	Weight per Unit (lb)	Yield, as Served (%)	Portion as Served or Used	Portions per Purchase Unit (no.)	Approximate Purchase Units for	
						25 Portions (no.)	100 Portions (no.)
Cheese							
cheddar	Pound	1.00	100	4 oz, grated, 1 cup	4.00	6¼	25
	Pound	1.00	100	2 oz	8.00	3¼	12½
	Pound	1.00	100	1 oz	16.00	1¾	6¼
	Longhorn	11–13	100	2 oz	88–104	a	1¼
	Daisies	20–25	100	2 oz	160–200	a	a
	Flats	32–37	100	2 oz	256–296	a	a
	Cheddars	70–78	100	2 oz	560–624	a	a
	Block	20	100	2 oz	160.00	a	a
	Block	40	100	2 oz	320.00	a	a
cottage, small or large curd, with pineapple or chive	Pound	1.00	100	4 oz	4.00	6¼	25
				2 oz	8.00	3¼	12½
	23-oz carton	2.00	100	4 oz	8.00	3¼	12½
	Tin	30.00	100	4 oz	120.00	a	a
cream	8-oz package	0.50	100	1 oz	8.00	3¼	12½
	12-oz package	0.75	100	1 oz	12.00	2¼	8½
	16-oz package	1.00	100	1 oz	16.00	1¾	6¼
processed, cheese food	Pound	1.00	100	2 oz	8.00	3¼	12½
				1 oz, 1 slice	16.00	1¾	6¼
	Package	2.00	100	2 oz	16.00	1¾	6¼
	Package	5.00	100	2 oz	40.00	a	2½
Cream							
half and half	Pint	1.07	100	1½ Tbsp	21.33	1¼	4¾
	Quart	2.14	100	1½ Tbsp	42.67	a	2½
light	Pint	1.06	100	1½ Tbsp	21.33	1½	4¾
	Quart	2.13	100	1½ Tbsp	42.67	a	2½
sour	½ pint	0.53	100	1 Tbsp	16.00	1¾	6¼
	¾ pint	0.80	100	1 Tbsp	24.00	1¼	4¼
whipping (volume doubles when whipped)	Pint	1.05	100	1¼ Tbsp	25.60	1	4
	Quart	2.10	100	1¼ Tbsp	51.20	a	2
Ice cream							
brick	Quart	1.25	100	1 slice (½ cup)	8.00	3¼	12½
bulk	Gallon	4.50	100	No. 12 scoop (sundae)	22–26	1	4
				No. 16 scoop	31–35	a	3
				No. 20 scoop (a la mode)	38–42	a	2½
				No. 24 scoop	47–51	a	2

Table E-8. (Continued)

Dairy Products as Purchased	Unit of Purchase	Weight per Unit (lb)	Yield, as Served (%)	Portion as Served or Used	Portions per Purchase Unit (no.)	Approximate Purchase Units for	
						25 Portions (no.)	100 Portions (no.)
Ice cream							
cups	3-oz	0.19	100	1 cup	1.00	25	100
	5-oz	0.31	100	1 cup	1.00	25	100
Sherbet	Gallon	6.00	100	No. 12 scoop	25.00	1	4
				No. 16 scoop	35.00	a	3
				No. 20 scoop	42.00	a	2½
				No. 24 scoop	50.00	a	2
Milk							
fluid[b]	Quart	2.15	100	1 cup	4.00	6¼	25
	Gallon	8.60	100	1 cup	16.00	1¾	6¼
	5-gal.	43.00	100	1 cup	80.00	a	1¼
condensed	14-oz can	0.88	100	1 cup	1.24	c	c
	15-oz can	0.94	100	1 cup	1.33	c	c
evaporated	14½-oz can	0.91	100	1 cup as is	1.67	c	c
		0.91	200	1 cup reconstituted	3.33	c	c
	No. 10 can	8.00	100	1 cup as is	14.00	c	c
		8.00	200 (measure)	1 cup reconstituted	28.00	c	c
Dry							
nonfat							
instant	Pound (about 6½ cups)	1.00	100	1 cup as is	6.50	c	c
		1.00	267 (measure)	1 cup reconstituted	17.06	c	c
regular (USDA)	Pound (about 3¼ cups)	1.00	100	1 cup as is	3.25	c	c
		1.00	533 (measure)	1 cup reconstituted	17.06	c	c
whole	Pound (about 3½ cups)	1.00	100	1 cup as is	3.50	c	c
		1.00	400 (measure)	1 cup reconstituted	14.22	c	c

[a]Number of purchase units needed is less than one.
[b]Skim milk and buttermilk weigh slightly more than whole fluid milk.
[c]Number of purchase units needed is determined by use.

Table E-9. Vegetables—Fresh

Fresh Vegetables as Purchased	Unit of Purchase	Weight per Unit[a] (lb)	Yield, as Served (%)	Portion as Served	Portions per Purchase Unit (no.)	Approximate Purchase Units for	
						25 Portions (no.)	100 Portions (no.)
Asparagus	Pound	1.00	—	4 medium spears, cooked	3.38	7½	29¾
	Pound	1.00	49	3 oz cut spears, cooked	2.61	9¾	38½
	Crate	28.00	49	3 oz cut spears, cooked	73.17	b	1½
Beans, lima, green							
in pod	Pound	1.00	40	3 oz cooked	2.13	11¾	47
	Bushel	32.00	40	3 oz cooked	68.27	b	1½
shelled	Pound	1.00	102	3 oz cooked	5.44	4¾	18½
Beans, snap, green or wax	Pound	1.00	84	3 oz cooked	4.48	5¾	22½
	Bushel	30.00	84	3 oz cooked	134.40	b	b
Beet greens, untrimmed	Pound	1.00	44	3 oz cooked	2.35	10¾	42¾
	Bushel	20.00	44	3 oz cooked	46.93	b	2¼
Beets							
with tops	Pound	1.00	43	3 oz sliced or diced, cooked	2.29	11	43¾
without tops	Pound	1.00	76	3 oz sliced or diced, cooked	4.05	6¼	24¾
	Burlap bag	50.00	76	3 oz sliced or diced, cooked	202.67	b	b
Blackeye peas, shelled	Pound	1.00	93	3 oz cooked	4.96	5¼	20¼
Broccoli	Pound	1.00	—	2 medium spears, cooked	4.57	5½	22
	Pound	1.00	62	3 oz cut spears, cooked	3.31	7¾	30¼
	Crate	40.00	62	3 oz cut spears, cooked	132.27	b	b
Brussels sprouts	Pound	1.00	77	3 oz cooked	4.11	6¼	24½
Cabbage	Bulk	1.00	79	2 oz coleslaw	6.32	4	16
	Bulk	1.00	75	3 oz sliced, cooked	4.00	6¼	25
	Bulk	1.00	80	3-oz wedge, cooked	4.27	6	23½
	Crate or sack	50.00	80	3-oz wedge, cooked	213.33	b	b
Cabbage, Chinese	Pound	1.00	88	2 oz raw	7.04	3¾	14¼
Carrots, without tops	Pound	1.00	82	2 oz shredded or grated, strips or diced, raw	6.56	4	15¼
	Pound	1.00	75	3 oz sliced or diced, cooked	4.00	6¼	25
	Bushel	50.00	75	3 oz sliced or diced, cooked	200.00	b	b
Cauliflower	Pound	1.00	45	2 oz sliced, raw	3.60	7	28
	Pound	1.00	44	3 oz cooked	2.35	10¾	42¾
	Crate	37.00	44	3 oz cooked	86.83	b	1¼
	Crate, large	50.00	44	3 oz cooked	117.33	b	b
Celery	Pound	1.00	70	3 oz chopped, cooked	3.73	6¾	27
	Pound	1.00	75	3 oz sliced, raw	4.00	6¼	25
	Pound	1.00	75	2 oz strips, raw	6.00	4¼	16¾
	Crate	60.00	75	3 oz chopped, raw	240.00	b	b
Celery hearts (24 pack)	Crate or box	30.00	95	2 oz strips, raw	228.00	b	b
Chard, untrimmed	Pound	1.00	56	3 oz	2.99	8½	33½
Collards	Pound	1.00	81	3 oz cooked	4.32	6	23¼
	Bushel	20.00	81	3 oz cooked	86.40	b	1¼
Corn, in husks	Dozen	8.00	37	3 oz cooked kernels	15.79	1¾	6½
	Dozen	8.00	—	1 ear, cooked	12.00	2¼	8½
	5-dozen crate or bag	40.00	—	1 ear, cooked	60.00	b	1¾
Cucumber	Pound	1.00	73	3 oz sliced, peeled, raw	3.89	6½	25¾
	Pound	1.00	95	3 oz sliced, unpeeled, raw	5.07	5	19¾

Table E-9. (Continued)

Fresh Vegetables as Purchased	Unit of Purchase	Weight per Unit[a] (lb)	Yield, as Served (%)	Portion as Served	Portions per Purchase Unit (no.)	Approximate Purchase Units for	
						25 Portions (no.)	100 Portions (no.)
Cucumber							
	Bushel	48.00	95	3 oz sliced, unpeeled, raw	243.20	b	b
Eggplant	Pound	1.00	75	4 oz cooked	3.00	8½	33½
	Bushel	33.00	75	4 oz cooked	100.00	b	1
Endive, escarole, chicory	Pound	1.00	75	1 oz raw	12.00	2¼	8½
	Bushel	25.00	75	1 oz raw	300.00	b	b
Kale, untrimmed	Pound	1.00	81	3 oz cooked	4.32	6	23¼
	Bushel	18.00	81	3 oz cooked	77.76	b	1½
Kohlrabi	Pound	1.00	50	3 oz cooked	2.67	9½	37½
Lettuce							
head	Pound	1.00	74	2 oz raw	5.92	4¼	17
iceberg	Carton	2 doz. heads	—	⅙ head, raw	144.00	4¼ heads	17 heads
Romaine	Pound	1.00	64	1 oz raw	10.24	2½	10
Mushrooms	Pound	1.00	67	1 oz sliced, cooked	10.72	2½	9½
	Basket	3.00	67	3 oz sliced, cooked	10.72	2½	9½
	Basket	9.00	67	3 oz sliced, cooked	32.16	b	3¼
Mustard greens	Pound	1.00	59	3 oz cooked	3.15	8	31¾
	Bushel	20.00	59	3 oz cooked	62.93	b	1¾
Okra	Pound	1.00	96	3 oz cooked	5.12	5	19¾
	Bushel	30.00	96	3 oz cooked	153.60	b	b
Onions							
green, partly topped	Pound	1.00	60	3 oz raw	3.20	8	31¼
	Wirebound crate	50.00	60	3 oz raw	160.00	b	b
mature	Pound	1.00	89	1 oz chopped or grated, raw	14.24	2	7¼
	Pound	1.00	76	3 oz small whole or pieces, cooked	4.05	6¼	24¾
	Sack	50.00	76	3 oz small whole or pieces, cooked	202.67	b	b
Parsley	Pound	1.00	—	½ cup	16.00	c	c
	Crate	19.00	—	½ cup	304.00	c	c
Parsnips	Pound	1.00	84	3 oz cooked	4.48	5¾	22½
	Bushel	50.00	84	3 oz cooked	224.00	b	b
Peas, green							
in pod	Pound	1.00	36	3 oz cooked	1.92	13¼	52¼
	Basket	15.00	36	3 oz cooked	28.80	b	3½
	Bushel	28.00	36	3 oz cooked	53.76	b	2
shelled	Pound	1.00	96	3 oz cooked	5.12	5	19¾
Peppers, green	Pound	1.00	82	1 oz diced or strips, raw	13.12	2	7¼
	Bushel	25.00	82	1 oz diced or strips, raw	328.00	b	b
	Carton	30.00	82	1 oz diced or strips, raw	393.60	b	b
	Pound	1.00	75	2 oz strips, cooked	6.00	4¼	16¾
Potatoes							
to be pared by hand	Pound	1.00	—	1 medium boiled	3.00	8½	33½
	Pound	1.00	54	2 oz french fried	4.32	6	23¼
	Pound	1.00	80	3 oz cubed and diced, cooked	4.27	6	23½
	Pound	1.00	95	4 oz mashed	3.80	6¾	26½
to be pared by machine	Pound	1.00	—	1 medium, boiled	3.00	8½	33½
	Pound	1.00	52	2 oz french fried	4.16	6¼	24¼
	Pound	1.00	76	3 oz cubed and diced, cooked	4.05	6¼	24¾
	Pound	1.00	90	4 oz mashed	3.60	7	28

(*continued*)

Table E-9. Vegetables—Fresh (Continued)

Fresh Vegetables as Purchased	Unit of Purchase	Weight per Unit[a] (lb)	Yield, as Served (%)	Portion as Served	Portions per Purchase Unit (no.)	Approximate Purchase Units for	
						25 Portions (no.)	100 Portions (no.)
Potatoes							
ready-to-cook	Pound	1.00	—	1 medium, boiled	3.00	8½	33½
	Pound	1.00	68	2 oz french fried	5.44	4¾	18½
	Pound	1.00	119	4 oz mashed	4.76	5¼	21¼
to be cooked in jacket	Pound	1.00	—	1 medium, baked in jacket	3.00	8½	33½
	Pound	1.00	—	1 medium, boiled	3.00	8½	33½
	Pound	1.00	87	3 oz cubed and diced	4.64	5½	21¾
	Pound	1.00	104	4 oz mashed	4.16	6¼	24¼
Pumpkin	Pound	1.00	63	4 oz mashed, cooked	2.52	10	39¾
Radishes							
with tops	Pound	1.00	63	1 oz sliced, raw	10.08	2½	10
	Pound	1.00	—	4 small	11.34	2½	9
without tops	Pound	1.00	90	1 oz sliced, raw	14.40	1¾	7
Rutabagas	Pound	1.00	79	3 oz cubed, cooked	4.21	6	24
	Pound	1.00	77	4 oz mashed	3.08	8¼	32½
	Bushel	56.00	77	4 oz mashed	172.48	b	b
Spinach							
partly trimmed	Pound	1.00	92	1 oz raw for salad	14.72	1¾	7
untrimmed	Pound	1.00	72	1 oz raw for salad	11.52	2¼	8¾
	Pound	1.00	67	3 oz cooked	3.57	7¼	28¼
	Bushel	20.00	67	3 oz cooked	71.47	b	1½
Squash, summer	Pound	1.00	83	3 oz diced or sliced, cooked	4.43	5¾	22¾
	Bushel	35.00	83	3 oz diced or sliced, cooked	154.93	b	b
	Pound	1.00	83	4 oz mashed	3.32	7¾	30¼
Squash, winter							
acorn	Pound	1.00	—	½ medium, baked	2.00	12½	50
hubbard	Pound	1.00	58	4 oz cubed, cooked	2.32	11	43¼
	Pound	1.00	57	4 oz mashed	2.28	11	44
Sweetpotatoes	Pound	1.00	—	1 medium, cooked in jacket	2.00	12½	50
	Pound	1.00	83	3 oz sliced	4.43	5¾	22¾
	Pound	1.00	81	4 oz mashed	3.24	7¼	31
	Bushel	50.00	—	1 medium, cooked in jacket	100.00	b	1
Tomatoes (medium)	Pound	1.00	91	2 slices	7.50	3½	13½
	Pound	1.00	—	1 wedge	12.00	2¼	8½
	Lug	32.00	—	1 wedge	384.00	b	b
	Bushel	53.00	—	1 wedge	636.00	b	b
Turnip greens, untrimmed	Pound	1.00	48	3 oz cooked	2.56	10	39¼
	Bushel	20.00	48	3 oz cooked	51.20	b	b
Turnips, without tops	Pound	1.00	74	3 oz cubed, cooked	3.95	6½	25½
	Pound	1.00	73	4 oz mashed	2.92	8¾	34¼
	Bushel	50.00	73	4 oz mashed	146.00	b	b
Watercress	Bunch	1.00	92	½ cup	27.77	c	c

[a]Legal weights for contents of bushels, lugs, crates, and boxes vary among States.
[b]Number of purchase units needed is less than one.
[c]Number of purchase units needed is determined by use.

Table E-10. Vegetables—Canned

Canned Vegetables as Purchased	Unit of Purchase	Weight per Unit (lb)	Yield, as Served (%)	Portion as Served	Portions per Purchase Unit (no.)	Approximate Purchase Units for 25 Portions (no.)	100 Portions (no.)
Asparagus							
cuts and tips	No. 300 can	0.88	61	3 oz	2.86	8¾	35
	No. 10 can	6.31	60	3 oz	20.19	1¼	5
spears	No. 300 can	0.91	—	6 medium	2.57	9¾	39
	No. 10 can	6.44	—	6 medium	18.53	1½	5½
Beans, lima, green	No. 303 can	1.00	69	3 oz	3.68	7	27¼
	No. 10 can	6.56	69	3 oz	24.14	1¼	4¼
Beans, snap, green or wax	No. 303 can	.97	59	3 oz	3.05	8¼	33
	No. 2½ can	1.75	59	3 oz	5.51	4¾	18¼
	No. 10 can	6.31	62	3 oz	20.87	1¼	5
Beans, dry—kidney, lima, or navy	No. 303 can	1.00	80	6 oz	2.13	11¾	47
	No. 10 can	6.75	80	6 oz	14.40	1¾	6¾
Bean sprouts	No. 10 can	6.62	52	3 oz	18.37	1½	5½
Beets							
diced	No. 303 can	1.00	66	3 oz	3.52	7¼	28¼
	No. 10 can	6.50	69	3 oz	23.92	1¼	4¼
sliced	No. 303 can	1.00	61	3 oz	3.25	7¾	31
	No. 10 can	6.50	65	3 oz	22.53	1¼	4½
whole baby beets	No. 303 can	1.00	62	3 oz	3.31	7¾	30¼
	No. 10 can	6.50	66	3 oz	22.88	1¼	4½
Carrots							
diced	No. 303 can	1.00	62	3 oz	3.31	7¾	30¼
	No. 10 can	6.50	69	3 oz	23.92	1¼	4¼
sliced	No. 303 can	1.00	62	3 oz	3.31	7¾	30¼
	No. 10 can	6.50	66	3 oz	22.88	1¼	4½
Chop suey vegetables	No. 10 can	6.38	100	3 oz	34.00	[a]	3
Collards	No. 303 can	.94	72	4 oz	2.71	9¼	37
	No. 2½ can	1.69	70	4 oz	4.73	5½	21¼
	No. 10 can	6.12	61	4 oz	14.93	1¾	6¾
Corn							
cream style	No. 303 can	1.00	100	4 oz	4.00	6¼	25
	No. 10 can	6.62	100	4 oz	26.48	1	4
whole kernel	No. 303 can	1.00	66	3 oz	3.52	7¼	28½
	No. 10 can	6.62	66	3 oz	23.30	1¼	4½
Kale	No. 303 can	.94	72	4 oz	2.71	9¼	37
	No. 2½ can	1.69	70	4 oz	4.73	5½	21¼
	No. 10 can	6.12	61	4 oz	14.93	1¼	6¾
Mushrooms	8 oz	.78	64	3 oz	2.66	9½	37¼
	No. 10 can	0.44	66	3 oz	22.67	1¼	4½
Mustard greens	No. 303 can	.94	72	4 oz	2.71	9¼	37
	No. 2½ can	1.69	70	4 oz	4.73	5½	21¼
	No. 10 can	0.12	61	4 oz	14.93	1¾	6¾
Okra	No. 303 can	.97	68	3 oz	3.51	7¼	28½
	No. 10 can	6.19	61	3 oz	20.14	1¼	5
Okra and tomatoes	No. 303 can	.94	100	3 oz	5.01	5	20
	No. 10 can	6.31	100	3 oz	33.65	[a]	3
Olives, large							
ripe							
pitted	No. 1 tall	0.47[b]	—	2 olives	21.33	1¼	4¾
whole	No. 1 tall	0.56[b]	—	2 olives	25.60	1	4
	No. 10	4.12[b]	—	2 olives	187.69	[a]	[a]
green, whole	Gallon	5.50[b]	—	2 olives	250.25	[a]	[a]

(continued)

Table E-10. Vegetables—Canned (Continued)

Canned Vegetables as Purchased	Unit of Purchase	Weight per Unit (lb)	Yield, as Served (%)	Portion as Served	Portions per Purchase Unit (no.)	Approximate Purchase Units for	
						25 Portions (no.)	100 Portions (no.)
Onions, small, whole	No. 303 can	1.00	56	3 oz	2.99	8½	33½
	No. 10 can	6.31	59	3 oz	19.86	1½	5¼
Peas, green	No. 303 can	1.00	64	3 oz	3.41	7½	29½
	No. 10 can	6.56	64	3 oz	22.39	1¼	4½
Peas and carrots	No. 303 can	1.00	69	3 oz	3.68	7	27¼
	No. 10 can	6.56	69	3 oz	24.14	1¼	4¼
Pickles							
dill or sour							
sliced or cut	Quart jar	1.38[b]	100	1 oz	22.00	1¼	4¼
	No. 10 jar	4.50[b]	100	1 oz	72.00	[a]	1½
	Gallon jar	5.62[b]	100	1 oz	90.00	[a]	1¼
whole	No. 2½ jar	1.19[b]	100	1 oz	19.00	1½	5½
	Quart jar	1.31[b]	100	1 oz	21.00	1¼	5
sweet							
sliced or cut	Quart jar	1.50[b]	100	1 oz	24.00	1¼	4¼
	No. 10 jar	4.88[b]	100	1 oz	78.00	[a]	1½
	Gallon jar	5.94[b]	100	1 oz	95.00	[a]	1¼
whole	No. 2½ jar	1.28[b]	100	1 oz	20.50	1¼	5
	Quart jar	1.38[b]	100	1 oz	22.00	1¼	4¾
Pickle relish							
sour	Quart	1.61[b]	100	1 oz	25.75	1	4
	No. 10 jar	5.73[b]	100	1 oz	91.75	[a]	1¼
	Gallon jar	7.16[b]	100	1 oz	114.50	[a]	[a]
sweet	Quart	1.75[b]	100	1 oz	28.00	1	3¼
	No. 10 jar	6.25[b]	100	1 oz	100.00	[a]	1
	Gallon jar	7.81[b]	100	1 oz	125.00	[a]	[a]
Pimientos, chopped	No. 2½ can	1.75	73	½ cup	4.80	[c]	[c]
	No. 10 can	6.81	68	½ cup	17.39	[c]	[c]
Potatoes, small whole	No. 2 can	1.25	—	2–3 cups	4.00	6¼	25
	No. 10 can	6.38	—	2–3 cups	25.00	1	4
Pumpkin, mashed	No. 300 can	0.91	100	4 oz	3.64	7	27½
	No. 2½ can	1.81	100	4 oz	7.24	3½	14
	No. 10 can	6.62	100	4 oz	26.50	1	4
Sauerkraut	No. 303 can	1.00	82	3 oz	4.37	5¾	23
	No. 2½ can	1.69	85	3 oz	7.66	3½	13¼
	No. 10 can	6.19	81	3 oz	26.74	1	3¾
Soups							
condensed	No. 1 picnic	0.66–0.75	200	1 cup diluted	2.50	10	40
	No. 3 cylinder	3.12	200	1 cup diluted	11.50	2¼	8¾
ready-to-serve	12-fl-oz can	—	100	1 cup	1.50	16¾	66¾
	25-fl-oz can (No. 2½)	—	100	1 cup	3.12	8¼	32¼

Table E-10. (Continued)

Canned Vegetables as Purchased	Unit of Purchase	Weight per Unit (lb)	Yield, as Served (%)	Portion as Served	Portions per Purchase Unit (no.)	Approximate Purchase Units for 25 Portions (no.)	100 Portions (no.)
Spinach	No. 303 can	0.94	72	4 oz	2.71	9¼	37
	No. 2½ can	1.69	70	4 oz	4.73	5½	21¼
	No. 10 can	6.12	61	4 oz	14.93	1¾	6¾
Squash, summer	No. 303 can	1.00	69	4 oz	2.75	9¼	36½
	No. 10 can	6.62	69	4 oz	17.50	1½	5¼
Squash, winter	No. 300 can	0.91	100	4 oz	3.64	7	27½
	No. 2½ can	1.81	100	4 oz	7.24	3½	14
	No. 10 can	6.62	100	4 oz	26.48	1	4
Succotash	No. 303 can	1.00	65	3 oz	3.47	7¼	29
	No. 10 can	6.75	65	3 oz	23.40	1¼	4½
Sweetpotatoes	No. 3 vacuum or squat	1.44	65	4 oz	3.74	6¾	26¾
	No. 2½ can, with syrup	1.81	66	4 oz	4.78	5¼	21
	No. 10 can, with syrup	6.38	71	4 oz	18.00	1½	5¾
Tomatoes	No. 303 can	1.00	100	4 oz	4.00	6¼	25
	No. 2½ can	1.75	100	4 oz	7.00	3¾	14½
	No. 10 can	6.38	100	4 oz	25.52	1	4
Tomato products							
catsup	14-oz bottle	0.88	100	1 oz	14.00	2	7¼
	No. 10 can	6.94	100	1 oz	111.00	a	1
chili sauce	12-oz jar	0.75	100	1 Tbsp	20.27	1¼	5
	No. 10 can	6.56	100	1 Tbsp	177.30	a	a
juice, concentrate[a]	6-fl-oz can	0.43	400	4 fl oz	6.00	4¼	16¾
Turnip greens	No. 303 can	0.94	72	4 oz	2.71	9¼	37
	No. 2½ can	1.69	70	4 oz	4.73	5½	21¼
	No. 10 can	6.12	61	4 oz	14.93	1¾	6¾
Vegetable juices	23-fl-oz can	1.54	100	4 fl oz	5.75	4½	17½
	46-fl-oz can	3.07	100	4 fl oz	11.50	2¼	8¾
	96-fl-oz can	6.41	100	4 fl oz	24.00	1¼	4¼
Vegetables, mixed	No. 303 can	1.00	68	3 oz	3.63	7	27¾
	No. 10 can	6.50	68	3 oz	23.57	1¼	4¼

[a]Number of purchase units needed is less than one.
[b]Drained weight.
[c]Number of purchase units needed is determined by use.
[d]See vegetable juices for canned tomato juice.

Table E-11. Vegetables—Frozen

Frozen Vegetables as Purchased	Unit of Purchase	Weight per Unit (lb)	Yield, as Served (%)	Portion as Served	Portions per Purchase Unit (no.)	Approximate Purchase Units for	
						25 Portions (no.)	100 Portions (no.)
Asparagus							
spears	Pound	1.00	—	4 medium, cooked	3.38	7½	29¾
	Package	2.50	—	4 medium, cooked	8.44	3	12
cuts and tips	Pound	1.00	80	3 oz cooked	4.27	6	23½
	Package	2.50	80	3 oz cooked	10.67	2½	9½
Beans, butter (lima)	Pound	1.00	100	3 oz cooked	5.33	4¾	19
	Package	2.50	100	3 oz cooked	13.33	2	7½
	Package	3.00	100	3 oz cooked	16.00	1¾	6¼
Beans, lima, green	Pound	1.00	100	3 oz cooked	5.33	4¾	19
	Package	2.50	100	3 oz cooked	13.33	2	7½
Beans, snap, green or wax	Pound	1.00	91	3 oz cooked	4.85	5¼	20¾
	Package	2.50	91	3 oz cooked	12.13	2¼	8¼
Blackeye peas	Pound	1.00	111	3 oz cooked	5.92	4¼	17
	Package	2.50	111	3 oz cooked	14.80	1¾	7
	Package	3.00	111	3 oz cooked	17.76	1½	5¾
Broccoli							
spears	Pound	1.00	—	2 medium	4.57	5½	22
	Package	2.50	—	2 medium	11.43	2¼	8¾
cut or chopped	Pound	1.00	85	3 oz cooked	4.53	5¾	22¼
	Package	2.50	85	3 oz cooked	11.33	2¼	9
Brussels sprouts	Pound	1.00	96	3 oz cooked	5.12	5	19¾
	Package	2.50	96	3 oz cooked	12.80	2	8
Carrots, sliced or diced	Pound	1.00	96	3 oz cooked	5.12	5	19¾
	Package	2.50	96	3 oz cooked	12.80	2	8
Cauliflower	Pound	1.00	90	3 oz cooked	4.80	5¼	21
	Package	2.50	90	3 oz cooked	12.00	2¼	8½
Collards	Pound	1.00	89	3 oz cooked	4.75	5½	21¼
	Package	2.50	89	3 oz cooked	11.87	2¼	8½
Corn							
on cob	Pound (about three 5-in. ears)	1.00	—	1 ear, cooked	3.00	8½	33½
whole kernel	Pound	1.00	97	3 oz cooked	5.17	5	19½
	Package	2.50	97	3 oz cooked	12.93	2	7¾
Kale	Pound	1.00	77	3 oz cooked	4.11	6¼	24½
	Package	2.50	77	3 oz cooked	10.27	2½	9¾
	Package	3.00	77	3 oz cooked	12.32	2¼	8¼
Mustard greens, leaf or chopped	Pound	1.00	80	3 oz cooked	4.27	6	23½
	Package	2.50	80	3 oz cooked	10.67	2½	9½
	Package	3.00	80	3 oz cooked	12.80	2	8
Okra, whole	Pound	1.00	82	3 oz cooked	4.37	5¾	23
	Package	2.50	82	3 oz cooked	10.93	2½	9¼
	Package	3.00	82	3 oz cooked	13.12	2	7¾
Peas, green	Pound	1.00	96	3 oz cooked	5.12	5	19¾
	Package	2.50	96	3 oz cooked	12.80	2	8
	Package	3.00	96	3 oz cooked	15.36	1¾	6¾
Peas and carrots	Pound	1.00	98	3 oz cooked	5.23	5	19¼
	Package	2.50	98	3 oz cooked	13.07	2	7¾
Peppers, green							
whole	Package	1.00	—	½ pepper, cooked	12.00	2¼	8½
	Package	2.50	—	½ pepper, cooked	30.00	a	3½
diced or sliced	Pound	1.00	97	1 oz cooked	15.52	1¾	6½
	Package	2.50	97	1 oz cooked	38.80	a	2¾
Potatoes							
french fried	Package	1.00	—	10 pieces	8.00	3¼	12½
	Package	5.00	—	10 pieces	40.00	a	2½
small whole	Container	5.00	—	3 cooked	16.67	1½	6

Table E-11. (Continued)

Frozen Vegetables as Purchased	Unit of Purchase	Weight per Unit (lb)	Yield, as Served (%)	Portion as Served	Portions per Purchase Unit (no.)	Approximate Purchase Units for	
						25 Portions (no.)	100 Portions (no.)
Spinach	Pound	1.00	80	3 oz cooked	4.27	6	23½
	Package	2.50	80	3 oz cooked	10.67	2½	9½
	Package	3.00	80	3 oz cooked	12.80	2	8
Squash, summer, sliced	Pound	1.00	87	3 oz cooked	4.64	5½	21¾
	Package	2.50	87	3 oz cooked	11.60	2¼	8¾
	Package	3.00	87	3 oz cooked	13.92	2	7¼
Squash, winter, mashed	Pound	1.00	92	4 oz cooked	3.68	7	27¼
	Package	2.50	92	4 oz cooked	9.20	2¾	11
Sweetpotatoes							
whole	Pound	1.00	—	1 whole, cooked	2.63	9¾	38¼
	Pound	1.00	98	4 oz cooked	3.92	6½	25¾
sliced	Package	2.50	98	4 oz cooked	9.80	2¾	10¼
	Package	3.00	98	4 oz cooked	11.76	2¼	8¾
Succotash	Pound	1.00	106	3 oz cooked	5.65	4½	17¾
	Package	2.50	106	3 oz cooked	14.13	2	7¼
Turnip greens, leaf or chopped	Pound	1.00	80	3 oz cooked	4.27	6	23½
	Package	2.50	80	3 oz cooked	10.67	2½	9½
	Package	3.00	80	3 oz cooked	12.80	2	8
Turnip greens with turnips	Pound	1.00	89	3 oz cooked	4.75	5½	21¼
	Package	3.00	89	3 oz cooked	14.24	2	7¼
Vegetables, mixed	Pound	1.00	95	3 oz cooked	5.07	5	19¾
	Package	2.50	95	3 oz cooked	12.67	2	8

[a]Number of purchase units needed is less than one.

Table E-12. Vegetables—Dried

Vegetables, Dried, Regular and Low-Moisture, as Purchased	Unit of Purchase	Weight per Unit (lb)	Yield, as Served (%)	Portion as Served	Portions per Purchase Unit (no.)	Approximate Purchase Units for	
						25 Portions (no.)	100 Portions (no.)
Regular							
Beans (includes white beans, lima beans, kidney beans, blackeye beans or peas)	Pound	1.00	232	3 oz cooked	12.37	2¼	8¼
Peas (includes any type, whole peas, split peas, or lentils)	Pound	1.00	223	3 oz cooked	11.89	2¼	8½
	Bushel	60.00	223	3 oz cooked	713.60	a	a
Low-moisture							
Onions, sliced	Pound	1.00	417	3 oz cooked	22.24	1¼	4½
Potatoes, white							
flakes	Pound	1.00	521	4 oz cooked	20.84	1¼	5
	Package	2.50	521	4 oz cooked	52.10	a	2
granules	Pound	1.00	506	4 oz cooked	20.24	1¼	5
	Package	2.50	506	4 oz cooked	50.60	a	2
Sweetpotatoes, flakes	Pound	1.00	294	4 oz cooked	11.76	2¼	8¾

[a]Number of purchase units needed is less than one.

Table E-13. Fruits—Fresh

Fresh Fruits as Purchased	Unit of Purchase	Weight per Unit[a] (lb)	Yield, as Served (%)	Portion as Served	Portions per Purchase Unit (no.)	Approximate Purchase Units for	
						25 Portions (no.)	100 Portions (no.)
Apples	Pound	1.00	—	1 medium, baked or raw	3.00	8½	33½
	Bushel	40.00	—	1 medium, baked or raw	120.00	b	b
	Pound	1.00	76	2 oz raw, chopped or diced	6.08	4½	16½
	Pound	1.00	87	4 oz applesauce	3.48	7¼	28¾
	Pound	1.00	63	4 oz cooked, sliced or diced	2.52	10	39¼
	Pound	1.00	—	⅙ 9-in. pie (2.12 lb apples per pie)	2.83	9	35½
	Pound	1.00	—	⅛ 9-in. pie	3.77	6¾	26¾
Apricots	Pound	1.00	—	2 medium	6.00	4¼	16¾
	Lug	24.00	—	2 medium	144.00	b	b
Avocados	Pound	1.00	75	2 oz sliced, diced, or wedges	6.00	4¼	16¾
	Lug	12.00	75	2 oz sliced, diced, or wedges	72.00	b	1½
	Box (⅘ bushel)	36.00	75	2 oz sliced, diced, or wedges	216.00	b	b
Bananas	Pound	1.00	—	1 medium	3.00	8½	33½
	Box	25.00	—	1 medium	75.00	b	1½
	Pound	1.00	68	2 oz sliced for fruit cup	5.44	4¾	18½
	Pound	1.00	68	3 oz sliced for dessert	3.63	7	27¾
	Pound	1.00	68	4 oz mashed	2.72	9¼	37
Blackberries	Quart	1.42	95	1 oz salad garnish	21.53	1¼	4¾
	Quart	1.42	95	3 oz	7.18	3½	14
	Crate (24 quarts)	34.00	95	3 oz	172.22	b	b
	Quart	1.42	—	⅙ 9-in. pie (0.92 quart per pie)	6.54	4	15½
	Quart	1.42	—	⅛ 9-in. pie	8.70	3	11½
Blueberries	Quart	1.97	92	1 oz salad garnish	28.98	b	3½
	Quart	1.97	92	3 oz	9.66	2¾	10½
	Crate (24 quarts)	47.25	92	3 oz	231.84	b	b
	Quart	1.97	—	⅙ 9-in. pie (0.59 quart per pie)	10.20	2½	10
	Quart	1.97	—	⅛ 9-in. pie	13.51	2	7½
Cantaloupe	Pound	1.00	50	3 oz sliced or diced	2.67	9½	37½
	1 (No. 36)	2.50	—	½ medium	2.00	12½	50
	Crate (No. 36)	80.00	—	½ medium	64.00	b	1¾
Cherries	Pound	1.00	89	3 oz pitted, raw	4.75	5½	21¼
	Lug	16.00	89	3 oz pitted, raw	75.95	b	1½
	Pound	1.00	—	⅙ 9-in. pie (1.60 lb per pie)	3.75	6¾	26¾
	Pound	1.00	—	⅛ 9-in. pie	5.00	5	20
Cranberries	Pound	1.00	96	1 oz raw, chopped, for relish	15.36	1¾	6¾
	Pound	1.00	182	2 oz sauce, strained	14.56	1¾	7
	Pound	1.00	239	2 oz cooked, whole	19.12	1½	5¼
	Box	25.00	239	2 oz cooked, whole	478.00	b	b
Figs	Pound	1.00	—	3 medium	4.00	6¼	25
	Box	6.00	—	3 medium	24.00	1¼	4¼
Grapefruit	Pound	1.00	44	4 fl oz juice	1.61	15¾	62¼
	Dozen (No. 64)	15.00	44	4 fl oz juice	24.22	1¼	4¼
	Pound	1.00	47	4 oz segments	1.88	13½	53¼
	Dozen	15.00	47	4 oz segments	28.20	b	3¾
	Dozen	15.00	—	½ medium	24.00	1¼	4¼
Grapefruit segments	½-gal. jar	4.22	100	4 oz	16.88	1½	6
Grapes							
with seeds	Pound	1.00	89	4 oz, seed removed	3.56	7¼	28¼
seedless	Pound	1.00	94	4 oz	3.76	6¾	26¾
	Lug	24.00	94	4 oz	90.24	b	1¼
Honeydew melon	Pound	1.00	60	3 oz sliced or diced	3.20	8	31¼
	1 melon	4.00	—	Wedge, ⅛ melon	8.00	3¼	12½
	1 melon	4.00	60	3 oz sliced or diced	12.80	2	8
Lemons	1 lemon (medium)	0.23	—	1 slice	8.00	3¼	12½
	1 lemon (medium)	0.23	—	1 wedge	6.00	4¼	16¾

Table E-13. (Continued)

Fresh Fruits as Purchased	Unit of Purchase	Weight per Unit[a] (lb)	Yield, as Served (%)	Portion as Served	Portions per Purchase Unit (no.)	Approximate Purchase Units for 25 Portions (no.)	Approximate Purchase Units for 100 Portions (no.)
Lemons (*continued*)	Pound (about 4 lemons)	1.00	43	2 fl oz juice	3.16	8	31¾
	Carton	36.00	43	2 fl oz juice	113.76	[b]	[b]
Limes	1 lime (medium)	0.15	—	Wedge, ¼ lime	4.00	6¼	25
	Pound	1.00	48	2 fl oz juice	3.52	7¼	28½
	Box (⅘ bushel)	40.00	48	2 fl oz juice	140.80	[b]	[b]
Mangoes	Pound	1.00	67	3 oz sliced or diced	3.57	7¼	28¼
	Lug	24.00	67	3 oz sliced or diced	85.76	[b]	1¼
Oranges	Pound	1.00	50	4 fl oz juice	1.83	13¾	54¾
	Pound	1.00	56	4-oz sections (no membrane)	2.24	11¼	44¾
	Pound	1.00	70	4-oz sections (with membrane)	2.80	9	35¾
California	Carton	38.00	70	4-oz sections (with membrane)	106.40	[b]	[b]
Florida	Box	85.00	50	4 fl oz juice	155.55	[b]	[b]
medium no. 176	Pound	1.00	—	1 whole	2.00	12½	50
	Dozen	6.00	50	4 fl oz juice	11.01	2½	9¼
	Dozen	6.00	56	4-oz sections (no membrane)	13.44	2	7½
small no. 250	Pound	1.00	—	1 whole	3.00	8½	33½
	Dozen	4.00	50	4 fl oz juice	7.34	3½	13¾
	Dozen	4.00	56	4 oz sections (no membrane)	8.96	3	11¼
Orange segments	½-gal. jar	4.28	100	4 oz	17.12	1½	6
Peaches	Pound	1.00	—	1 medium	4.00	6¼	25
	Pound	1.00	76	3 oz sliced or diced	4.05	6¼	24¾
	Bushel	48.00	76	3 oz sliced or diced	194.56	[b]	[b]
	Pound	1.00	—	⅙ 9-in. pie (1.88 lb per pie)	3.19	8	31½
	Pound	1.00	—	⅛ 9-in. pie	4.26	6	23½
Pears	Pound	1.00	—	1 medium	3.00	8½	33½
	Pound	1.00	78	3 oz sliced or diced	4.16	6¼	24¼
	Bushel	46.00	78	3 oz sliced or diced	191.36	[b]	[b]
Pineapples	Pound	1.00	52	3 oz cubed	2.77	9¼	36¼
	½ crate	35.00	52	3 oz cubed	97.07	[b]	1¼
Pineapple chunks	½-gal. jar	4.36	100	4 oz	17.44	1½	5¾
Plums	Pound	1.00	—	3 medium	2.67	9½	37½
	Pound	1.00	94	3 oz halves pitted	5.01	5	20
	4-basket crate	28.00	94	3 oz halves pitted	140.37	[b]	[b]
Raspberries	Quart	1.47	97	1 oz salad garnish	22.87	1¼	4½
	Quart	1.47	97	3 oz	7.62	3½	13¼
	Crate (24 quarts)	35.00	97	3 oz	181.07	[b]	[b]
	Quart	1.46	—	⅙ 9-in. pie (0.68 quart per pie)	8.85	3	11½
	Quart	1.46	—	⅛ 9-in. pie	11.76	2¼	8¾
Rhubarb, trimmed	Pound	1.00	103	3 oz cooked	5.49	4¾	18¼
	Pound	1.00	—	⅙ 9-in. pie (1.44 lb per pie)	4.17	6	24
	Pound	1.00	—	⅛ 9-in. pie	5.56	4½	18
Strawberries	Quart	1.48	87	1 oz salad garnish	20.53	1¼	5
	Quart	1.48	87	3 oz	6.84	3¾	14¾
	Crate (24 quarts)	35.00	87	3 oz	162.40	[b]	[b]
	Quart	1.46	—	⅙ 9-in. pie (1 quart per pie)	6.00	4¼	16¾
	Quart	1.46	—	⅛ 9-in. pie	8.00	3¼	12½
Tangerines	Pound	1.00	—	1 medium	4.00	6¼	25
	Box	45.00	—	1 medium	180.00	[b]	[b]
	Pound	1.00	74	3 oz sections	3.95	6½	25½
Watermelon	Pound	1.00	46	3 oz	2.45	10¼	41
	1 melon	18 to 30	—	1/16 melon	16.00	1¾	6¼

[a]Legal weights for contents of bushels, lugs, crates, and boxes vary among states.
[b]Number of purchase units needed is less than one.

Table E-14. Fruits—Canned

Canned Fruits as Purchased	Unit of Purchase	Weight per Unit (lb)	Yield, as Served (%)	Portion as Served	Portions per Purchase Unit (no.)	Approximate Purchase Units for	
						25 Portions (no.)	100 Portions (no.)
Apples, solid pack	No. 2 can	1.12	100	4 oz	4.48	5¾	22½
	No. 2½ can	1.62	100	4 oz	6.48	4	15½
	No. 10 can	6.00	100	4 oz	24.00	1¼	4¼
				⅙ 9-in. pie	24.00	1¼	4¼
Apple juice	23-fl-oz can	1.57	100	4 fl oz	5.75	4½	17½
	46-fl-oz can	3.14	100	4 fl oz	11.50	2¼	8¾
	96-fl-oz can	6.56	100	4 fl oz	24.00	1¼	4¼
Applesauce	No. 303 can	1.00	100	4 oz	4.00	6¼	25
	No. 2½ can	1.81	100	4 oz	7.24	3½	14
	No. 10 can	6.75	100	4 oz	27.00	1	3¾
Apricots, halves	No. 303 can	1.00	—	3–5 medium	4.00	6¼	25
	No. 2½ can	1.88	—	3–5 medium	7.00	3¾	14½
	No. 10 can	6.62	—	3–5 medium	25.00	1	4
Blackberries	No. 303 can	1.00	100	4 oz	4.00	6¼	25
	No. 10 can	6.62	100	4 oz	26.48	1	4
Blueberries	No. 300 can	0.91	199	4 oz	3.64	7	27½
	No. 10 can	6.56	199	4 oz	26.24	1	4
Boysenberries	No. 303 can	0.94	100	4 oz	3.76	6¾	26¾
	No. 10 can	6.62	100	4 oz	26.48	1	4
Cherries							
red, sour, pitted	No. 303 can	1.00	100	4 oz	4.00	6¼	25
	No. 10 can	6.56	100	4 oz	26.24	1	4
				⅙ 9-in. pie	24.00	1¼	4¼
sweet	No. 303 can	1.00	100	4 oz	4.00	6¼	25
	No. 2½ can	1.81	100	4 oz	7.24	3½	14
	No. 10 can	6.75	100	4 oz	27.00	1	3¾
Cranberries, strained or whole	No. 300 can	1.00	100	2 oz	8.00	3¼	12½
	No. 10 can	7.31	100	2 oz	58.50	a	1¾
Cranberry juice	1 pint	1.11	100	4 fl oz	4.00	6¼	25
	1 quart	2.23	100	4 fl oz	8.00	3¼	12½
	1 gallon	8.92	100	4 fl oz	32.00	a	3¼
Figs	No. 303 can	1.06		3–4 figs	4.00	6¼	25
				3–4 figs	7.00	3¾	14½
	No. 2½ can	1.88		3–4 figs	25.00	1	4
	No. 10 can	7.00					
Fruit cocktail or salad	No. 303 can	1.06	100	4 oz	4.24	6	23¾
	No. 2½ can	1.88	100	4 oz	7.52	3½	13½
	No. 10 can	6.75	100	4 oz	27.00	1	3¾
Grapefruit juice	18-fl-oz can	1.24	100	4 fl oz	4.50	5¾	22¼
	46-fl-oz can	3.14	100	4 fl oz	11.50	2¼	8¾
	96-fl-oz can	6.57	100	4 fl oz	24.00	1¼	4¼

Table E-14. (Continued)

Canned Fruits as Purchased	Unit of Purchase	Weight per Unit (lb)	Yield, as Served (%)	Portion as Served	Portions per Purchase Unit (no.)	Approximate Purchase Units for 25 Portions (no.)	Approximate Purchase Units for 100 Portions (no.)
Grapefruit sections	No. 303 can	1.00	100	4 oz	4.00	6¼	25
	No. 3 cylinder	3.12	100	4 oz	12.48	2¼	8¼
Lemon juice	32-fl-oz can	2.16	100	2 fl oz	16.00	1¾	6¼
Lime juice	32-fl-oz can	2.17	100	2 fl oz	16.00	1¾	6½
Orange juice	18-fl-oz can	1.24	100	4 fl oz	4.50	5¾	22¼
	46-fl-oz can	3.16	100	4 fl oz	11.50	2¼	8¾
	96-fl-oz can	6.59	100	4 fl oz	24.00	1¼	4¼
Oranges, mandarin	No. 10 can	6.38	100	4 oz	25.50	1	4
Peaches							
halves or slices	No. 303 can	1.00	—	2 medium	3.00	8½	33½
	No. 2½ can	1.81	—	2 medium	7.00	3¾	14½
	No. 10 can	6.75	—	2 medium	25.00	1	4
				⅛ 9-in. pie	24.00	1¼	4¼
whole, spiced	No. 10 can	6.88	—	1 each	25.00	1	4
Pears, halves	No. 303 can	1.00	—	2 medium	3.00	8½	33½
	No. 2½ can	1.81	—	2 medium	7.00	3¾	14½
	No. 10 can	6.62	—	2 medium	25.00	1	4
Pineapple							
chunks and cubes	No. 2½ can	1.88	100	4 oz	7.52	3½	13½
	No. 10 can	6.75	100	4 oz	27.00	1	3¾
crushed	No. 2½ can	1.88	100	4 oz	7.52	3½	13½
	No. 10 can	6.81	100	4 oz	27.24	1	3¾
sliced	No. 2½ can	1.88	—	1 large	8.00	3¼	12½
	No. 10 can	6.81	—	1 large or 2 small	25.00	1	4
Pineapple juice	18-fl-oz can	1.24	100	4 fl oz	4.50	5¾	22¼
	46-fl-oz can	3.17	100	4 fl oz	11.50	2¼	8¾
	96-fl-oz can	6.62	100	4 fl oz	24.00	1¼	4¼
Plums	No. 2½ can	1.88	—	2–3 plums	7.00	3¾	14½
	No. 10 can	6.75	—	2–3 plums	25.00	1	4
Prunes	No. 2½ can	1.88	100	4 oz	7.52	3½	13½
	No. 10 can	6.88	100	4 oz	27.52	1	3¾
Raspberries	No. 303 can	1.00	100	4 oz	4.00	6¼	25
	No. 10 can	6.75	100	4 oz	27.00	1	3¾
Strawberries	No. 303 can	1.00	100	4 oz	4.00	6¼	25
	No. 10 can	6.75	100	4 oz	27.00	1	3¾

aNumber of purchase units needed is less than one.

Table E-15. Fruits—Frozen

Frozen Fruits as Purchased	Unit of Purchase	Weight per Unit (lb)	Yield, as Served (%)	Portion as Served	Portions per Purchase Unit (no.)	Approximate Purchase Units for 25 Portions (no.)	Approximate Purchase Units for 100 Portions (no.)
Apples, sliced	Pound	1.00	106	4 oz	4.24	6	23¾
				⅙ 9-in. pie (1.50 lb per pie)	4.00	6¼	25
	Package	2.50	106	4 oz	10.60	2½	9½
	Package	5.00	106	4 oz	21.20	1¼	4¾
	Can	30.00	106	4 oz	127.20	*a*	*a*
Apricots	Pound	1.00	95	4 oz	3.80	6¾	26½
	Can	25.00	95	4 oz	95.00	*a*	1¼
	Can	30.00	95	4 oz	114.00	*a*	*a*
Blackberries	Pound	1.00	103	4 oz	4.12	6¼	24½
	Can	30.00	103	4 oz	123.60	*a*	*a*
Blueberries	Pound	1.00	108	4 oz	4.32	6	23½
	Package	2.50	108	4 oz	10.80	2½	9½
	Can	25.00	108	4 oz	108.00	*a*	1
	Can	30.00	108	4 oz	129.60	*a*	*a*
Cherries, red, sour, pitted	Pound	1.00	100	4 oz	4.00	6¼	25
				⅙ 9-in. pie (1.50 lb per pie)	4.00	6¼	25
	Can	30.00	100	4 oz	120.00	*a*	*a*
Grapefruit sections	Pound	1.00	100	4 oz	4.00	6¼	25
	Package	3.00	100	4 oz	12.00	2¼	8½
Grapefruit juice, concentrate	6-fl-oz can	0.46	400	4 fl oz	6.00	4¼	16¾
	32-fl-oz can	2.46	400	4 fl oz	32.00	*a*	3¼
Grape juice, concentrate	6-fl-oz can	.48	400	4 fl oz	6.00	4¼	16¾
	32-fl-oz can	2.54	400	4 fl oz	32.00	*a*	3¼
Lemon juice, concentrate	4-fl-oz can	0.31	500	2 fl oz	10.00	2½	10
	6-fl-oz can	0.47	500	2 fl oz	15.00	1¾	6¾
Lemonade, concentrate	6-fl-oz can	0.49	700	2 fl oz	21.00	1¼	5
	18-fl-oz can	1.46	700	2 fl oz	63.00	*a*	1¾
Melon scoops	Pound	1.00	100	3 oz	5.33	4¾	19
	Package	6.50	100	3 oz	34.67	*a*	3
Orange juice, concentrate	6-fl-oz can	.46	400	4 fl oz	6.00	4¼	16¾
	12-fl-oz can	.93	400	4 fl oz	12.00	2¼	8½
	32-fl-oz can	2.48	400	4 fl oz	32.00	*a*	3¼
Peaches, sliced	Pound	1.00	95	4 oz	3.80	6¾	26½
				⅙ 9-in. pie (1.33 lb per pie)	4.50	5¾	22¼
	Can	6.50	95	4 oz	24.70	1¼	4¼
	Can	10.00	95	4 oz	38.00	*a*	2¾
	Can	30.00	95	4 oz	114.00	*a*	*a*
Pineapple							
chunks	Pound	1.00	100	4 oz	4.00	6¼	25
	Can	10.00	100	4 oz	40.00	*a*	2½
crushed	Can	30.00	100	4 oz	120.00	*a*	*a*
Pineapple juice, concentrate	6-fl-oz can	.47	400	4 fl oz	6.00	4¼	16¾
	32-fl-oz can	2.53	400	4 fl oz	32.00	*a*	3¼
Raspberries	Pound	1.00	100	4 oz	4.00	6¼	25
	Can	6.50	100	4 oz	26.00	1	4
	Can	10.00	100	4 oz	40.00	*a*	2½
	Can	30.00	100	4 oz	120.00	*a*	*a*
Rhubarb	Pound	1.00	106	4 oz	4.24	6	23¾
				⅙ 9-in. pie (1.50 lb per pie)	4.00	6¼	25
	Package	2.50	106	4 oz	10.60	2½	9½
	Can	10.00	106	4 oz	42.40	*a*	2½
	Can	25.00	106	4 oz	106.00	*a*	1
	Can	30.00	106	4 oz	127.20	*a*	*a*

Table E-15. (Continued)

Frozen Fruits as Purchased	Unit of Purchase	Weight per Unit (lb)	Yield, as Served (%)	Portion as Served	Portions per Purchase Unit (no.)	Approximate Purchase Units for 25 Portions (no.)	Approximate Purchase Units for 100 Portions (no.)
Strawberries	Pound	1.00	100	4 oz	4.00	6¼	25
	Can	6.50	100	4 oz	26.00	1	4
	Can	10.00	100	4 oz	40.00	[a]	2½
	Can	30.00	100	4 oz	120.00	[a]	[a]
Tangerine juice, concentrate	6-fl-oz can	0.47	400	4 fl oz	6.00	4¼	16¾
	32-fl-oz can	2.48	400	4 fl oz	32.00	[a]	3¼

[a]Number of purchase units needed is less than one.

Table E-16. Fruits—Dried

Fruits, Dried, Regular and Low-Moisture, as Purchased	Unit of Purchase	Weight per Unit (lb)	Yield, as Served (%)	Portion as Served	Portions per Purchase Unit (no.)	Approximate Purchase Units for 25 Portions (no.)	Approximate Purchase Units for 100 Portions (no.)
Regular							
Apple slices	Pound	1.00	412	4 oz	16.48	1¾	6¼
				⅙ 9-in. pie (½ lb per pie)	18.00	1½	5¼
	Carton	5.00	412	4 oz	82.40	[a]	1¼
Apricots	11-oz package	0.69	344	4 oz	9.46	2¾	10¾
	Pound	1.00	344	4 oz	13.76	2	7½
	Carton	30.00	344	4 oz	412.80	[a]	[a]
Dates	12-oz package	0.75	100	3 oz	4.00	6¼	25
	Pound	1.00	100	3 oz	5.33	4¾	19
	Carton	15.00	100	3 oz	80.00	[a]	1¼
Peaches	11-oz package	0.69	422	4 oz	11.60	2¼	8¾
	Pound	1.00	422	4 oz	16.88	1½	6
				⅙ 9-in. pie (⅓ lb per pie)	18.00	1½	5¾
	Carton	30.00	422	4 oz	506.40	[a]	[a]
Prunes	Pound	1.00	253	4 oz	10.12	2½	10
	2-lb package	2.00	253	4 oz	20.24	1¼	5
	Carton	30.00	253	4 oz	303.60	[a]	[a]
Raisins	Pound	1.00	100	½ cup	6.00	4¼	16¾
Low-moisture							
Apples	Pound	1.00	584	4 oz	23.36	1¼	4½
				⅙ 9-in. pie (¼ lb per pie)	24.00	1¼	4¼
	No. 10 can	1.50	584	4 oz	35.04	[a]	3
Applesauce	Pound	1.00	911	4 oz	36.44	[a]	2¾
	No. 10 can	2.50	911	4 oz	91.10	[a]	1¼
Apricots	Pound	1.00	505	4 oz	20.20	1¼	5
	No. 10 can	3.50	505	4 oz	70.70	[a]	1½
Fruit cocktail	Pound	1.00	558	4 oz	22.32	1¼	4½
	No. 10 can	2.75	558	4 oz	61.38	[a]	1¾
Peaches	Pound	1.00	534	4 oz	21.36	1¼	4¾
				⅙ 9-in. pie (¼ lb per pie)	24.00	1¼	4¾
	No. 10 can	3.00	534	4 oz	64.08	[a]	1¾
Prunes, whole, pitted	Pound	1.00	462	4 oz	18.48	1½	5½
	No. 10 can	3.00	462	4 oz	55.44	[a]	2

[a]Number of purchase units needed is less than one.

Table E-17. Flour, Cereals, and Mixes

Flour, Cereals, and Mixes as Purchased	Unit of Purchase	Weight per Unit (lb)	Yield, as Served (%)	Portion as Served or Used	Portions per Purchase Unit (no.)	Approximate Purchase Units for	
						25 Portions (no.)	100 Portions (no.)
Flour	5-lb bag	5.00	—	1 cup	20.00	a	a
	25-lb bag	25.00	—	1 cup	100.00	a	a
	100-lb sack	100.00	—	1 cup	400.00	a	a
Cereals, uncooked							
bulgur, cracked wheat (USDA)	Pound	1.00	401	¾ cup cooked	10.67	2½	9½
				1 cup uncooked	2.67	a	a
cornmeal	1-lb box	1.00	628	¾ cup cooked	15.33	1¾	6¾
	5-lb bag	5.00	628	¾ cup cooked	76.65	b	1½
	10-lb bag	10.00	628	¾ cup cooked	153.30	b	b
	1-lb box	1.00	100	1 cup uncooked	3.00	a	a
corn grits	1-lb box	1.00	628	¾ cup cooked	16.43	1¾	6¼
	1-lb box	1.00	100	1 cup uncooked	2.75	a	a
farina	1-lb box	1.00	855	¾ cup cooked	21.92	1¼	4¾
	5-lb bag	5.00	855	¾ cup cooked	109.60	b	1
macaroni	1-lb box	1.00	311	¾ cup cooked	12.00	2¼	8½
	20-lb box	20.00	311	¾ cup cooked	240.00	b	b
	1-lb box	1.00	100	1 cup uncooked	3.75	a	a
noodles	1-lb box	1.00	329	¾ cup cooked	10.67	2½	9½
	20-lb box	20.00	329	¾ cup cooked	213.40	b	b
	1-lb box	1.00	100	1 cup uncooked	7.25	a	a
rice	1-lb box	1.00	320	¾ cup cooked	11.27	2¼	9
	10-lb box	10.00	320	¾ cup cooked	112.70	b	b
	100-lb sack	100.00	320	¾ cup cooked	1,127.00	b	b
	1-lb box	1.00	100	1 cup uncooked	2.75	a	a
rolled oats	1-lb box	1.00	610	¾ cup cooked	15.33	1¾	6¾
	3-lb box	3.00	610	¾ cup cooked	46.00	b	2¼
	50-lb sack	50.00	610	¾ cup cooked	766.50	b	b
	1-lb box	1.00	100	1 cup uncooked	4.50	a	a
rolled wheat (USDA)	1-lb box	1.00	375	¾ cup cooked	8.89	3	11¼
	3-lb box	3.00	375	¾ cup cooked	26.67	b	3¾
spaghetti	1-lb box	1.00	359	¾ cup cooked	12.12	2¼	8¼
	20-lb box	20.00	359	¾ cup cooked	242.40	b	b
	1-lb box	1.00	100	1 cup uncooked	6.06	a	a
whole wheat	1-lb box	1.00	608	¾ cup cooked	15.20	1¾	6¾
	4½-lb box	4.50	608	¾ cup cooked	68.40	b	1½
	50-lb sack	50.00	608	¾ cup cooked	760.00	b	b
Cereals, ready-to-eat							
bran flakes (25–40%)	Pound	1.00	100	1 oz	16.00	1¾	6¼
	14½-oz package	0.91	100	1 oz	14.50	1¾	7
	10-lb package	10.00	100	1 oz	160.00	b	b
bran flakes with raisins	Pound	1.00	100	1¼ oz	12.80	2	8
	14-oz package	0.88	100	1¼ oz	11.20	2¼	9
	200 individuals	15.62	100	1¼ oz	200.00	b	b
corn flakes	Pound	1.00	100	1 oz	16.00	1¾	6¼
	12-oz package	0.75	100	1 oz	12.00	2¼	8½
	10-lb package	10.00	100	1 oz	160.00	b	b
puffed rice	Pound	1.00	100	⅜ oz	25.60	1	4
	8-oz package	0.50	100	⅜ oz	12.80	2	8
	10-oz package	10.00	100	⅜ oz	256.00	b	b

Table E-17. (Continued)

Flour, Cereals, and Mixes as Purchased	Unit of Purchase	Weight per Unit (lb)	Yield, as Served (%)	Portion as Served or Used	Portions per Purchase Unit (no.)	Approximate Purchase Units for	
						25 Portions (no.)	100 Portions (no.)
puffed wheat	Pound	1.00	100	½ oz	32.00	b	3¼
	8-oz package	0.50	100	½ oz	16.00	1¾	6¼
	10-lb package	10.00	100	½ oz	320.00	b	b
puffed wheat, pre-sweetened	Pound	1.00	100	⅝ oz	18.29	1½	5½
	9-oz package	0.56	100	⅝ oz	10.29	2½	9¾
	200 individuals	10.94	100	⅝ oz	200.00	b	b
rice flakes	Pound	1.00	100	⅝ oz	18.29	1½	5½
	9½-oz package	0.59	100	⅝ oz	10.86	2½	9¼
	10-lb package	10.00	100	⅝ oz	182.86	b	b
shredded wheat	Pound	1.00	100	1⅗ oz	10.00	2½	10
	12-oz package	0.75	100	1⅗ oz (2 small)	7.50	3½	13½
	200 individuals	20.00	100	1⅗ oz	200.00	b	b
wheat flakes	Pound	1.00	100	1 oz	16.00	1¾	6¼
	10-oz package	0.62	100	1 oz	10.00	2½	10
	10-lb package	10.00	100	1 oz	160.00	b	b
Mixes^c							
cake							
angel food	Pound	1.00	—	¹⁄₁₂ 10-in. cake	12.00	2¼	8½
	12-cake case	12.00	—	¹⁄₁₂ 10-in. cake	144.00	b	b
other	Pound	1.00	—	{ 2 in. × 3 in. cut	15.20	1¾	6¾
				{ Cupcake	20.00	1¼	5
	5-lb box	5.00	—	{ 2 in. × 3 in. cut	75.100	b	1½
				{ Cupcake	100.00	b	1
frosting	Pound	1.00	—	{ 2 in. × 2 in.	38–39	b	2¾
				{ Cupcake	36–37	b	3
	5-lb box	5.00	—	{ 2 in. × 2 in.	190–195	b	b
				{ Cupcake	180–185	b	b
Cookie							
basic sugar	Pound	1.00	—	2½-oz cookies	17–20	1½	6
	5-lb box	5.00	—	2½-oz cookies	85–100	b	1¼
brownie	Pound	1.00	—	2 in. × 2 in.	20–30	1¼	5
	5-lb box	5.00	—	2 in. × 2 in.	100–150	b	1
Hot bread							
biscuit	Pound	1.00	—	2-in. biscuit	20.00	1¼	5
	5-lb box	5.00	—	2-in. biscuit	100.00	b	1
muffins	Pound	1.00	—	1½-oz muffin	14–16	2	7¼
	5-lb box	5.00	—	1½-oz muffin	70–80	b	1½
rolls							
sweet	Pound	1.00	—	1¼-oz roll	18–19	1½	5¾
	5-lb box	5.00	—	1¼-oz roll	90–95	b	1¼
yeast	Pound	1.00	—	1-oz roll	23–25	1¼	4½
	5-lb box	5.00	—	1-oz roll	115–120	b	b
Piecrust	Pound	1.00	—	9-in. shell	3.00	8½	33½
	5-lb box	5.00	—	9-in. shell	16.00	1¾	6¼

^aNumber of purchase units needed is determined by use.

^bNumber of purchase units needed is less than one.

^cYields of mixes vary widely, depending on manufacturer, size of pan, and baking time and temperature. See instructions on package or box.

Table E-18. Bakery Foods

Bakery Foods as Purchased	Unit of Purchase	Weight per Unit (lb)	Portion as Served	Portions per Purchase Unit (no.)	Approximate Purchase Units for 25 Portions (no.)	Approximate Purchase Units for 100 Portions (no.)
Breads[a]						
raisin	1-lb loaf	1.00	1 slice	18.00	1½	5¾
	2-lb loaf	2.00	1 slice	36.00	[b]	3
rye	1-lb loaf	1.00	1 slice	23.00	1¼	4½
	1½-lb loaf	1.50	1 slice	28.00	1	3¾
	2-lb loaf	2.00	1 slice	33.00	[b]	3¼
white and whole wheat	1-lb loaf	1.00	⅝-in. slice	16.00	1¾	6¼
			1 cup soft cubes or crumbs	18.00	1½	5¾
			1 cup toasted cubes	13.50	2	7½
			1 cup dry crumbs	6.00	4¼	16¾
	1¼-lb loaf	1.25	⅝-in. slice	19.00	1½	5½
	1½-lb loaf	1.50	⅝-in. slice	24.00	1¼	4¼
	2-lb loaf	2.00	½-in. slice	28.00	1	4
			⅜-in. slice	36.00	[b]	3
	3-lb loaf	3.00	½-in. slice	44.00	[b]	2½
			⅜-in. slice	56.00	[b]	2
Cake						
layer	8-in.	—	1/12 cake	12.00	2¼	8½
	9-in.	—	1/16 cake	16.00	1¾	6¼
	12-in.	—	1/30 cake	30.00	[b]	3½
	14-in.	—	1/40 cake	40.00	[b]	2½
loaf	Pound	1.00	⅛ cake	8.00	3¼	12½
sheet	8-in. square	—	2 in. × 2 in. (small)	16.00	1¾	6¼
	9 in. × 13 in.	—	3 in. × 3 in. (regular)	12.00	2¼	8½
	12 in. × 18 in.	—	2 in. × 2 in.	54.00	[b]	2
			3 in. × 3 in.	24.00	1¼	4¼
	16 in. × 24 in.	—	2 in. × 2 in.	96.00	[b]	1¼
			3 in. × 3 in.	40.00	[b]	2½
Cookies						
brownies	Pound	1.00	2 cookies	18.00	1½	5¾
butter	Pound	1.00	2 cookies	46.50	[b]	2¼
chocolate chip	Pound	1.00	2 cookies	21.50	1¼	4¾
cream filled	Pound	1.00	2 cookies	19.50	1½	5¼
fig bars	Pound	1.00	2 cookies	15.50	1¾	6½
gingersnaps	Pound	1.00	2 cookies	30.00	[b]	3½
shortbread	Pound	1.00	2 cookies	29.00	[b]	3½
sugar	Pound	1.00	2 cookies	10.50	2½	9¾
vanilla	Pound	1.00	2 cookies	46.50	[b]	2¼
Crackers						
graham	Pound	1.00	2 crackers	32.50	[b]	3¼
saltines	Pound	1.00	2 crackers	65–70	[b]	1¾
soda	Pound	1.00	2 crackers	30–35	[b]	3½
Rolls						
frankfurter	Pound	1.00	1 roll (1⅓ oz)	12.03	2¼	8½
hamburger	Pound	1.00	1 roll (1¾ oz)	9.14	2¾	11
hard, round	Pound	1.00	1 roll (1⅝ oz)	8.74	3	11½
plain, pan	Pound	1.00	1 roll (1⅓ oz)	12.03	2¼	8½
sweet, pan	Pound	1.00	1 roll (1½ oz)	10.67	2½	9½
Pie	8-in.	—	⅛ pie	6.00	4¼	16¾
	9-in.	—	½ pie	7.00	3¾	14½
	10-in.	—	⅛ pie	8.00	3¼	12½

[a] End crusts of bread were excluded in determining portions per purchase unit.
[b] Number of purchase units needed is less than one.

Table E-19. Fats and Oils

Fats and Oils as Purchased	Unit of Purchase	Weight per Unit (lb)	Portion as Served or Used	Portions per Purchase Unit (no.)	Approximate Purchase Units for	
					25 Portions (no.)	100 Portions (no.)
Butter or margarine						
pound print	Carton	1.00	1 cup	2.00	a	a
			1 pat	72.00	b	1½
¼-lb print	Carton	1.00	1 pat	72.00	b	1¼
chips	Case	5.00	1 pat	360.00	b	b
Lard	Carton	1.00	1 cup	2.00	a	a
	Can	50.00	1 cup	100.00	a	a
Salad dressing (oil or mayonnaise type)	Pint	1.00	1 Tbsp	32.00	b	3¼
	Quart	2.00	1 Tbsp	64.00	b	1¾
	Gallon	8.00	1 Tbsp	256.00	b	b
Salad oil	Pint	0.97	1 cup	2.00	a	a
	Quart	1.94	1 cup	4.00	a	a
	Gallon	7.76	1 cup	16.00	a	a
Shortening (hydrogenated)	Can	1.00	1 cup	2.50	a	a
	Can	3.00	1 cup	7.50	a	a
	Can	50.00	1 cup	125.00	a	a

aNumber of purchase units needed is determined by use.
bNumber of purchase units needed is less than one.

Table E-20. Sugar and Sweets

Sugar and Sweets as Purchased	Unit of Purchase	Weight per Unit (lb)	Portion as Served or Used	Portions per Purchase Unit (no.)	Approximate Purchase Units for 25 Portions (no.)	Approximate Purchase Units for 100 Portions (no.)
Sugar						
brown, dark or light	Carton	1.00	1 cup	2.00	a	a
		25.00	1 cup	50.00	a	a
cubes	Carton	1.00	2 cubes	40.00	b	2½
	Bulk	25.00	2 cubes	1000.00	b	b
granulated						
bulk	Carton	1.00	2 level or 1 rounded tsp	54.00	b	2
			1 cup	2.25	a	a
	Bag	5.00	1 cup	11.25	a	a
	Bag	25.00	1 cup	56.25	a	a
	Sack	100.00	1 cup	225.00	a	a
individuals	Package	1.50	1 packet	100.00	b	1
	Carton	45.00	1 packet	3000.00	b	b
powdered (confec-tioners)	Carton	1.00	1 cup	3.50	a	a
	Sack	25.00	1 cup	87.50	a	a
Syrup						
blends	12-fl-oz bottle	1.03	2 Tbsp	12.00	2¼	8½
	Quart	2.83	2 Tbsp	32.00	b	3¼
	No. 10 can	8.50	2 Tbsp	96.00	b	1¼
	Gallon	11.00	2 Tbsp	128.00	b	b
corn	Pint	1.50	2 Tbsp	16.00	1¾	6¼
	5-lb can	5.00	2 Tbsp	53.33	b	2
	No. 10 can	8.79	2 Tbsp	93.76	b	1¼
			1 cup	11.72	a	a
maple	Pint	1.38	2 Tbsp	16.00	1¾	6¼
	Gallon	11.00	2 Tbsp	128.00	b	b
molasses	Pint	1.50	2 Tbsp	16.00	1¾	6¼
	Jar	2.00	2 Tbsp	21.00	1¼	5
	No. 10 can	9.31	2 Tbsp	99.00	b	1
Jam, jelly, marmalade						
bulk	Jar	1.00	1 Tbsp	23.00	1¼	4½
	No. 10 can	8.38	1 Tbsp	192.00	b	b
individuals	Carton	—	1 packet	200.00	b	b
Other sweets						
apple butter	Jar	1.00	1 packet	11.00	2½	9¼
	No. 10 can	7.50	1 packet	81.00	b	1¼
honey	Jar	1.00	1 packet	11.00	2½	9¼
	2-lb can	2.00	1 packet	22.00	1¼	4¾
	5-lb can	5.00	1 packet	54.00	b	2
Desserts, dry						
gelatin, flavored	3-oz package	0.19	½ cup	4.00	6¼	25
	6-oz package	0.38	½ cup	8.00	3¾	12½
	Pound	1.00	½ cup	21.33	1¼	4¾
Pudding, pie filling						
chocolate	4-oz package	0.25	½ cup	4.00	6¼	25
	Pound	1.00	4 oz	20.00	1¼	5
			Fill for ⅛ 9-in. pie	18.67	1½	5½
lemon chiffon	Pound	1.00	Fill for ⅛ 9-in. pie	32.00	b	3¼
vanilla	3-oz package	0.19	½ cup	4.00	6¼	25
	Pound	1.00	4 oz	25.60	1	4
			Fill for ⅛ 9-in. pie	24.00	1¼	4¼
Pudding, instant						
chocolate	4½-oz package	0.28	½ cup	4.00	6¼	25
	Pound	1.00	½ cup	14.29	1¾	7
vanilla	3¾-oz package	0.23	½ cup	4.00	6¼	25
	Pound	1.00	½ cup	17.39	1½	5¾

aNumber of purchase units needed is determined by use.
bNumber of purchase units needed is less than one.

Table E-21. Beverages

Beverages as Purchased	Unit of Purchase	Weight per Unit (lb)	Portion as Served	Portions per Purchase Unit (no.)	Approximate Purchase Units[a] for	
					25 Portions (no.)	100 Portions (no.)
Carbonated drinks						
6-oz bottles	Case (24)	—	6 fl oz	24.00	—	—
12-oz bottles	Case (24)	—	6 fl oz	48.00	—	—
16-oz bottles	Case (24)	—	6 fl oz	64.00	—	—
Cocoa						
regular, unsweetened	Pound	1.00	1 measuring cup, prepared	50.00	½	2
instant, sweetened						
bulk	8-oz carton	0.50	1 cup	28.00	(1½ cup)	(6 cup)
	38-oz carton	2.38	1 cup	133.00	(1½ cup)	(6 cup)
individuals	Carton (50)	—	1 packet	50.00	½	2
syrup, sweetened	16-oz can	1.00	1 cup	29.00	1	3½
Coffee						
ground	Pound	1.00	1 measuring cup, prepared	37.00[b]	—	—
instant						
bulk	6-oz jar	0.38	1 level tsp	180.00	(½ cup + 1 tsp)	(2 cup + 4 tsp)
			1 rounded tsp	90.00	(½ cup + 1 tsp)	(2 cup + 4 tsp)
	10-oz jar	0.62	1 level tsp	300.00	(½ cup + 1 tsp)	(2 cup + 4 tsp)
individuals	Carton (72)	—	1 packet	72.00	—	—
Tea						
bulk	Pound	1.00	1 measuring cup, prepared	256.00	—	(6¼ oz)
bags	Package (48)	0.24	1 measuring cup or more	48.00	—	—
	Carton (100)	0.50	1 measuring cup or more	100.00	¼	1
instant	1½-oz jar	0.09	1 cup hot tea	96.00	(½ cup + 1 cup)	(2 cup + 4 tsp)
			1 cup iced tea	64.00	(¾ cup)	(3 cup)

[a]Numbers in parentheses refer to approximate measure to serve 25 and 100 portions: tsp, teaspoon; oz, ounces.
[b]Varies depending on brand of coffee used and method of preparation.

Appendix F. Rounding Off Weights and Measures

Table F-1. Guide for Rounding Off Weights and Measures[a]

Item	If Total Amount of an Ingredient Is	Round It to
Weights	less than 2 oz	measure unless wt is in ¼, ½, or ¾ oz amounts
Various miscellaneous ingredients	2–10 oz	closest ¼ oz or convert to measure
	more than 10 oz, but less than 2 lb 8 oz	closest ½ oz
	2 lb 8 oz to 5 lb	closest full oz
	more than 5 lb	closest ¼ lb
Measures		
Primarily spices, seasonings, flavorings, condiments, leavenings, and similar items	less than 1 Tbsp	closest ⅛ tsp
	more than 1 Tbsp but less than 3 Tbsp	closest ¼ tsp
	3 Tbsp to ½ cup	closest ½ tsp or convert to weight
	more than ½ cup but less than ¾ cup	closest full tsp or convert to weight
	more than ¾ cup but less than 2 cups	closest full Tbsp or convert to weight
	2 cup to 2 qt	nearest ¼ cup
Primarily milk, water, eggs, juice, oil, syrup, molasses, etc.	more than 2 qt but less than 4 qt	nearest ½ cup
	1 gal. to 2 gal.	nearest full cup or ¼ qt
	more than 2 gal. but less than 10 gal.	nearest full qt
	more than 10 gal. but less than 20 gal.	closest ½ gal.
	over 20 gal.	closest full gal.

[a]From American Dietetic Association. 1967. Standardizing Recipes for Institutional Use. ADA, Chicago, IL.

Appendix G. Decimal Equivalents of a Pound

Table G-1. Ounces and Decimal Equivalents of a Pound[a]

Ounces	Decimal Part of a Pound	Ounces	Decimal Part of a Pound
¼	0.016	8¼	0.516
½	0.031	8½	0.531
¾	0.047	8¾	0.547
1	0.063	9	0.563
1¼	0.078	9¼	0.578
1½	0.094	9½	0.594
1¾	0.109	9¾	0.609
2	0.125	10	0.625
2¼	0.141	10¼	0.641
2½	0.156	10½	0.656
2¾	0.172	10¾	0.672
3	0.188	11	0.688
3¼	0.203	11¼	0.703
3½	0.219	11½	0.719
3¾	0.234	11¾	0.734
4	0.250	12	0.750
4¼	0.266	12¼	0.766
4½	0.281	12½	0.781
4¾	0.297	12¾	0.797
5	0.313	13	0.813
5¼	0.328	13¼	0.828
5½	0.344	13½	0.844
5¾	0.359	13¾	0.859
6	0.375	14	0.875
6¼	0.391	14¼	0.891
6½	0.406	14½	0.906
6¾	0.422	14¾	0.922
7	0.438	15	0.938
7¼	0.453	15¼	0.953
7½	0.469	15½	0.969
7¾	0.484	15¾	0.984
8	0.500	16	1.000

[a]From American Dietetic Association. 1967. Standardizing Recipes for Institutional Use. ADA, Chicago, IL.

Appendix H. Factors for Metric Conversion

Table H-1. Factors for Metric Conversion of Units Commonly Used in Food Preparation[a]

English Unit		Multiply by			Metric Unit
		Exact	Soft		
Weight					
ounces (oz)	×	28.35	or 28.00	=	grams (g)[b]
pounds (lb or #)	×	0.453	or 0.45	=	kilograms (kg)
Volume					
teaspoons (tsp)	×	4.97	or 5.00	=	milliliters (ml)
tablespoons (Tbsp)	×	14.8	or 15.00	=	ml
fluid ounces (fl oz)	×	29.575	or 30.00	=	ml
cups (C)	×	236.6	or 0.240	=	ml
pints (pt)	×	0.473	or 0.47	=	liters (L)
quarts (qt)	×	0.946	or 0.95	=	L
gallons (gal.)	×	3.786	or 3.80	=	L
Pressure					
pounds per square inch (psi)	×		6.90	=	kilopascals (kPa)
Temperature					
degrees Fahrenheit (°F)		5/9 (after subtracting 32)		=	degrees Celsius (°C)

[a]From American Dietetic Association. 1967. Standardizing Recipes for Institutional Use. ADA, Chicago, IL.

Appendix I. JCAH Standards for Dietary Services

Standard

DT.1   The dietetic department/service is organized, directed and staffed, and integrated with other units and departments/services of the hospital in a manner designed to assure the provision of optimal nutritional care and quality foodservice.*

Required Characteristics

DT.1.1 The relationship of the dietetic department/service to other units and departments/services of the hospital is either specified in the overall hospital organization plan or described in writing elsewhere.

DT.1.2 The scope of the dietetic services provided to inpatients and, as appropriate, to ambulatory care patients and patients in a hospital-administered home care program, is defined in writing.

DT.1.3 The dietetic department/service is directed on a full-time basis by an individual who, by education or specialized training and experience, is knowledgeable about foodservice management.
    DT.1.3.1   The director is responsible to the chief executive officer or his designee.
    DT.1.3.2   The director has the authority and responsibility for assuring that
        DT.1.3.2.1   established policies are implemented;
        DT.1.3.2.2   overall coordination and integration of the therapeutic and administrative aspects of dietetic services are maintained; and
        DT.1.3.2.3   the quality, safety, and appropriateness of the dietetic department/service functions are monitored and evaluated and that appropriate actions based on findings are taken.*

DT.1.4 Dietetic services are provided by a sufficient number of qualified personnel under competent supervision.*

DT.1.5 A qualified dietitian supervises the nutritional aspects of patient care and assures that quality nutritional care is provided to patients.*
    DT.1.5.1   Qualified dietitians or qualified designees participate in committee activities concerned with nutritional care.
    DT.1.5.2   When the services of a qualified dietitian are used on a part-time basis, this individual provides such services on the premises on a regularly scheduled basis.*
    DT.1.5.3   The regularly scheduled visits are sufficient to provide for at least the following:
        DT.1.5.3.1   Liaison with the hospital administration, medical staff, and nursing staff;
        DT.1.5.3.2   Patient/family counseling as needed;
        DT.1.5.3.3   Approval of menus, including modified diets;*
        DT.1.5.3.4   Any required nutritional assessments;*
        DT.1.5.3.5   Participation in the development of policies and procedures;
        DT.1.5.3.6   Participation in continuing education programs; and;
        DT.1.5.3.7   Evaluation of the dietetic services provided.*

---

*The asterisked items are key factors in the accreditation decision process. For an explanation of the use of the key factors, see page ix of "Using the Manual."

DT.1.5.4   When a qualified dietitian serves only in a consultant status, this individual regularly submits written reports to the chief executive officer concerning the extent of services provided.*

DT.1.5.5   When dietetic services are provided by an outside food-management company, the company complies with all applicable requirements of this *Manual,* and the contract specifies the compliance requirements.*

Standard

DT.2   Dietetic services personnel are prepared to conduct their assigned responsibilities through appropriate orientation, education, and training.

Required Characteristics

DT.2.1 The education, training, and experience of personnel who provide dietetic services are documented and are related to each individual's level of participation in the provision of dietetic services.
DT.2.1.1   A formal training program may be required as a prerequisite to employment.

DT.2.2 New personnel receive an orientation of sufficient duration and substance before providing dietetic services without direct supervision.
DT.2.2.1   The orientation is documented.

DT.2.3 As appropriate to their level of responsibility, new personnel receive instruction and demonstrate competence in the following:
DT.2.3.1   Personal hygiene and infection control;
DT.2.3.2   The proper inspection, handling, preparation, serving, and storing of food;
DT.2.3.3   The proper cleaning and safe operation of equipment;
DT.2.3.4   General foodservice sanitation and safety;
DT.2.3.5   The proper method of waste disposal;
DT.2.3.6   Portion control;
DT.2.3.7   The writing of modified diets using the diet manual/handbook;
DT.2.3.8   Diet instruction; and
DT.2.3.9   The recording of pertinent dietetic information in the patient's medical record.

DT.2.4 Dietetic services personnel participate in relevant in-service education programs.
DT.2.4.1   Personnel from all work shifts participate.

DT.2.5 The director of the dietetic department/service or qualified designee participates in planning and conducting in-service education for dietetic personnel and, as appropriate, for other hospital personnel.
DT.2.5.1   In-service education includes safety and infection control requirements described elsewhere in this Manual.
DT.2.5.2   Outside educational opportunities are provided as feasible, at least for supervisory dietetic personnel.

DT.2.6 The extent of participation of dietetic personnel in continuing education is realistically related to the size of the staff and the scope and complexity of the dietetic services provided.
DT.2.6.1   Participation in continuing education is documented.

DT.2.6.2 Education programs for dietetic services personnel are based, at least in part, on the results of dietetic department/service evaluations.

DT.2.7 The training of dietetic students and dietetic interns is conducted only in programs accredited by the appropriate professional educational organization.

DT.2.7.1 Individuals in student status are directly supervised by a qualified dietitian when engaged in patient care activities.

DT.2.7.2 When the hospital provides clinical facilities for the education and training of dietetic students from an outside program, the respective roles and responsibilities of the dietetic department/service and the outside educational program are defined in writing.

Standard

DT.3 Written policies and procedures specify the provision of dietetic services.*

Required Characteristics

DT.3.1 There are written policies and procedures concerning the scope and conduct of dietetic services.

DT.3.1.1 Administrative policies and procedures concerning food procurement, preparation, and service are developed by the director of the dietetic department/service.

DT.3.1.2 Nutritional care policies and procedures are developed by a qualified dietitian.

DT.3.1.2.1 When appropriate, concurrence or approval should be obtained from the medical staff through its designated mechanism and from the nursing department/service.

DT.3.2 Policies and procedures are subjected to timely review, revised as necessary, dated, and enforced.

DT.3.3 The policies and procedures relate to at least the following:

DT.3.3.1 The responsibilities and authority of the director of the dietetic department/service and, when the director is not a qualified dietitian, the qualified dietitian.

DT.3.3.2 Food purchasing, storage, inventory, preparation, and service.

DT.3.3.3 Diet orders, which are recorded in the patient's medical record by an authorized individual before the diet is served to the patient.

DT.3.3.4 The proper use of and adherence to standards for nutritional care, as specified in the diet manual/handbook.

DT.3.3.5 Nutritional assessment and counseling, and diet instruction.

DT.3.3.6 Menus.

DT.3.3.7 The role, as appropriate, of the dietetic department/service in the preparation, storage, distribution, and administration of enteric tube feedings, and total parenteral nutrition programs.

DT.3.3.8 Alterations in diets or diet schedules, including the provision of foodservice to persons who do not receive the regular meal service.

DT.3.3.9 Ancillary dietetic services, as appropriate, including food storage and kitchens on patient care units, formula supply, cafeterias, vending operations, and ice making.

DT.3.3.10   An identification system designed to assure that each patient receives the appropriate diet as ordered.

DT.3.3.11   Personal hygiene and health of dietetic personnel.

DT.3.3.12   Infection control measures to minimize the possibility of contamination and transfer of infection.*

    DT.3.3.12.1   These measures include

        DT.3.3.12.1.1   the establishment of a monitoring procedure to assure that dietetic personnel are free from infections and open skin lesions;

        DT.3.3.12.1.2   the establishment of sanitation procedures for the cleaning and maintenance of equipment and work areas; and

        DT.3.3.12.1.3   the washing and storage of utensils and dishes.

DT.3.3.13   Pertinent safety practices, including the control of electrical, flammable, mechanical, and, as appropriate, radiation hazards.*

DT.3.3.14   Compliance with applicable law and regulation.*

DT.3.4   The role of the dietetic department/service in the hospital's internal and external disaster plans is clearly defined.

    DT.3.4.1   The dietetic department/service is able to meet the nutritional needs of patients and staff during a disaster, consistent with the capabilities of the hospital and community served.

    DT.3.4.2   For requirements of the hospital's disaster plans, refer to the "Plant, Technology, and Safety Management" chapter of this Manual.

DT.3.5   A qualified dietitian develops or adopts a diet manual/handbook in cooperation with representatives of the medical staff and with other appropriate dietetic staff.*

    DT.3.5.1   The standards for nutritional care specified in the diet manual/handbook should be at least in accordance with those of the Recommended Dietary Allowances (1980) of the Food and Nutrition Board of the National Research Council of the National Academy of Sciences.

    DT.3.5.2   The nutritional deficiencies of any diet that is not in compliance with the recommended dietary allowances are specified.

    DT.3.5.3   The diet manual/handbook serves as a guide to ordering diets, and the served menus should be consistent with the requirements in the diet manual/handbook.

    DT.3.5.4   The diet manual/handbook is reviewed annually and revised as necessary by a qualified dietitian, dated to identify the review and any revisions made, and approved by the medical staff through its designated mechanism.

    DT.3.5.5   A copy of the diet manual/handbook is located in each patient care unit.

    DT.3.5.6   All master menus and modified diets are approved by a qualified dietitian.*

DT.3.6   Current reference material is available to all dietetic personnel and is conveniently located.

Standard

DT.4   The dietetic department/service is designed and equipped to facilitate the safe, sanitary, and timely provision of foodservice to meet the nutritional needs of patients.*

Required Characteristics

DT.4.1 Sufficient space and equipment are provided for the dietetic department/service to accomplish the following:

DT.4.1.1   Store food and nonfood supplies under sanitary and secure conditions.

DT.4.1.2   Store food separately from nonfood supplies.

DT.4.1.2.1   When storage facilities are limited, paper products may be stored with food supplies.

DT.4.1.3   Prepare and distribute food, including modified diets.

DT.4.1.4   Clean and sanitize utensils and dishes apart from food preparation areas.

DT.4.1.5   Allow supportive personnel to perform their duties.

DT.4.2 The facilities and equipment of the dietetic department/service are in compliance with applicable sanitation and safety law and regulations.*

DT.4.3 The following sanitation precautions are taken in the handling and preparation of food:*

DT.4.3.1   Food is protected from contamination and spoilage.*

DT.4.3.2   Foods are stored at proper temperatures, utilizing appropriate thermometers and maintaining temperature records.

DT.4.3.3   Lighting, ventilation, and humidity are controlled to prevent the condensation of moisture and growth of molds.

DT.4.3.4   Methods to prevent contamination are used for making, storing, and dispensing ice.

DT.4.3.5   Separate cutting boards are provided for meat, poultry, fish, and raw fruits and vegetables.

DT.4.3.5.1   Cooked foods should not be cut on the same boards used for preparing raw food.

DT.4.3.5.2   Separate cutting boards may not be required when there are boards in use that are nonabsorbent and can be cleaned and sanitized adequately, and when the cleaning and sanitizing procedure is performed properly between usage for different food categories.

DT.4.3.6   All working surfaces, utensils, and equipment are cleaned thoroughly and sanitized after each period of use.

DT.4.3.7   Adequate hand-washing and hand-drying facilities are conveniently located throughout the department/service.

DT.4.3.8   Dishwashing and utensil-washing equipment and techniques that result in sanitized serviceware and that prevent recontamination are used.

DT.4.3.9   Plasticware, china, and glassware that have lost their glaze or are chipped or cracked are discarded.

DT.4.3.10   Disposable containers and utensils are discarded after one use.

DT.4.3.11   Traffic of unauthorized individuals through food preparation and service areas is controlled.

DT.4.3.12   Garbage is held, transferred, and disposed of in a manner that does not create a nuisance or a breeding place for insects, rodents, and vermin or otherwise permit the transmission of disease.*

DT.4.3.12.1   Garbage containers are leakproof and nonabsorbent with close-fitting covers.

DT.4.3.12.1.1   The use of impervious plastic liners is desirable.

DT.4.4 The following safety precautions are implemented:

DT.4.4.1   Walk-in refrigerators and freezers can be opened from the inside.

DT.4.4.2   Insulation or protection from hot-water and cold-water pipes, water heaters, refrigerator compressors, condensing units, and heat-producing equipment is provided.

DT.4.4.3   Food and nonfood supplies are clearly labeled.

DT.4.4.4   A review is conducted of the hospital's preventive and corrective maintenance and safety program as they relate to the dietetic department/service.*

DT.4.4.4.1   Actions are taken based on the findings of the review.*

DT.4.4.4.2   The review and actions taken are documented.*

DT.4.4.5   All food is procured from sources that process food under regulated quality and sanitation controls.

DT.4.4.5.1   The use of local produce is not precluded:

Standard

DT.5   Dietetic services are provided in accordance with a written order by the individual responsible for the patient, and appropriate dietetic information is recorded in the patient's medical record.

Required Characteristics

DT.5.1 The qualified dietitian or authorized designee enters dietetic information into the medical record as specified, and in the location determined, by those performing the medical record review function.

DT.5.1.1   These determinations are made by the medical record committee when one exists.

DT.5.2 At the request of the appropriate medical staff member, the qualified dietitian or authorized designee documents appropriate nutritional information in the medical record.

DT.5.2.1   Such documentation may include the following:

DT.5.2.1.1   A summary of the dietary history and/or nutritional assessment when the past dietary pattern is known to have a bearing on the patient's condition or treatment;

DT.5.2.1.2   Timely and periodic assessments of the patient's nutrient intake and tolerance to the prescribed diet modification, including the effect of the patient's appetite and food habits on food intake and any substitutions made;

DT.5.2.1.3   A description of the diet instructions given to the patient or family and an assessment of their diet knowledge; and

DT.5.2.1.4   A description or copy of the diet information forwarded to institution when a patient is discharged.

DT.5.2.1.4.1   If nutritional care follow-up reverts to the practitioner's office practice or a health care agency, this should be noted in the patient's medical record.

DT.5.3 Within 24 hours of admission and within 24 hours after any subsequent orders for diet modification, the diet order is confirmed by the practitioner responsible for the patient receiving oral alimentation.

Standard

DT.6   Appropriate quality control mechanisms are established.*

Required Characteristics

DT.6.1 At least the following quality control mechanisms are implemented.*

DT.6.1.1   All menus are evaluated for nutritional adequacy.

DT.6.1.2   There is a means of identifying patients who are not receiving oral intake.

DT.6.1.3   Special diets are monitored.

DT.6.1.4   Not more than 15 hours should elapse between the serving of the evening meal and the next substantial meal for patients who are on oral intake and do not have specific dietary requirements.

DT.6.1.5   As appropriate, the nutrient intake of patients is assessed and recorded.

DT.6.1.6   As appropriate, patients with special dietary needs receive instructions relative to their diets, and an indication of the patient's (or family's) understanding of these instructions is recorded in the patient's medical record.

DT.6.1.7   As appropriate, patients who are discharged from the hospital on modified diets receive written instructions and individualized counseling before discharge.

DT.6.1.8   Before discharge, patients are given instructions about and are counseled on potential drug-food interactions.

DT.6.1.9   A maximum effort is made to assure an appetizing appearance, palatability, proper serving temperature, and retention of the nutrient value of food.

DT.6.1.9.1   Whenever possible, patient food preferences are respected, and appropriate dietary substitutions are made available.

DT.6.1.9.2   Surveys to determine patient acceptance of food are encouraged, particularly in the case of long-stay patients.

Standard

DT.7   As part of the hospital's quality assurance program, the quality and appropriateness of patient care services provided by the dietetic department/service are monitored and evaluated, and identified problems are resolved.*

Required Characteristics

DT.7.1   The dietetic department/service has a planned and systematic process for the monitoring and evaluation of the quality and appropriateness of patient care services and for resolving identified problems.*

DT.7.1.1   The director of the dietetic department/service, with medical and nursing participation, is responsible for assuring that the process is implemented.*

DT.7.2   The quality and appropriateness of patient care services are monitored and evaluated in all major functions of the dietetic department/service.*

DT.7.2.1   Such monitoring and evaluation are accomplished through the following means:

DT.7.2.1.1   Routine collection in the dietetic department/service or through the hospital's quality assurance program, of information about important aspects of dietetic services;* and

DT.7.2.1.2   Periodic assessment by the dietetic department/service of the collected information in order to identify important problems in patient care services and opportunities to improve care.*

DT.7.2.1.2.1   In DT.7.2.1.1 and DT.7.2.1.2, the dietetic department/service agrees on objective criteria that reflect current knowledge and clinical experience.*

DT.7.2.1.2.1.1   These criteria are used by the dietetic department/service or by the hospital's quality assurance program in the monitoring and evaluation of patient care service.*

DT.7.3 When important problems in patient care services or opportunities to improve care are identified,

DT.7.3.1   actions are taken;* and

DT.7.3.2   the effectiveness of the actions taken is evaluated.*

DT.7.4 The findings from and conclusions of the monitoring, evaluation, and problem-solving activities are documented and, as appropriate, are reported.*

DT.7.5 The actions taken to resolve problems and improve patient care services, and information about the impact of the actions taken, are documented and, as appropriate, are reported.*

DT.7.6 As part of the annual reappraisal of the hospital's quality assurance program, the effectiveness of the monitoring, evaluation, and problem-solving activities in the dietetic department/service is evaluated.*

DT.7.7 When an outside source(s) provides dietetic services, or when there is no designated dietetic department/service, the quality and appropriateness of patient care services provided are monitored and evaluated, and identified problems are resolved.*

DT.7.7.1   The chief executive officer is responsible for assuring that a planned and systematic process for such monitoring, evaluation, and problem-solving activities is implemented.*

Note: For other standards related to dietetic services, refer to the following chapters of this Manual: "Home Care Services," "Infection Control," "Medical Record Services," "Pharmaceutical Services," "Plant, Technology, and Safety Management," and "Quality Assurance."

Notes and Comments:

_____

_____

_____

_____

_____

_____

_____

_____

_____

_____

_____

_____

_____

_____

_____

_____

_____

Appendix J. Long-Term Care Survey Guidelines for Dietary Services

Survey Area A: Menus and Nutritional Adequacy. F176, SNF(405.1125(b), F177, ICF(442.332(a)(1), F196.

Menus are planned and followed to meet the nutritional needs of each resident in accordance with the physician's orders and, to extent possible, based on the recommended dietary allowances of the Food and Nutrition Board of the National Research Council, National Academy of Science. The intent is to ensure that each resident receives food in the amount, kind, and consistency to support optimal nutritional status.

Observation. Specific observations that might be indicative of possible nutrition problems are: underweight, overweight, dehydration, edema, cracked lips, pallor, dull or dry hair, swollen or red tongue, bleeding gums, decubitus ulcers, and infections.

Physiological factors that may affect food intake include: vomiting, food intolerance, poor dentition, sore mouth, constipation, diarrhea, inability to feed self, decreased visual and olfactory acuity, unable to communicate, and loss of appetite. Psychological and social factors include: confusion, excessive food likes and dislikes, and refusal to eat. Selected biochemical changes that might indicate changes in nutritional status. Observe laboratory data for visceral protein status of serum albumin, transferrin, BUN, and serum electrolytes.

During mealtime observe the resident for: adherence to food preferences, adequate space for eating, self-feeding skills, proper position for eating, ability to eat foods served, use of adaptive feeding devices, amount of food actually eaten, protection of resident's clothes, amount of time resident is allowed to chew and swallow, assistance provided as needed to and from dining area, all beverages covered, assistance provided in case of choking, incontinence, falling, or other emergencies. Observe nursing staff in the supervision of dining areas including resident's rooms during meal times.

Observe serving portion sizes on all menu items and compare to the following:

1. Milk Group—1 pint daily. Source of protein, calcium, phosphorus, and B complex.
2. Meat Group—5 lean meat equivalents daily (1 meat equivalent equals 1 oz. meat, poultry, fish, cheese or egg; also dried peas, beans, and nuts). Source of protein, iron, and vitamin B12.
3. Vegetable and Fruit Group—5 servings or more daily (½ cup = 1 serving). Source of vitamin A, C, B6, folacin, and fiber.
4. Bread–Cereal–Potato–Legume–Pasta Group—7 servings daily (1 serving = 1 slice bread, ½ cup other; and ¾ cup flake-type cereal).

Observe menu for fats and sweets (to increase caloric intake); use of iodized salt (unless contraindicated), and adequate fiber.

Interview. Ask manager to explain the procedure for making substitutions and recording the changes. Is menu usually followed? Ask residents the following: How are your meals? Are there foods you are not allowed to have? Are you on a special diet? Do you receive foods that are not appropriate for your diet? If so, what do you and the staff do about that? What time do you receive breakfast, lunch, and supper? Do you always receive a meal at mealtime? If not, why? What happens then? Do you like the taste of your food? Is the temperature appropriate (i.e., milk chilled, coffee hot)? Do you get enough to eat? What do you do if you are still hungry after a meal? Do you receive nourishment in the evening?

Do you have a choice about what you want to eat? Do you receive medicine during meals? If yes, do you know what it is or what it is for? Do you get food from outside the facility that you buy or family brings? How often? What kind of food? How often does anyone from the kitchen come to ascertain your feelings and opinions on the food service and your portion size? Where do you eat (i.e., dining room, your room)? Is this your choice? Do you have a choice of where you eat? How often have you seen a therapist for your swallowing difficulties? How has the therapist instructed you, staff, and family on methods to improve your swallowing? Ask dietitian to describe the meal planning input you received from residents.

Record Review. Review nutrition assessment for the following documentation: usual body weight, ideal body weight, and height; dietary allergies, sensitivities, ability to chew and swallow regular food without difficulty; full or partial dentures; mental and emotional condition; physical appearance and skin condition; appetite and food preference; vitamin and mineral supplements; food and fluid intake in measurable terms and frequency of meals; degree of assistance needed in eating, related mobility, vision, or other identified problems; medications (i.e., diuretics, insulin, antibiotics); related laboratory findings (i.e.; fasting blood sugar, cholesterol, sodium, potassium, hemoglobin, BUN, serum albumin, transferrin or creatinine-height index if available); food-drug interactions; mental-emotional assessment as it relates to resident's food habits.

Review plan of care and nursing notes. Review physicians' orders, progress notes, and notes from other professional disciplines as appropriate. Nutritional status depends not only on adequacy of menu planning but also whether the resident eats the food and how the body uses it. While the surveyor is not responsible for individual nutritional assessments of residents, when specific information is needed during the survey to make a compliance decision, the surveyor will utilize the following minimum assessment guidelines:

- Menu evaluated for adequate energy and nutrients: calories, protein, vitamin C, and calcium.
- Selected evaluation of residents for in-depth review.
- Check list can be used to evaluate daily menus for basic foods (using standard serving portions).
- Check daily food plan for: 1 pint milk; 5 meat equivalents (1 equivalent = 1 oz edible portion, weighed after cooking); 5 servings or more of fruits and vegetables, including a dark green or deep yellow vegetable for vitamin A value every other day and a citrus fruit or other fruit rich in vitamin C daily; 7 servings from the bread-cereal-potato-legume-pasta group; and fats and sweets. Without fats and sweets, the diet contains 1,415 Kcal.
- Diets are adapted from facility's currently approved diet manual.
- Menus are dated and contain minimum portion sizes.
- Substitutions are noted on file copy.
- Substitutions are made within the same food group i.e., meat for another source of protein in the meat group, or vegetable of similar nutritional value.
- Documentation of decision to withdraw or begin artificial feeding and hydration.
- Check menu for variety. Are they specific (i.e., states kind of fruit, juice, or vegetable)?

Selected nutritional requirement record review include the basal energy expenditure (BEE) and caloric requirement using Harris-Benedic formula. NOTE: The following sample formulas and guidelines are not the only acceptable guides available. The surveyor should ask to use the assessment guidelines used by the facility before using the ones provided here.

1. Anthropometry—Weight/Height. An important indicator of nutritional outcome. Disease state can have adverse effect on desired body weight.
2. Weight for height calculation formula. For females, allow 100 lbs. for first 5 ft. of height plus 5 lbs. for each additional inch. For males, allow 106 lbs. for first 5 ft. of height plus 6 lbs. for each additional inch.
3. Estimating caloric needs, using Harris-Benedict equation:

$$
\begin{aligned}
\text{Men:} \quad 66 \ &+ \ (13.7 \times \text{wt. in kg}) \\
&+ \ (5 \times \text{ht. in cm}) \\
&- \ (6.8 \times \text{age}) = \text{BEE}
\end{aligned}
$$

$$
\begin{aligned}
\text{Women:} \quad 65.5 \ &+ \ (9.6 \times \text{wt. in kg}) \\
&+ \ (1.7 \times \text{ht. in cm}) \\
&- \ (4.7 \times \text{age}) = \text{BEE}
\end{aligned}
$$

Parenteral Anabolic: $1.75 \times$ BEE
Oral Anabolic: $1.5 \times$ BEE (Kcals)
Oral Maintenance: $1.20 \times$ BEE (Kcals)

Metric conversions (approx.): pound (lb) $\times$ 0.45 = kilograms (kg). Inches (in) $\times$ 2.5 = centimeters (cm).

4. Estimating protein needs. Allow 0.8 gram protein per kilogram of ideal body weight. Increase to $1.2 - 1.5$ gm/kg for patients with depleted protein stores (decubitus, draining wounds, fractures)
5. Fluid requirement, based on actual body weight. Over 55 years with no major cardiac or renal diseases, the following example is offered:

Note: 2.2 lbs. equals 1 kg of body weight.

120 lbs/2.2 lbs = 54.5 kg (55 kgs)
55 kg $\times$ 30 cc = 1,650 cc/day

Note: Isotonic Standard Tube Feeding = approximately 80% water.

6. Percentage of body weight allowed for amputation:

Leg	20%
Below knees	10%
Arm	6
At elbow	3.6

7. Suggested standards for evaluating significance of weight loss:

Interval	Significant Loss	Severe Loss
1 week	1–2%	2%
1 month	5	5
3 months	7½	7½
6 months	10	10

8. Laboratory indices for visceral protein:

	Mild Deficiency	Moderate Deficiency	Severe Deficiency
Albumin (g/d)	3.5–3.2	3.2–2.8	2.8
Total lymphocyte count (cu/mm)	1800–1500	1500–900	900
Transferrin (if available)	200–100	180–160	160

Evaluation Factors. Were physician diet orders followed? Did nursing plan for feeding and assistance at mealtime? Is there rehabilitative use of assistive devices, if appropriate? Is modification of consistency of meals made if resident has a problem or change in condition? Are between meal and bedtime snacks provided as needed? Is socialization at meals provided? Has dietitian provided counseling of resident and family as needed (related to diet)? Is usual body weight maintained and supported? Is there evidence that the plan is being carried out (e.g., documentation in the patient's chart, observation by the surveyor, and resident/staff interviews)? If the resident refuses meals or does not respond to intervention, do notes in the chart indicate efforts to intervene or provide counseling? Is there evidence that the resident's progress is regularly observed (e.g., awareness of food and fluid intake such as acceptance of foods, food consumed, and resident's appetite)? Is fluid intake for resident encouraged; Foley catheter and problem feeders monitored? Is there general evidence as to whether poor resident conditions are due to poor care or whether the facility has taken appropriate measures to prevent or resolve problems? Is there indication of progress toward desired outcomes? If not, is the evidence of reevaluation available within specified time frames? *Note:* When the anthropometric and clinical data do not correlate with dietary data (food intake, dietary supplements) the supervisor should take note that the problem may not be nutritional.

Survey Area B: Therapeutic Diets. F179, SNF(405.1125(c), F180, ICF(442.332(b)(1)

F181: Therapeutic diets are prescribed by the attending physician.

F182: Therapeutic menus are planned in writing, prepared, and served as ordered with supervision from the dietitian and advice from the attending physician whenever necessary.

Observation. Observe system for the provision of diets: dietetic service kardex or file; therapeutic menus; nourishment preparation and service; adequacy of nourishment; and individual menus or diet cards. The surveyor should also attempt to observe that staff use proper technique in administering feedings and medications; that staff checks for location of tube before feeding and that tubing is irrigated before and after addition of medication; and that unused milk-based tube feeding is discarded in a timely manner.

Observe tray and meal service to determine if low sodium diets are palatable (taste); if sugar sources on diabetic trays are proper; and if salt sources on sodium restricted diet trays are proper. Observe functioning of system to provide needed nutrients: resident's general appearance; meal service (food acceptance, adherence to food preferences); food supplements (type of support, method of service, assistance provided, and timely provision as ordered); portion sizes; and if diet conforms with physician's orders. Observe to determine if system is in place for the correct provision of renal diets: individualized menus; dietary staff; and if menus are utilized when serving diets.

Interview. Ask staff: How many and what type of therapeutic diets served? When is nourishment prepared and served? Who is responsible? What nourishment is provided for day of survey? The surveyor should interview staff regarding their knowledge of the feeding schedule and training in administering tube feedings. Some residents having difficulty in speaking and swallowing with tube in place (i.e., poor toleration). The surveyor should inquire if mouth feeding was attempted.

If the resident is able to be interviewed, suggested questions may be: How long have you been fed by this tube? When was the last time you tried to eat by mouth? What happened? How often do you receive the feeding? Is this consistent? Does the staff help you in feeding? Do you feel comfortable and safe with all the staff who perform the feeding? If not, what happens? Are you losing or gaining weight? What is your goal? How often is the tube changed? Who does this? Do you feel comfortable and safe with all staff who perform this procedure?

Interview staff regarding knowledge of diabetic diets as follows: What nourishment does the diabetic patient receive? If diabetic patient refuses the meal, what is done to supplement the meal? If resident is able to be interviewed, the following questions are suggested: How long have you been on your diabetic diet? Do you know some of the foods you must avoid? What are they?

For the resident with decubitus ulcers, ask staff the following questions regarding knowledge of dietary needs: What do you do when this resident refuses milk, meats, bread? What nourishments are provided to this resident? How often? What happens when a weight loss is noticed with this resident? Ask resident: Has anyone talked with you about the importance of eating your meals? Do you get foods that you don't eat on your tray? When do you feel hungry? Do you get between meal nourishments?

Interview staff regarding knowledge of renal diets as follows: What foods should be restricted when a patient has kidney problems? What nourishments are given to these patients? Ask resident: Are you on a special diet? What foods must you avoid? Do you feel hungry? Do you eat everything at mealtimes? Are the foods served to you the correct ones for your diet? Has the dietitian explained your diet to you?

Record Review. Surveyor should review physician diet orders in medical record, nurses' kardex, dietary kardex, therapeutic diet menu, and diet cards. Surveyor should consider appropriateness of special diet that has been up-dated and reviewed since admission; and progress notes that reflect reevaluation of resident's progress on diet. Selected number of residents on therapeutic diets should be considered for in-depth review.

For residents on tube feeding, the review should include: plan of care; frequency and amount of feeding based on the physician's order and the time span over which each feeding is accomplished; medication and treatment records; fluid intake records; number of calories as well as amount of additional water; periodic reassessment of ability to swallow; and measures taken to prevent diarrhea, and constipation and to treat if they have developed.

For diabetic diets, the review should include: pertinent laboratory data on urinary glucose and serum glucose; and weight gain or loss. For the resident with decubitus ulcers, the record review should include: identity of residents with conditions that immobilize or prevent voluntary body movement; identity of location, number, size, and depth of decubitus ulcers; calculations of kilocaloric and protein levels as needed; micronutrient need assessment and recommendation; progress notes on weight and healing of ulcers; pertinent laboratory data on hemoglobin, hematocrit, serum albumin, total lymphocyte count; and fluid intake sufficient to maintain hydration.

Renal patient diet review should include: pertinent laboratory data on serum sodium, BUN, serum potassium, albumin, hematocrit, and creatinine; pertinent medications such as vitamins, minerals, and supplements; and weight gains or losses.

Evaluation Factors. Evaluate pureed diets as follows: ordered by physician; prepared fresh daily; same calories and/or food groups as if served whole; and pureed foods are coordinated with regular menu. Evaluate tube feeding as follows: Has the feeding been ordered by physician? Is tube feeding nutritionally adequate? Have attempts been made to progress tube feeding if necessary? Have changes in resident condition been noted and addressed (weight loss, constipation, diarrhea, skin condition)? Have observed problems been coordinated with other departments and resolved? Is feeding being monitored to ensure that feeding is occuring at the ordered/appropriate rate? Are nourishments varied as preferences allow?

Evaluate diabetic diet and other therapeutic diets as follows: ordered by physician; varied, nutritionally adequate; individualized to suit resident; re-evaluation indicates diet meets objectives; laboratory results support diagnosis; and between meals nourishment provided as needed and recorded in measurable amounts.

Evaluate renal diets as follows: ordered by physician; written menu is nutritionally complete in so far as medically possible, including calories; individualized to suit resident; laboratory testing as needed; and coordinated with dialysis unit to determine effectiveness of diet.

Survey Area C: Food Preparation. F204, SNF 405.1125(e).

F205: Food is prepared by methods that conserve its nutritive value and flavor.

F206: Meals are palatable, served at proper temperatures. They are cut, ground, chopped, pureed, or in a form which meets individual resident needs.

F207: If a resident refuses food served, appropriate substitutes of similar nutritive value are offered. The intent is to provide foods that are safe and nutritious.

Observation. Surveyor should observe the following: feeding assistance provided or not provided by staff; length of time residents sit and wait for meal service; length of time between cooking and service; trays are free of spilled food or liquid; foods are appropriately covered and kept at a proper temperature; cooking and service utensils are clean, sanitary, and greaseless; refrigerated foods covered; leftover and precooked foods dated and labeled; all cooked food stored above raw meat in refrigerator; temperature gauge on or in refrigerator to record temperature; shelving to allow air circulation; food stored off the floor (this applies to food stored in walk-in and freezer); no rust on shelves; no dripping or spillage on shelves and floors; degree to which diet modification is commensurate with residents tolerance and capability; observe residents for meal satisfaction; observe appearance of food color, texture, aroma, and flavor; less than 75% of meal is consumed; and type of substitutions provided.

Record Review. The surveyor should review: plan of care; progress notes; notes from other professional disciplines to determine rehabilitation potential to self-feed, use of assistance devices; record of food substitution to determine alternate choice provided, standardized recipes; progress notes; diet cards; and day's menu substitute record.

Evaluation Factors. The facility has kitchen and dietetic service areas adequate to meet the foodservice needs. These areas are properly ventilated, arranged, and equiped for sanitary refrigeration, storage, and preparation of food. Equipment and storage areas are clean, well maintained, within proper temperature ranges, and safe. Proper temperatures (Fahrenheit) are as follows:

Frozen food storage	0 or below
Cold food storage	40–45 degrees
Hot food holding equipment	140 degrees minimum
Dishwasher wash cycle	150–160 degrees
Dishwasher rinse cycle	160–180 degrees or a color change in thermo paper; or adherence to manufacturers recommendations.

Dietary personnel are clean and free of infectious disease. They practice acceptable techniques and procedures to keep food at proper temperatures and protected against contamination. Has resident been assessed for eating program to maintain independence? The food substitute is of similar nutritive value as the refused item (e.g., milk refused, alternate of calcium rich food should be provided).

Survey Area D: Frequency of Meals. F208, SNF 405.1124(d), F209, ICF 442.331(a).

F210: At least three meals are served daily at regular hours with not more than a 14-hour span between a substantial evening meal and breakfast.

F211: To the extent medically possible, bedtime nourishments are offered to all residents.

Observation. The surveyor should observe the following: all factors listed under menus and nutritional adequacy; who serves nourishments; and the nourishment list and schedule.

Interview. The surveyor should interview various residents about the nourishment service as follows: Are nourishments offered routinely? At what time are they offered? By whom? What kind of nourishment are offered?

Record Review. The surveyor should review menus as under Survey Area A, and the nourishment list.

Evaluation Factors. The surveyor should determine if three meals or their equivalent are served daily with not more than a 14-hour span between the evening meal and breakfast; and must find evidence that patients are offered nourishments on a planned basis and documented.

Survey Area E: Staffing. F212, SNF 405.1125(a)

F213: Foodservice personnel are on duty daily over a period of 12 or more hours. The intent is that persons are providing services commensurate with their level of training; and at the level of sophistication needed by the residents.

Observation. The surveyor should observe if foodservice personnel are on duty for all defined dietary responsibilities: supervision, food preparation, dishwashing, and cleaning. Observe duty schedules.

Interview. Interview personnel to verify that they are aware of their responsibilities and job descriptions.

Evaluation Factors. The surveyor will use the following factors to evaluate: an assessment of the total dietetic service operation; the capabilities of the dietetic supervisor to manage and supervise dietetic services; dietetic personnel are on duty over a 12-hour period and demonstrate ability to perform tasks adequately; dietetic personnel receive appropriate orientation and training consistent with their duties and responsibilities; there is evidence that the dietetic staff are knowledgeable about foodservice policies and procedures and apply these accepted professional practices in their daily work; and services provided are consistent with the size, scope, and facilities available.

Appendix K. Conditions of Participation for Patient Rights

Table K-1. Indicators for Patient Rights[a]

Code		Conditions of Participation
		Governing Body (Condition of Participation)
F50		SNF (405.1121)
		Resident Rights
F51		SNF (405.1121(d)) (Standard) Indicators A thru K apply to this standard for SNFs.
F52		ICF (442.311) (Standard) Indicators A thru K apply to this standard for ICFs.
	A.	*Information*
F53		1. The facility informs each resident, before or at the time of admission, of his/her rights and responsibilities.
F54		2. The facility informs each resident, before or at the end of admission, of all rules governing resident conduct.
F55		3. The facility informs each resident of amendments to their policies on residents' rights and responsibilities and rules governing conduct.
F56		4. Each resident acknowledges in writing receipt of residents' rights information and any amendment to it.
F57		5. The resident must be informed in writing of all services and charges for services.
F58		6. The resident must be informed in writing of all changes in services and charges before or at the time of admission and on a continuing basis.
F59		7. The resident must be informed of services not covered by Medicare or Medicaid and not covered in the basic rate.
	B.	*Medical Condition and Treatment*
F60		1. Each resident is informed by a physician of his/her health and medical condition unless the physician decides that informing the resident is medically contraindicated.
F61		2. Each resident is given an opportunity to participate in planning his/her total care and medical treatment.
F62		3. Each resident is given an opportunity to refuse treatment.
F63		4. Each resident gives informed, written consent before participating in experimental research.
F64		5. If the physician decides that informing the resident of his/her health and medical condition is medically contraindicated, the physician has documented this decision in the resident's medical record.
	C.	*Transfer and Discharge*
		Each resident is transferred or discharged only for:
F65		1. Medical reasons.
F66		2. His/her welfare or that of other residents.
F67		3. Nonpayment except as prohibited by the Medicare or Medicaid program.

[a]From Health Care Financing Administration (1988).

Table K-1.   Indicators for Patient Rights (Continued)

Code	Conditions of Participation
F68	4. Each resident is given reasonable advance notice to ensure orderly transfer or discharge. Exception: Not required for ICF residents.
	D. Exercising Rights
F69	1. Each resident is encouraged and assisted to exercise his/her rights to a resident of the facility and as a citizen.
F70	2. Each resident is allowed to submit complaints and recommendations concerning the policies and services of the facility to staff or to outside representatives of the resident's choice or both.
F71	3. Such complaints are submitted free from restraint, coercion, discrimination, or reprisal.
	E. Financial Affairs
F72	1. Residents are allowed to manage their own personal financial affairs.
F73	2. The facility establishes and maintains a system that assures full and complete accounting of residents' personal funds. An accounting report is made to each resident in a skilled nursing facility at least on a quarterly basis.
F74	3. The facility does not commingle resident funds with any other funds.
F75	4. If a resident requests assistance from the facility in managing his/her personal financial affairs, resident's delegation is to be in writing.
	5. The facility system of accounting includes written receipts for:
F76	All personal possessions and funds received by or deposited with the facility.
F77	All disbursements made to or for the resident.
F78	6. The financial record must be available to the resident and his/her family.
	F. Freedom from Abuse and Restraints
F79	1. Each resident is free from mental and physical abuse.
F80	2. Chemical and physical restraints are only used when authorized by a physician in writing for a specified period of time or in emergencies.
F81	3. If used in emergencies, they are necessary to protect the resident from injury to himself/herself or others.
F82	4. The emergency use is authorized by a professional staff member identified in the written policies and procedures of the facility.
F83	5. The emergency use is reported promptly to the resident's physician by the staff member.
	G. Privacy
F84	1. Each resident is treated with respect, consideration and full recognition of his/her dignity and individuality.
F85	2. Each resident is given privacy during treatment and care of personal needs.
F86	3. Each resident's record, including information in an automated data bank, are treated confidentially.
F87	4. Each resident must give written consent before the facility releases information from his/her record to someone not otherwise authorized to receive it.
F88 F89	5. Married residents are given privacy during visits by their spouse. Married residents are permitted to share a room.

Table K-1. **(Continued)**

Code	Conditions of Participation
	H. *Work*
F90	No resident may be required to perform services for the facility.
	I. *Freedom of Association and Correspondence*
F91	1. Each resident is allowed to communicate, associate and meet privately with individuals of his/her choice unless this infringes upon the rights of another resident.
F92	2. Each resident is allowed to send and receive personal mail unopened.
	J. *Activities*
F93	Each resident is allowed to participate in social, religious, and community group activities.
	K. *Personal Possessions*
F94	Each resident is allowed to retain and use his/her personal possessions and clothing as space permits.
	L. *Delegation of Rights and Responsibilities*
F95	ICF (442.312) (Standard)
F96	1. All the rights and responsibilities of a resident pass to the resident's guardian, next of kin or sponsoring agency or agencies if the resident is adjudicated incompetent under State law or is determined by his/her physician to be incapable of understanding his/her rights and responsibilities.
F97	2. Physician determinations of incapability and the specific reasons thereof are recorded by the physician in the resident's record.
	Staff Development
F98	SNF(405.1121(h)) (Standard)
F99	ICF (442.314) (Standard)
F100	1. Facility staff is knowledgeable about the problems and needs of the aged, ill, and disabled.
F101	2. Facility staff practices proper techniques in providing care to the aged, ill, and disabled.
F102	3. Facility staff practices proper technique for prevention and control of infection, fire prevention and safety, accident prevention, confidentiality of resident information, and preservation of resident dignity, including protection of privacy and personal and property rights.

Appendix L.   Material Safety Data Sheet

Section I.	
Manufacturer's Name	Emergency Telephone Number
Address (Number, City, State & Zip Code)	
Chemical Name and Synonyms	Trade Name and Synonyms
Chemical Family	Formula

Section II. Hazardous Ingredients			
Carcinogen	Material	Percent	TLV (units)

Section III. Physical Data			
Boiling Point		Specific Gravity (water = 1)	
Vapor Pressure (mm Hg)		Percent Volatile by Volume	
Vapor Density (air = 1)		Evaporation Rate	
Solubility in Water			
Appearance and Odor			

Section IV. Fire and Explosion Hazards			
Flash Point	Flammable Limits	LE	LE
Extinguishing Media			
Special Fire Fighting Procedures			
Unusual Fire and Explosion Hazards			

Section V. Health Hazard Data			
Threshold Limit Value			
Effects of Overexposure			
Emergency and First Aid Procedures			

Section VI. Reactivity Data			
Stability	Stable		Conditions to Avoid
	Unstable		
Incompatibility (materials to avoid)			
Hazardous Decomposition Products			
Hazardous Polymerization	May Occur		Conditions to Avoid
	Will Not Occur		

Section VII. Spill or Leak Procedures		
Steps to Be Taken if Material is Released or Spilled		
Waste Disposal Method		

Section VIII. Special Protection Information			
Respiratory Protection			
Ventilation	Local Exhaust		Special
	Mechanical (General)		Other
Protective Gloves		Eye Protection	
Other Protective Equipment			

Section IX. Special Precautions
Precautions to Be Taken in Handling and Storing
Other Precautions

Appendix M.   Label Format for Containers

Product Name or Material Identity

Safe Use Category* _____

W A R N I N G !

Overexposure may result in respiratory, skin, or eye irritation.

Check Appropriate Box(es):

☐   Do Not Use in Confined Space Without
       Appropriate Protective Equipment

☐   Flammable

Health Hazards:

☐   Harmful if Inhaled or Swallowed

☐   Harmful if Absorbed Through Skin

☐   Cancer-Suspect Agent (C)

_____

Specific Chemicals with Additional Health Hazards—See Safe Use
Instructions:

_____

_____

_____

_____

*Employees have the right and are encouraged to review the MSDS
and Safe Use Instructions for additional chemical and health hazard
information.

Index

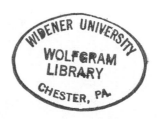
WIDENER UNIVERSITY
WOLFGRAM
LIBRARY
CHESTER, PA.